Early Start Denver Model for Young Children with Autism

Early Start Denver Model for Young Children with Autism

PROMOTING LANGUAGE, LEARNING, AND ENGAGEMENT

Sally J. Rogers and Geraldine Dawson

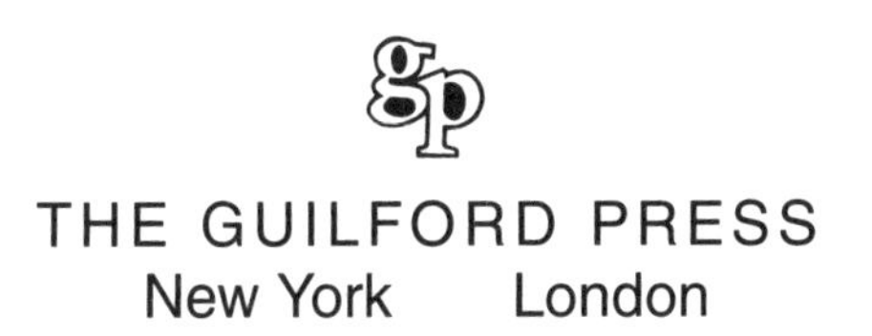

THE GUILFORD PRESS
New York London

A Division of Guilford Publications, Inc.
72 Spring Street, New York, NY 10012
www.guilford.com

Printed in the United States of America

This book is printed on acid-free paper.

Last digit is print number: 9 8 7 6 5 4 3 2

Library of Congress Cataloging-in-Publication Data

Rogers, Sally J.
Early start Denver model for young children with autism : promoting language, learning, and engagement / Sally J. Rogers and Geraldine Dawson.
p. cm.
Includes bibliographical references and index.
ISBN 978-1-60623-631-4 (pbk.: alk. paper); ISBN 978-1-60623-632-1 (hardcover)
1. Autism in children—Treatment. 2. Autistic children—Behavior modification. 3. Autistic children—Means of communication. 4. Social interaction in children. 5. Toddlers—Development. 6. Child development. I. Dawson, Geraldine. II. Title.
RJ506.A9R64 2010
618.92′85882—dc22

2009033627

The *Early Start Denver Model Curriculum Checklist for Young Children with Autism,* which appears here in Appendix A, is sold separately in sets of ready-to-use booklets (ISBN 978-1-60623-633-8).

To Michael Bucci and his family, and all the other children and parents who taught me how to help

—S. J. R.

In memory of Eric Schopler, a pioneer

—G. D.

About the Authors

Sally J. Rogers, PhD, is Professor of Psychiatry at the M.I.N.D. Institute, University of California, Davis. A developmental psychologist, she is involved at the international level in major clinical and research activities on autism, including one of the 10 Autism Centers of Excellence network projects funded by the National Institutes of Health/ National Institute of Child Health and Human Development, involving a multisite, randomized, controlled trial of an infant–toddler treatment for autism. She is also the director of an interdisciplinary postdoctoral training grant for autism researchers. Dr. Rogers is on the executive board of the International Society for Autism Research, is an editor of the journal *Autism Research*, and is a member of the DSM-V workgroup on autism, pervasive developmental disorder, and other developmental disorders. She has spent her entire career studying cognitive and social-communicative development and intervention in young children with disabilities and has published widely on clinical and developmental aspects of autism, with a particular interest in imitation problems. As a clinician, she provides evaluation, treatment, and consultation to children and adults with autism and their families.

Geraldine Dawson, PhD, is Chief Science Officer at Autism Speaks, Research Professor of Psychiatry at the University of North Carolina at Chapel Hill, Professor Emeritus at the University of Washington (UW), and Adjunct Professor of Psychiatry at Columbia University. Previously, she was Professor of Psychology and Psychiatry at UW and Founding Director of the UW Autism Center, which has been designated a National Institutes of Health Autism Center of Excellence since 1996. While at UW, Dr. Dawson led a multidisciplinary autism research program focusing on genetics, neuroimaging, diagnosis, and treatment. She received continuous funding from the National Institutes of Health for her research from 1980 until 2008, when she left UW to join Autism Speaks. She was Founding Director of the UW Autism Center's multidisciplinary clinical services program, which is the largest of its kind in the northwestern United States. Dr. Dawson has testified before the U.S. Senate on behalf of individuals with autism and played a key role on the Washington State Autism Task Force. Her research and publications focus on early detection and treatment of autism, early patterns of brain dysfunction (electrophysiology), and, more recently, the development of endophenotypes for autism genetic studies.

Acknowledgments

This book is the product of many people's input over a very long period. The most important contributors to the work are the children, parents, and clinicians from Denver, Seattle, and Sacramento over the past 25 years or more who participated in our research studies or sought clinical services. What is presented here was learned, not so much in graduate school or from textbooks, but primarily from the children and their families who shared their lives with us and gave us so many opportunities to learn about the children's abilities, interests, and challenges. Parents allowed us to join with them to help shape their children's development, told us what worked and what didn't, and trusted us to become part of their support network and work with their children. They have been our teachers, and this book is a compilation of what parents, clinicians, and children have taught us.

Next, we acknowledge the many colleagues from many disciplines with whom we have worked side by side for so many years, learning about the needs of young children with autism spectrum disorders (ASD) and their families, trying one way after another to help each one grow and progress. Special recognition is due to Amy Donaldson, Terry Hall, Jean Herbison, Diane Osaki, Milani Smith, Laurie Vismara, Chris Whalen, and Jamie Winter. These people were fundamental in developing specific parts of the intervention approach described here. In addition, Renee Charlifue, Marybeth Garel, Deborah Hayden, Susan Hepburn, Terry Katz, Hal Lewis, Jeff Munson, Judy Reaven, Kathy Reis, and Chris Wilcox had important input into the clinical model and the research that has been generated from the model over the years. We particularly appreciate Laura Schreibman's ongoing support, enthusiasm, and guidance for bringing together pivotal response training and the Denver Model.

We also want to acknowledge the support and generosity of many colleagues over the years, colleagues who had special expertise in the development and treatment of young children with ASD and were so willing to share their work and their knowledge with us: Marie Bristol, Annette Groen, Cathy Lord, Ivar Lovaas, Gail McGee, Gary Mesibov, Sam Odom, Eric Schopler, Laura Schreibman again, Tris Smith, Amy Wetherby, and Paul Yoder.

The Early Start Denver Model (ESDM) Curriculum Checklist (Appendix A) is the product of many years of clinical development and use, first at the University of Colorado Health Sciences Center in Denver, Colorado, and later at the University of Washington and the University of California, Davis. The Curriculum Checklist has been developed by an expert team of clinicians across these three sites. Special acknowledgments go to the following people for their seminal contributions to this tool: Amy Donaldson, S-LP, PhD; Terry Hall, MA, S-LP; Jean Herbison, MA; Diane Osaki, OTR; Laurie Vismara, PhD; and Jamie Winter, PhD. We also express our appreciation to several colleagues at the University of Washington whose contributions were essential to the study that tested the efficacy of the ESDM intervention: Cathy Brock, MA; Jessica Greenson, PhD; Jeff Munson, PhD; and Milani Smith, PhD.

Special thanks go to our editor at The Guilford Press, Rochelle Serwator, whose enthusiasm for this project never waned and who provided energy and encouragement to sometimes very tired and tardy authors. Barbara Watkins did a masterful job of organizing and clarifying the manuscript and helping us communicate clearly and succinctly.

And, finally, we want to acknowledge the support of our families, both children and spouses, who valued the work we were trying to do and who supported the lifetime of time and energy we have spent in work in early autism. Our children, from the time they seemed too young to have really understood, somehow felt that it was right that their moms needed to help other kids too, and generously shared their moms with many. Thanks to our children and our husbands for participating in the many, many autism-related activities that we have brought them to, across the decades and the globe, with enthusiasm and commitment.

Preface

The child is both the artist and the painting.
—ALFRED ADLER

This book describes an approach for working with very young children with autism spectrum disorders (ASD) that fosters children's spontaneous tendency to approach and interact with others (termed *initiative*) and their ability to engage with others. The approach, called the Early Start Denver Model (ESDM), follows each child's interests and proclivities and provides a "scaffold" for his or her communication and interaction. The ESDM deeply embraces both "constructionist" and "transactional" models of child development. The constructionist approach views infants as active beings who construct their own mental and social world out of their motor, sensory, and interpersonal–affective experiences. In other words, the child is the artist creating his or her own "picture" of the world. The transactional approach views infants and the other people in their caregiving environment as affecting and influencing the development of each other. The caregiver's temperament, behavior, and emotions help to shape and change the infant's behavior and representations of people and of the world, while at the same time the infant's temperament, behavior, and skills alter the behavior patterns of the caregivers, and this goes on continuously throughout the developmental period—which is one's entire life. Through this interactive process, the painting is co-created.

The ESDM seeks to empower children with ASD to become active participants in the world, initiating interactions with other people. Autism often affects a child's initiative. In particular, children with autism often are less inclined to initiate interaction with people and tend to focus on a narrow range of activities. This characteristic is present from the very beginning and continues throughout the individual's life; it is one hallmark of autism. For a young child, fewer social initiations result in fewer learning opportunities, and a narrowed and repetitive range of activities also results in a narrowed range of learning opportunities. The nature of autism constricts learning opportunities, affecting every hour of the child's life and resulting in a greater and greater number of lost opportunities month by month and year by year. The young child with autism thus has far fewer experiences with which to construct his or her understanding of the people and events in the world.

However, autism not only affects the individual child; it affects every person who interacts with that child. From the first cries, coughs, and fusses of a newborn, infants behave in ways that adults respond to with caregiving, smiles, play, and soothing. Each of these social interactions offers multiple learning opportunities for the infant, whose responses to caregivers tend to elicit additional interactions. Infants thus actively shape the amount and type of social exchanges with caregivers from their first moment of life, and this child-initiated social exchange continues throughout the child's waking hours each day, resulting in hundreds of daily opportunities for language, social, play, and cognitive learning. The young child with autism is not likely to be initiating these ongoing social exchanges at anywhere near the rate of other children—not with caregivers, not with siblings, and not with other children—which decreases learning opportunities tremendously. However, an additional insidious effect of autism is that even when others initiate social exchanges with the young child with autism, as parents and siblings and other children often do, the child with autism may not respond with pleasure, eye contact, and laughter. Lacking a clear, interpretable response that tells the partner that the child enjoys the interaction and wants it to continue, the caregivers may not receive a response from the child that reinforces their own social initiation. If social partners feel as if their initiations are not positive for the child, they may well decrease their initiations. In behavioral language, their initiations are being extinguished due to lack of positive reinforcement from the child. So now the child with autism is in double indemnity: The child is not initiating frequently enough and thus creating learning opportunities, and the social partners are decreasing their initiations, with further resulting loss of learning opportunities.

The ESDM begins by addressing the child's social interaction with others—it provides a means of priming, scaffolding, rewarding, and increasing children's initiations, and helps parents and other partners interpret the child's cues and continue in interactions. The immediate effect of these techniques is to increase dramatically the number of social learning opportunities the child is experiencing, hour by hour and day by day. While this increase in learning opportunities also occurs in other intervention methods, such as discrete trial teaching, often these methods put the child in the role of the responder and the child's initiations are suppressed. We understand the lack of initiative that is core to autism as one of the most detrimental aspects of the disorder for child learning and progress, and the ESDM begins by building the child's social initiative and social engagement.

The ESDM is not unique in this approach; a number of other developmental and social-communicative models of early intervention for ASD also foster this kind of initiative: DIR (Developmental, Individual difference, Relationship-based model)/Floortime, RDI (Relationship Development Intervention), and SCERTS (Social Communication, Emotional Regulation, Transactional Support) quickly come to mind. However, the ESDM differs from these other approaches in several ways:

1. The ESDM predates other models that focus on facilitating the relationship between the child with ASD and his or her caregiver. In fact, the first papers on the Denver Model date from the 1980s, and many of the main aspects of the model—the focus on positive child affect, balanced social interactions, the "one-up rule," the use of sensory social routines to develop social initiative, the approach to language develop-

ment beginning with natural gestures—were already in place and described in the first 1986 paper, well before the other approaches first appeared in print.

2. There is a body of peer-reviewed, published empirical work supporting the model. At this time, there are eight data-based outcome papers in press or published, including both single-subject and group designs, and a randomized controlled trial. Thus, the ESDM is probably the best studied of any of the developmentally based early interventions for ASD.

3. The model is very well articulated. Both the teaching content and the teaching procedures are thoroughly described, with fidelity measures and data collection systems provided. When used as described, it provides a comprehensive and carefully detailed program of activities and teaching objectives that can be used by anyone, anywhere. That is another of its strengths.

4. The model does not require a particular setting for its delivery. It is designed to be used by parents, teachers, therapists, at home, in preschool, and in a clinical office—anywhere that adults are interacting with children.

5. The model is data based and stresses the importance of data collection to evaluate teaching efficacy and to adjust and maximize progress.

6. The model is comprehensive. It addresses all the developmental skills of early childhood: language, play, social interaction, and joint attention, but also imitation, motor skills, self-care, and behavior.

7. The model provides a systematic way of altering the intervention when children are not progressing well—a decision tree for clinicians to use when the child is not making progress—and by so doing it allows for the full range of empirically supported practices to be brought into use, in a thoughtful and step-by-step fashion.

Thus, while the ESDM shares some common features with other social-developmental approaches, it also has distinctive features.

The ESDM shares features with approaches that are based on applied behavior analysis (ABA). Teaching procedures follow the principles of operant learning and are based on powerful ABA teaching tools—prompting, fading, shaping, and chaining—in a clearly articulated manner. However, the ESDM differs from some ABA approaches, such as a discrete trials approach, in several ways:

1. It uses a curriculum that is based on the most current concepts derived from the scientific literature focusing on children's development.

2. There is an explicit focus on the quality of relationships, affect, and adult sensitivity and responsivity, a feature that is often missing in many ABA programs.

3. The strategies and curriculum that are used to facilitate language development are based on the most current scientific understanding of how language develops, rather than a Skinnerian model.

The ESDM has currently been found to be effective in enhancing development in children with ASD from ages 18 months to 48 months, and initial studies of efficacy have been carried out both for short-term parent delivery and for longer-term, intensive, home-therapy delivery. Research in the model is ongoing. We are currently funded by the National Institutes of Health to conduct a multisite, randomized, independent replication study of the ESDM. While further research is needed, the amount of public interest in the model, the huge need for infant–toddler interventions in ASD, and the strength of the initial data have justified the need to publish this manual for the ESDM now.

Just as the Denver Model has changed over the years, the ESDM will also change in the future. Intervention approaches need to reflect the most recent science of the times, and as we learn more, the model will be altered to reflect new understanding. However, this manual defines the model as it is currently being studied and taught. We hope that parents, early interventionists, early special educators, occupational therapists, speech–language pathologists, and psychologists, among others, will find this helpful in their work in early ASD.

Contents

Chapter 1 Current Understanding of Infant Learning and Autism 1

How Infants Learn 2

How Brain Development Supports the Acquisition of Social-Communicative Skills 4

How Autism Likely Affects Brain Development and Learning 8

Brain Changes in Early Childhood and Beyond 12

The Role of Early Intervention in Shaping Early Brain Development and Outcome in Autism 13

Chapter 2 An Overview of the Early Start Denver Model 14

Foundations of the ESDM 14

The ESDM Curriculum 17

ESDM Teaching Procedures 19

Evidence of Effectiveness 29

Similarities and Differences between the ESDM and Other Intervention Models for Toddlers with ASD 33

Conclusion 34

Chapter 3 Using the Early Start Denver Model 35

Delivery Settings 35

Delivery to Whom? 36

Delivery by Whom? 36

ESDM Procedures 37

Using the Generalist Model to Deliver Intervention 39

The Interdisciplinary Treatment Team 40

Partnering with Families 50

Transitioning Out of the ESDM Intervention 55

Conclusion 57

Chapter 4 Developing Short-Term Learning Objectives 58

Assessment Using the ESDM Curriculum Checklist 58

Constructing the Learning Objectives 68

Balancing Objectives across Domains 68
How Many Objectives? 68
Selecting Skill Content 69
Elements of the Objective 70
Writing Functional Objectives 75
Isaac's 12-Week Learning Objectives 76
Conclusion 79

Chapter 5 Formulating Daily Teaching Targets and Tracking Progress 80
Mapping Out Learning Steps for Each Objective 80
Tracking Progress 87
Summary 94
Appendix 5.1. Learning Objectives and Learning Steps for Isaac 95

Chapter 6 Developing Plans and Frames for Teaching 101
Becoming a Play Partner 102
Joint Activity Routines: Frames for Teaching 108
Managing Unwanted Behaviors 120
Organizing and Planning the Session 123
When Children Aren't Progressing: A Decision Tree 130
Conclusion 134

Chapter 7 Developing Imitation and Play 136
Teaching Imitation 136
Teaching Play Skills 146
Conclusion 153

Chapter 8 Developing Nonverbal Communication 154
Coordinating Attention Underlies Communication 155
Developing Use and Understanding of Natural Gestures 156
Teaching Conventional Gesture Use 160
Conclusion 166

Chapter 9 Developing Verbal Communication 168
Stimulating Development of Speech Production 169
Receptive Language 179
Conclusion 182

Chapter 10 Using the Early Start Denver Model in Group Settings 184
Considering Characteristics of Autism in Classroom Organization 185
Physical Organization 186
Planning the Daily Schedule and Routines 189
Choreography of the Classroom 192
Staff Planning and Communication 192

Small- and Large-Group Instruction **194**
Classroom Behavior Management **197**
Transitions and Individual Schedule Systems **198**
Curriculum for Peer Relations and Self-Care **202**
Kindergarten Transition **206**
Conclusion **207**

Appendix A Early Start Denver Model Curriculum Checklist and Item Descriptions **209**
Introduction **209**
Administration **210**
Scoring **211**
Translating Items into Teaching Objectives **211**
Materials Needed **212**
Early Start Denver Model Curriculum Checklist for Young Children with Autism **213**
Early Start Denver Model Curriculum Checklist: Item Descriptions **230**

Appendix B Early Start Denver Model Teaching Fidelity Rating System: Administration and Coding **259**
Procedure for Coding Fidelity of Treatment Implementation **259**
Early Start Denver Model **261**
Early Start Denver Model Fidelity Coding Sheet **271**

References **273**

Index **287**

Early Start Denver Model for Young Children with Autism

Chapter 1

Current Understanding of Infant Learning and Autism

The last several decades have witnessed an explosion of knowledge about how infants and toddlers learn. Given that the symptoms of autism spectrum disorders (ASD) often appear before the first birthday, this new knowledge can be brought to bear in our understanding of how best to intervene with young infants and toddlers who are at risk for autism. The Early Start Denver Model (ESDM) is a comprehensive, early intervention approach for toddlers with autism ages 12–36 months and continuing until ages 48–60 months. It refines, adapts, and extends downward in age, the original Denver Model for preschoolers with ASD ages 24–60 months. ESDM uses the knowledge of how the typical baby develops to facilitate a similar developmental trajectory in young infants who are at risk for autism.

The earliest symptoms of autism suggest that the brain systems that support social and language development are affected. Motor symptoms are also likely to be affected in many infants. Studies of home videotapes taken of infants who later develop autism (Osterling & Dawson, 1994; Palomo, Belinchon, & Ozonoff, 2006) show that these infants spend less time looking at other people, are less responsive when their names are called, and often fail to develop early gestures, such as pointing, which are important for setting the stage for language development. The rapid learning capacity of infants, however, suggests the infant–toddler years are a period of great plasticity and change. In fact, infants who have sustained a brain injury often show dramatic recovery, especially if early stimulation is provided. This frames the challenge and promise of early intervention for infants and toddlers with ASD: We need to capitalize on the tremendous plasticity of the infant period so we can minimize the disabilities that often characterize ASD.

The ESDM aims to do this, starting early and incorporating findings from developmental research into its teaching curriculum and techniques. The ESDM is defined by (1) a specific developmental curriculum that defines the skills to be taught at any given time, and (2) a specific set of teaching procedures used to deliver the curriculum. The ESDM is not tied to a specific delivery setting, but can be applied in group programs or home programs by therapy teams and/or parents, and in individual therapy sessions in clinic settings or home delivered by several different disciplines. It is an intervention approach that is highly specified and yet quite flexible in terms of teaching contexts, goals, and materials. A variety of studies, including a new, large, randomized controlled trial, indicate that the ESDM is effective for increasing children's cognitive and language abilities, social interaction and initiative, decreasing the severity of their ASD symptoms, and improving their overall behavior and adaptive skills.

In this book we describe the ESDM and show how to implement it with young children with ASD. In this first chapter we review findings from the research on typical infant development that have influenced the ESDM. Chapter 2 presents the foundations for the ESDM and overviews its curriculum, core teaching procedures, and evidence of effectiveness. Chapter 3 describes practical aspects of ESDM delivery including the range of settings, the interdisciplinary team, and partnering with families. Chapters 4 and 5 detail ESDM evaluation and treatment planning, respectively, including how to plan for daily teaching and track progress within and across sessions. Chapter 6 shows readers step-by-step how to become a play partner and develop joint activity play routines with the child. Joint activity routines provide the platform for teaching in the ESDM. The next three chapters explain how to teach the child imitation and play skills (Chapter 7), nonverbal communication (Chapter 8), and verbal communication (Chapter 9). The teaching of key social behaviors is embedded throughout the curriculum and throughout these chapters. In the final chapter (Chapter 10), we describe special considerations when implementing the ESDM in group settings such as preschool programs. Included in Chapter 10 is a discussion of peer relations and self-care skills, curriculum areas relevant to any ESDM setting.

In the sections below, we provide a brief review of research findings on (1) how infants learn, (2) how brain development supports the acquisition of social-communicative skills, (3) how autism likely affects brain development and learning, (4) brain plasticity in early childhood and beyond, and (5) the role of early intervention in shaping early brain development and outcome in autism.

HOW INFANTS LEARN

Many interventionists—early childhood special educators, clinical psychologists, occupational therapists (OTs), speech–language pathologists (S-LPs), and others—have been schooled in the constructionist theory of early cognition, as articulated by the French developmental psychologist, Jean Piaget (1963). The constructionist view suggests that infants essentially construct their own knowledge base and representational models (mental pictures) of the physical environment through their own sensorimotor explorations of objects and the physical world. This sensory motor knowledge gradually becomes internalized and evolves into cognitive representations of actions, objects, and events in the world. These higher-order cognitive capacities develop in the latter half of the second year through the infant's ability to internalize imitation. The hallmarks of representational thought in infancy involve object permanence, insightful problem solving, symbolic play, deferred imitation, and symbolic speech.

Over the past 20 years, however, a revolution in our understanding of infant learning has required that we give up the constructionist model of representational development. We now understand that infants have many ways and levels of "knowing." Interpreting infants' immature motor actions as evidence of what they know has misled us and we have underestimated their knowledge about people, objects, and events. A good example is the concept of object permanence, better known in the research literature as the *A*-not-*B* task. Decades ago, Piaget (1963) noted that infants as old as 1 year of age show a lack of "object permanence" as evidenced by their failure to correctly search for an object that had been hidden in front of them. This failure in reaching for a hidden object was thought to reflect an inability of the infant to form a memory or representation of the object when it was no longer in sight. In other words, "out of sight—out of mind." Later, however, scientists decided to study where infants *look,* rather than where they *manually search,* to discover what infants know about the physical world (Baillargeon, 2004). For example, they showed infants two barriers a short distance apart on the right end of a platform. They then hid the barriers and placed a ball at one end of the platform, hitting the ball so that it rolled behind the screen. When they raised the screen, the ball was resting *between* the two barriers rather than *in front* of the first barrier. They found that infants looked longer and showed surprise when violation of their expectation occurred, suggesting that the 2- to 3-month-old infant had maintained a mental representation of the object when it was out of sight.

Current research on infant learning in the first year of postnatal life has illuminated learning capacities that would not have been predicted from constructionist models. Infants' abilities to understand how objects work in the physical environment, recognition of the similarity between their own actions and those of others, ability to remember information, and their perception and responses to the social world far exceed what one might predict from their immature motor skills. To assess the abilities of young infants, scientists have used innovative methods such as examining how the infant's sucking rates, eye gaze patterns, and electrical brain responses change when a stimulus is altered.

Furthermore, infants are active learners who are interested in forming and testing hypotheses about the world. Their knowledge grows as they interact with objects and people. Current research suggests that as infants interact with the world, their brains rely on "statistical learning" to detect patterns and make meaning (Saffran, Aslin, & Newport, 1996). Infants are "intuitive statisticians," making inferences and predictions based on the data they are constantly gathering about the world. For example, Saffran et al. (1996) found that infants use statistical information in the speech stream to detect the boundaries between words. In fact, statistical learning—that is, the ability to detect the way information is distributed and make inferences from this information—appears to play a role in many aspects of language, cognitive, and social development. When an infant is interacting with the world in an unusual way, such as focusing primarily on objects and not people, we assume that the infant's knowledge and construction of the world is also unusual. This infant may fail to develop typical language, in part, because he or she is not paying attention to speech and its distributional properties. Thus, a key goal of intervention is to help the infant pay attention to key information such as speech and people's faces and actions, and to "boost," or make more salient, certain patterns or types of information so that the infant is able to easily make sense of the information that is essential for typical language and social development.

Finally, the last few decades of infant research have shown that although infants are "statistical learners," they are simply not like little computers that are input with whatever information is in their surroundings. Instead, for inferences to be made and learning to occur, the infant must be actively and *affectively engaged* with his or her environment. It is now recognized, for example, that the typical development of speech perception occurs within an affective-rich social interactive context where the infant's attention is directed toward information that he or she finds socially rewarding. This was demonstrated in an experiment conducted by Pat Kuhl (Kuhl, Tsao, & Liu, 2003), which demonstrated that simple exposure to language does not necessarily facilitate the development of speech and language development. Rather, language needs to be experienced by the infant with a social interactive contact for typical speech perception to develop. Thus, an intervention that is designed for an infant who may show little interest in the social environment must address this fundamental requirement for learning as one of the first steps of the treatment strategy.

In sum, decades of research on infant cognition and learning have taught us that infants use their visual and auditory systems to process a great deal of information about their physical environment, long before their motor capacities permit much sensory motor exploration. Infants are quite sensitive to patterns, contingencies, and statistical regularities, and this sensitivity allows them to integrate information across sensory systems. This sensitivity also allows them to detect mismatches and novelty. Their preference for novelty allows them to focus their attention on these unexpected events to process them. Socially, infants are aware of other people's actions and relationships between certain stimuli and certain actions. This is true both for causal actions and for emotional responses. This makes human behavior predictable and meaningful for infants. The infant motor system develops more slowly than visual and auditory systems, and infant motor acts on objects tell us more about the motor system than about the infant's underlying learning capacity and existing knowledge base. Furthermore, infants' affective engagement with the social environment provides a necessary context in which perceptual, cognitive, language, and social development occur.

HOW BRAIN DEVELOPMENT SUPPORTS THE ACQUISITION OF SOCIAL-COMMUNICATIVE SKILLS

The early symptoms of autism suggest that the brain systems that support social and language learning are not developing normally. Some scientists (Kennedy & Courchesne, 2008; Williams & Minshew, 2007; Pinkham, Hopfinger, Pelphrey, Piven, & Penn, 2008) believe that this reflects a more general problem in the development of brain systems that support complex behavior, particularly those involving the coordination of several higher-order brain regions. Other scientists (Mundy, 2003) believe that autism affects the social-communicative brain circuits specifically and that many other higher-order regions are relatively spared. These two points of view are not mutually exclusive as the development of social and communicative behavior requires the coordination among several brain regions (Dawson, 2008). Therefore, it is helpful to consider how the "social brain network" works so we can design interventions that will promote its normal development.

The social brain network involves a number of structures that have been demonstrated through animal and human studies to be actively involved in processing social information, emotion, and social behavior (see Figure 1.1). Brain activation occurs in these areas in response to social stimuli; damage in these areas results in abnormalities in social behavior. Key parts of the social brain network include parts of the temporal

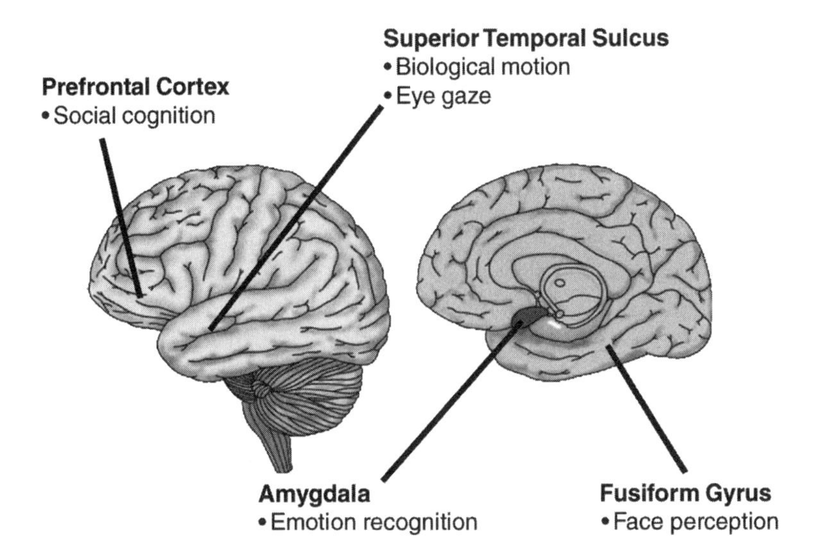

FIGURE 1.1. Social brain circuitry.

lobe (fusiform gyrus and superior temporal sulcus), the amygdala, and parts of the prefrontal cortex. Both the fusiform gyrus (specialized for face perception) and the superior temporal sulcus (STS; specialized for perception of animate movement, also referred to as "biological motion") are important in detecting and interpreting social information, such as facial expressions.

The amygdala is involved in assigning emotional value to various stimuli—both positive (reward) values and negative (e.g., fear or punishment) values. Imagine how a child might behave if all the stimuli around him or her were assigned the same emotional value or if unusual stimuli were assigned value. Rather than focusing attention on the meaningful things in the environment (such as other people), his or her attention might wander or get stuck on irrelevant stimuli (such as background noise or a piece of fuzz on the carpet). This decreased focus on key aspects of the social environment is often seen in children with autism. Difficulties in assigning negative values to stimuli (such as fear) help explain why some children with autism have an apparent lack of awareness of danger.

When an infant's attention is drawn to another's face and voice and the infant experiences positive emotion (e.g., interest, joy), the fusiform, STS, and amygdala are activated. The prefrontal cortex (particularly the orbitofrontal or ventromedial prefrontal cortex) is important for many aspects of social behavior, including inhibiting inappropriate responses, monitoring one's own behavior, and engaging in planned behavior. When we engage in social interactions, if we are socially skilled, we are constantly monitoring how the other person is responding to what we are doing and adjusting our behavior according to those responses. This ability to flexibly change our behavior in response to differing feedback is a core function of the ventromedial prefrontal cortex. When this area is not functioning properly, the person becomes insensitive to the needs of others and tends to perseverate on topics of one's own interest. This failure to be sensitive to social feedback is a common feature found in people with autism.

Researchers have studied social brain activities during infancy, both by using tasks that they know activate certain brain areas and using brain imaging methods to examine whether those brain regions are responding normally when exposed to social stimuli. The methods used to gather this information in young infants and children include measuring electrical brain activity (EEG [electroencephalography] and MEG [magnetoencephalography]) and blood flow in the brain (FMRI [functional magnetic resonance imaging]) as infants and children are exposed to visual and auditory social stimuli (Cassuam, Kuefner, Weterlund, & Nelson, 20056; Rivera-Gaziola, Silva-Pereyra, & Kuhl, 2005; Kylliainen, Braeutigan, & Hietanen, 2006; Pelphrey & Carter, 2008). In the next section, we provide more detail about the different parts of the social brain.

What's in a Face?

Many of the brain areas that adults use to extract information from faces are active in infants within the first few months of postnatal life, though greater specialization and integration of brain regions will change with development. Specific brain regions respond to various facial stimuli, including direction of eye gaze and eye contact, and facial and vocal emotional displays.

Face Recognition

The human brain is wired from the beginning to notice and respond to others' faces. Newborn infants show rapid face recognition and a visual preference for faces over other complex visual stimuli. By 4 months, infants show a sensitivity to the orientation of faces, responding more readily to upright than inverted faces. By 6–7 months of age, infants show different brain responses when they see a familiar versus an unfamiliar face.

Eye Gaze

Sensitivity to eye contact and gaze direction is present very early in life. Infants as young as 4 months of age differentially respond to eye gaze and emotion. This sensitivity to gaze may be more entwined with the fusiform face-processing brain areas earlier in infancy, with greater activation of STS appearing later as brain specialization proceeds.

Joint Attention

Infants as young as 3 months of age appear to be sensitive to the occurrence of joint attention, marked by gaze patterns that coordinate looks to an object or event and looks to a social partner. By 8–9 months of age, brain responses to these referential gaze patterns show adult-like patterns involving STS and the dorsal part of the medial prefrontal cortex in adults.

Emotion Perception

Infants by 7 months of age discriminate facial expressions, as shown by their orienting and habituation responses during visual attention paradigms in which they are exposed to faces showing the same or different emotions. By 6–7 months of age, infants show a different electrical brain response to different emotional faces. Infants show a specific response pattern to negative emotions, compared to positive emotions. Such facial emotion stimuli also activate regions of the prefrontal cortex. Similarly, infants by 7 months of age discriminate vocal expressions of emotion in similar research paradigms, including differential reactions to positive versus negative emotions. Infants of this age also integrate emotional information from two different sensory domains—visual and auditory. They show this by responding differently to stimuli that show both facial and vocal emotions that either correspond or do not correspond to each other (e.g., a happy face with a happy voice vs. a happy face with an angry voice). The brain regions involved in these responses in infants of this age involve the amygdala within the temporal lobe, and these brain activation patterns are quite similar to those seen in adults experiencing the same kinds of stimuli.

Interpreting Others' Behavior

Infants also discriminate aspects of others' social behavior that involve body action and movement patterns.

Biological Motion

As mentioned earlier, this term refers to the movement patterns of living things. It involves spontaneous movement and spontaneous changes in direction of movement. This contrasts to the movement patterns of objects, which always occur in response to an external force (thus not spontaneous or self-initiated) and maintain a specific direction unless another force redirects the line of motion. Infants' ability to discriminate these differing motion patterns of people versus things is present from the first few months, as demonstrated by their visual looking patterns. Furthermore, infants appear to use adult-like processes for discriminating biological motion. Thus, infants can determine animate from inanimate stimuli very early.

Understanding Others' Actions

By 8 months of age, infants appear to predict the effects of others' goal-directed actions, shown by their different responses to people acting on objects in conventional, or expected, versus unconventional, or unexpected, ways. Infants also demonstrate awareness of what the effect of conventional actions should be. For instance, they show a differential response when people direct a comment to an object, as opposed to a person. Infants are aware of the meaning of these action–effect patterns long before they are physically able to carry out such acts themselves. Such findings demonstrate well infants' ability to learn a considerable amount about people from observing them in natural environments, and they also demonstrate infants' tendency to extract predictable patterns from experiences and then use those to interpret new experiences (statistical learning).

Thus, from birth, infants are sensitive to social and emotional stimuli. Many parts of the adult's "social brain" are active in infants before their first birthdays. Brain regions that respond to social stimuli, especially those involving older brain structures (subcortical) rather than the prefrontal cortex, are active at birth. However, within a few months after birth, infants also use cortical processes in their responses to social stimuli. These findings suggest that preference for social stimuli, and automatic attention to social stimuli, are basic properties of the human brain. What is more, the infant brain may be *more* responsive to social stimuli than the adult brain. Johnson and colleagues (Johnson et al., 2005) suggest that in infants, the social brain is more broadly "tuned," more sensitive and responsive to input, more "ready" to respond, than in adults. Infant brain responses to social input and to other types of input are more diffusely distributed across the brain and become more specialized and localized over time. This specialization requires interaction with the social environment. Thus, the human infant brain is exquisitely responsive to the social world and rapidly learns about many aspects of people.

HOW AUTISM LIKELY AFFECTS BRAIN DEVELOPMENT AND LEARNING

Although autism has many different causes involving both genetic and environmental factors, each of these causes ultimately affects the core brain regions involved in social and communicative development. There is currently no autism signature in the brain—no difference that is universally present in people who have autism, and only in them. However, there are some brain differences that are found in the majority of people with autism, and researchers have suggested how those differences might help explain some of the unusual behavior we see in people with autism. We next briefly review our current knowledge about brain differences in autism (see Geschwind & Levitt, 2007, for a current, detailed review). The parts of the brain that have been found to be affected in some people with autism include the cerebellum (attention and motor behavior), the amygdala (emotion), parts of the temporal lobe (language and social perception), and the prefrontal cortex (attention, planning, abstract thought, and social behavior).

Brain structures don't operate independently; rather, they "team up" to form complex networks that support complex behaviors like motor functioning, attention, cognition, language, and social behavior. Complex behaviors require several parts of the brain to act in a coordinated, synchronous fashion, much like the instruments in an orchestra must be coordinated in order to create music. Many brain regions have to be connected through networks of neurons to accomplish such behaviors. Such connections, particularly long-range connections that allow different parts of the brain to act in a coordinated fashion, appear impaired in autism.

Abnormal Connectivity in Autism

Studies suggest that autism affects how the connections between different neurons (called *synapses*) are made, and how connections between different brain regions are made (Garber, 2007). Early in typical development, a profusion of neurons and synapses develops, allowing different brain regions to communicate with each other through these webs of connecting neurons. This is followed by a thinning out of this dense network, so that the networks are "leaner"; that is, more selective, efficient, and fast. This selection process is guided, in part, by experience; those connections that are utilized become strengthened and more responsive, and those that are underutilized die away. Thus, the neural networks that remain are those that have been actively used; stimulating these cell connections strengthens them, makes them faster, and also makes them more responsive to the stimuli that caused their initial activation.

In autism, evidence suggests that this process of developing neural networks is faulty and results in poor connectivity, particularly affecting brain regions that are farther away from each other (Murias, Webb, Greenson, & Dawson, 2007). Genetic studies have shown that the genes that increase risk for autism are those that regulate the excitatory and inhibitory balance in neural networks (Geschwind, 2008). Maintaining this balance is critical for neural networks to function properly.

When there is poor connectivity between the different parts of the brain, such as appears to be the case in autism, it is much more difficult for the child to learn to carry out complex behaviors that require integrated functioning across brain regions. Consider, for example, the apparently simple behavior of an infant pointing to a favorite toy in order to share interest in that toy with his or her parent. This joint attention behavior can be performed by most 10- to 12-month-old infants. In this act of pointing to share interest, the brain regions involved in visual perception (looking at the toy), attention (shifting attention from the toy to the parent), motor behavior (both the eyes and the hands), and emotion (expressing joy or interest) must act in a coordinated fashion. Lack of normal brain connectivity will affect the development of this type of complex skill.

Larger-Than-Average Head Size

Many children with autism show an unusual pattern of head growth. Studies indicate that the infant who later develops autism has a normal size head at birth, but then shows accelerated growth beginning around 4 months of age (Courchesne et al., 2007). This accelerated growth pattern is particularly evident in early life; after that, the rate decelerates to a more normal rate. How might large heads affect children's development? The size of the head is driven by the size of the growing brain inside it, so bigger head size reflects bigger brain size. Brains grow by adding both gray matter (the neurons) and white matter (involving the myelin sheath that surrounds and insulates the neurons), and glial cells, which are part of the underlying cellular structure of the brain.

As we described above, during infancy there is a period of cell proliferation followed by a period of cell reduction, or "pruning," in which it is assumed that neurons that are not part of active information networks die off (apoptosis), reducing "noise" in the system and making for a more efficient, better organized, neural organization. Some researchers have suggested that unusually rapid head growth reflects unusually rapid cell proliferation without the accompanying pruning, with the end result that there are too many neurons that are not well organized, resulting in an inferior general learning "machine" (Redclay & Courchesne, 2005). A second current theory to explain large head size in autism involves inflammation of the brain. This theory arose when scientists found evidence of inflammation in the brains of individuals with autism in postmortem studies (Pardo, Vargas, & Zimmerman, 2005). This is a very active area of work right now, and the answers to the question about what causes the brain growth and what it means for autism lie in the future.

Cerebellar Differences

One of the most consistent findings in autism is the decreased number of a certain type of cell in the cortex of the cerebellum—the Purkinje cells (Bauman & Kemper, 1994). In autism, there are 35–50% fewer Purkinje cells than normal, and autopsy studies have suggested that these missing cells have never formed, further suggesting that the abnormality occurs during prenatal brain development. The Purkinje neurons inhibit the excitation of other neurons all through the brain. They have very long axons that connect all the way forward to areas within the frontal lobes. The cerebellar neurons are in fact massively connected to widespread areas of the cortex in all the brain lobules: the frontal, parietal, temporal, and occipital lobes; and they connect via intermediate connections with the thalamus, which is part of the limbic system. This represents another brain structure abnormality that can affect brain connectivity in autism. Research involving people who have abnormal cerebellar activity demonstrates effects on attention, emotion, and cognition as well as motor functions. Thus, abnormal connectivity due to the Purkinje cell decrease could affect many neural pathways that appear involved in the many symptoms seen in autism.

Social Brain Network Differences

Brain imaging studies that allow scientists to view the activity of different brain regions while a person is engaged in different tasks (e.g., while looking at a face or listening to words with emotional content) have demonstrated that the social brain is not functioning properly in individuals with autism. The most common finding is reduced activity in the social brain regions while a person is engaged in social tasks. For example, Dawson, Carver, Meltzoff, Panagiotides, and McPartland (2002) found that preschool-age children with autism did not show the typical level of brain response to facial and emotional stimuli. This was striking because such brain responses are typically evident by 6–7 months of age. This study suggests that autism affects social brain structures that develop in the first year of life.

Another finding in autism is the failure of one part of the social brain (e.g., amygdala) to be functioning in coordination with another part (e.g., fusiform) during a social task. Several brain imaging studies have suggested abnormal functioning of the amygdala, which is involved in assigning reward value to stimuli and is a particularly salient feature of autism. Studies have shown that the amygdala is particularly enlarged early on (Sparks et al., 2002) and that neurons in the amygdala are reduced in number and size (Schumann & Amaral, 2006). It has been proposed that a failure to assign reward value to social stimuli, such as faces, voices, gestures, and other social stimuli, is a fundamental impairment in autism that has downstream consequences (Dawson, Webb, & McPartland, 2005). The lack of sensitivity to "social reward" would explain why the child with autism fails to look at others. If a young toddler with autism is failing to look at others, then he or she is missing the opportunity to learn about social communication, facial expressions, and a wide range of other social and communicative behaviors. Such studies have helped us understand why children with autism have such difficulty responding appropriately in social situations.

Mirror Neuron System

The mirror neuron system involves several brain areas: the inferior parietal lobe, inferior frontal cortex, Broca's area in the temporal lobe, the STS, and the motor cortex. This system activates when a person (or primate) carries out an intentional action and when observing another person (or primate) carry out an intentional action. In humans, the mirror neuron system also fires when making and when observing gestures and facial expressions that do not have a particular goal in terms of actions on objects. The mirror neuron system, including Broca's area (the language area) is activated by observing imitation and gesture and by imitating another person. This suggests that developing imitation skills, nonverbal gestural communication, and verbal communication heavily involves the mirror neuron system. Empathic reactions and theory of mind problems also activate the mirror neuron system, and these are all tasks that involve coordinating representations of one's own experience and those of another person's experience. Thus, the mirror neuron system is considered extremely important for developing social behavior, especially behaviors that allow one to coordinate with another person's experience.

It has been suggested that mirror neuron system dysfunction could underlie autism (Williams, Whiten, Suddendorf, & Perrett, 2001). A number of studies have demonstrated that the mirror neuron systems of people with autism do not respond normally to watching other people's gestures and expressions and imitating them. Since the mirror neuron system does not involve a single area or circuit, but rather is a very widespread property of the human brain (Iacoboni & Mazziotta, 2007), abnormal functioning of the mirror neuron system is thought to reflect problems with overall brain connectivity.

Neurochemistry Differences

Neurons in the brain respond to chemical signals, and signals from one neuron to the next are conveyed through chemical changes in the synapse—the space between the sending and receiving dendrites of the neurons. Thus, abnormal levels of these neurotransmitters can affect both brain function and overt behavior. The possibility that brain chemistry differences underlie autism has been discussed ever since abnormal levels of serotonin one neurotransmitter were first reported. It is now a well-replicated finding that group studies of persons with autism demonstrate increased levels of serotonin in the bloodstreams of both affected people and their first-degree relatives. However, it is not clear that this reflects differences in brain levels of serotonin, and studies that have examined the effects of changing serotonin levels in autism have not found the marked behavioral effects one would expect if this was a major cause (Posey, Erickson, Stigler, & McDougle, 2006). Another theory of abnormal neurochemistry involves two peptides, oxytocin and vasopressin, which are closely related and affect social behavior and repetitive behavior in a wide number of mammals (Insel, O'Brien, & Leckman, 1999). There is evidence of decreased oxytocin levels in persons with ASD, and evidence of abnormalities in the gene associated with vasopressin, though no reports of decreased vasopressin levels have yet been reported. Some small experimental studies suggest enhanced social effects of oxytocin treatment in both persons with typical development and those with ASD.

BRAIN CHANGES IN EARLY CHILDHOOD AND BEYOND

In their landmark autopsy studies involving brain tissue from persons with ASD, Bauman and Kemper (1994) noted that the differences they observed in brain cells and structures did not appear to be limited to differences present from infancy. Their observations of brain differences related to age variables suggested ongoing brain changes over time, from early childhood into adulthood. What might cause continued brain changes? Certainly, exposure to neurotoxic influences could account for ongoing brain changes, as could immune abnormalities; research continues in these areas. However, altered experiences can also alter brain function. Experience is important for establishing neural connections, as explained above. It also plays a role in "turning on" certain gene functions. For example, studies with animals have shown that certain social behaviors, such as a mother licking her pup, can influence the expressions of genes that regulate cortisol, a stress hormone. Other studies have shown that exposure to an enriched environment reduces poor outcomes in animals that have sustained brain injury or have a genetic propensity to develop seizures.

In the past few years, we have learned a great deal about how quickly the human brain responds to changes in experiences. Beginning to learn a new skill, like playing a string instrument, causes measurable effects on brain function in a matter of days. Brain regions that did not respond to the stimulus before practice begin to respond. Brain regions that had previously responded during a different stimulus are "recruited" by the new skill and now begin to respond to the new stimulus. Our mirror neuron system responds much more actively to observation of skills that we can ourselves perform than to those that we recognize but cannot perform. Experiences sculpt the brain, stimulating the formation of networks of responsive neurons and neural regions that allow for increasingly skilled and automatic performance. Our brains develop neural networks based on our ongoing behavior; that is, networks that support and enhance response patterns to frequently encountered stimuli. The experience of reward and feedback from the environment is an integral part of this process.

Consider, then, how having autism might affect how the brain develops. Infants with autism respond differently to the environment, many from the first year of life. The infant is less responsive to social stimuli and doesn't initiate social interaction. Thus, he or she has many fewer social interactions over the course of a day than would be typical. At the same time, the infant may be overly fixated on objects and engage in repetitive play with objects. These daily experiences and response patterns are sculpting his or her brain, developing reward expectations, stimulating the formation of increasingly developed neural networks stimulated by and supporting object-related events, and not developing neural networks or attentional systems oriented toward social events. As the day-to-day life of a child with autism becomes increasingly different from that of a nonautistic peer, the brain connections and neural response patterns are likely also diverging, and this may be another source of ongoing brain differences. These brain changes, though, are considered to be "reactive," not part of the core neural features of autism, but secondary and associated to the altered life patterns that accompany infant autism, and that are, perhaps, preventable (Dawson, 2008).

THE ROLE OF EARLY INTERVENTION IN SHAPING EARLY BRAIN DEVELOPMENT AND OUTCOME IN AUTISM

As described earlier, infancy is considered to be a period of marked plasticity in brain development and learning potential. Given this plasticity of young brains, and the effect of experience in shaping brain function and structure, we should expect that intervention experiences will contribute to brain changes as well as behavior changes. The activities children engage in across their day are not neutral—they are either building a more social and communicative brain or building a more object-oriented brain. In the ESDM, we use a style of interaction in which adults capture children's attention to faces and bodies (social orienting) and then provide extremely clear social and communicative behavior signals that represent optimum parenting techniques for developing elaborated language, social and symbolic play, and social initiations from children. Addressing the fundamental social orienting and initiation deficiencies that mark early autism are core features of the ESDM. We discuss those core features and the ESDM's theoretical foundations in the next chapter.

Chapter 2

An Overview of the Early Start Denver Model

The ESDM was developed for intensive delivery of comprehensive early intervention to toddlers as young as 12 months of age. It is a refined and adapted extension of the Denver Model intervention for preschoolers with autism ages 24–60 months. Throughout this text, we refer to the ESDM when we discuss interventions for children younger than 3 years of age. We refer to the Denver Model when we discuss use of the model across the entire preschool age period, encompassing 3- and 4-year-olds as well.

The ESDM is grounded in current empirical knowledge of infant–toddler learning, and of the effects of autism on early development, as reviewed in Chapter 1. Its aim is to reduce the severity of autism symptoms and accelerate children's developmental rates in all domains, but particularly cognitive, social–emotional, and language domains. In this chapter, we present an overview of the ESDM, describe how it accomplishes its goals, and describe its similarities and differences from other well-known models. We begin with a brief discussion of the key approaches that underlie the ESDM.

FOUNDATIONS OF THE ESDM

Several different, complementary approaches come together to provide the foundations of the ESDM. These include the original Denver Model developed by Rogers and colleagues beginning in 1981 (Rogers, Herbison, Lewis, Pantone, & Reis, 1986); Rogers and Pennington's (1991) model of interpersonal development in autism; Dawson and colleagues' (2004) model of autism as a disorder of social motivation; and pivotal response training (PRT), a teaching approach based in applied behavior analysis (ABA) that highlights child initiative and spontaneity and can be delivered in natural contexts (Schreibman & Pierce, 1993; Koegel & Koegel, 1988).

The Denver Model

The Denver Model began in the 1980s, as a developmentally based group preschool program for young children with autism ages 24–60 months (Rogers et al., 1986; Rogers & Lewis, 1989; Rogers, Hall, Osaki, Reaven, & Herbison, 2000). Seeing autism primarily as a failure of social-communicative development, the program focused on building close relationships with children as a foundation for social and communication development. It primarily emphasized lively, dynamic interactions involving a strong positive affect that would lead children to seek out social partners as participants in favorite activities. The technique of "sensory social routines" was developed that highlighted the highly engaging dyadic exchanges that children initiated and continued through nonverbal, and later, verbal communications. As described in more detail in Chapter 6, sensory social routines are a core feature of the ESDM. Experience in the Denver Model also taught that most of the children treated had developmental delays across all domains, thus necessitating a multidisciplinary team approach. Of equal importance, a developmental curriculum systematically assessed all aspects of children's development, and short-term developmental objectives defined the individual curriculum for each child, intensively taught in individual and small-group settings throughout the day. Teaching followed children's leads and emphasized language, nonverbal communication, cognition, and play.

Core features of the Denver Model that are retained in the ESDM include (1) an interdisciplinary team that implements a developmental curriculum addressing all domains; (2) focus on interpersonal engagement; (3) development of fluent, reciprocal, and spontaneous imitation of gestures, facial movements and expressions, and object use; (4) emphasis on both nonverbal and verbal communication development; (5) focus on cognitive aspects of play carried out within dyadic play routines; and (6) partnership with parents.

Work over the first 10 years of the Denver Model led Rogers and colleagues to appreciate the profound deficits in imitation that typify young children with autism. This deficit was not mentioned in theories of autism at the time, and there were few studies of imitation in autism. However, the lack of imitation in these little children presented a huge barrier to child learning, and it led to deeper thinking about the role of imitation in early development. Writings by Daniel Stern (1985), Andrew Meltzoff (Meltzoff & Moore, 1977), and others provided compelling arguments for the centrality of imitation in social-communicative development in infancy.

Rogers and Pennington's Model of Interpersonal Development in Autism

Rogers and Pennington (1991) published a heuristic developmental model of autism strongly influenced by the work of Daniel Stern (1985) and the infant research that occurred in the 1970s and 1980s. In this model, Rogers and Pennington (1991) hypothesized that an early impairment in imitation, a capacity normally available to infants from birth (Meltzoff & Moore, 1977), is present in autism from the beginnings of life and disrupts the early establishment of bodily synchrony and coordination. Such bodily synchrony is the first way in which the infant and caregiver attune to each other's feelings and states, and impairment in such synchrony was suggested to affect the emotional coordination between them. Emotional coordination may be further affected by the atypical expressions of facial emotion in the infant with autism (Yirmiya, Kasari, Sigman, & Mundy, 1989); and this may prevent the parent from easily mirroring the infant's emotional states. Impairments in imitation and affective sharing at this level between infant and caregiver create barriers to developing an understanding of both the infant's and the partner's feelings and mental states. It also severely affects the development of the infant's awareness of and use of intentional communication, for the same reasons. These impediments are seen in toddlers with autism in the behavioral landmarks of intersubjective development that Stern described: delayed and decreased imitation, joint attention, emotion sharing, and intentional communication (Rogers, Hepburn, Stackhouse, & Wehner, 2003; Charman et al., 1998; Seibert, Hogan, & Mundy, 1982; Mundy, Sigman, & Kasari, 1990; Kasari, Sigman, Mundy, & Yirmiya, 1990; Wetherby & Prutting, 1984; Uzgiris, 1973; Stone & Caro-Martinez, 1990; Stone, Ousley, Yoder, Hogan & Hepburn, 1997). A main focus of ESDM treatment is to address these critical developments in the social–emotional–communicative domain, within emotionally rich relationships with responsive, sensitive others. In Stern's (1985) model (and those of many others: Ainsworth, Blehar, Waters, & Wall, 1978; Carpenter & Tomasello, 2000), a sensitive and responsive relationship provided by caregivers is critical for these developments to come about.

The Social Motivation Hypothesis of Autism

The ESDM also has been strongly influenced by research on another core feature of autism: impaired social motivation, discussed at length in Chapter 1. Persons with autism of all ages spend less time than other persons attending to and interacting with other people. This pattern of behavior is present even before imitation and joint attention deficits discriminate infants with autism. Dawson and colleagues (Dawson, Webb, et al., 2002; Dawson et al., 2004; Dawson, Webb, & McPartland, 2005) have hypothesized that the biology of autism involves a fundamental deficiency in social motivation due to the young child's relative lack of sensitivity to social reward. This lack results in a failure of the young child with autism to have a normal preference for and active attention to social information in his or her environment, including other's faces, voices, gestures, and speech. This failure to actively attend to and engage with others contributes to impairments in imitation, emotional sharing, and joint attention, and is a major obstacle to the child's development of social–emotional and communicative skills. As a result, the child with autism becomes more and more removed from the social world around him or her, and from all the crucial learning experiences that exist inside that world. The child falls farther and farther behind because he or she lacks the interactive skills needed to access the ongoing social learning environment in which typical infants, toddlers, and young children are completely immersed. Dawson and colleagues have suggested that this early lack of engagement in the social environment not only alters the course of behavioral development in children with autism, but it also affects the way neural systems underlying the perception and representation of social and linguistic information are developed and organized (Dawson et al., 2005; Dawson & Zanolli, 2003). Several of the strategies utilized in the ESDM, such as the sensory social techniques of the Denver Model and the PRT techniques developed by Koegel, Schreibman, and colleagues (Koegel & Koegel, 1995; Koegel, 2000; Schreibman, 1988), are designed to increase the salience of social rewards and thus enhance the child's social attention and motivation for social interaction.

Pivotal Response Training

A particular method of teaching children with autism using the principles of ABA was developed by Schreibman and Koegel (Schreibman & Pierce, 1993; Koegel & Koegel,

1988) and first published in the 1980s. PRT differs greatly from discrete trial teaching (the method publicized by Lovaas [1987] and described later in this chapter), even though the same core ABA teaching principles underlie both. PRT techniques were developed to optimize children's motivation to interact with adults and engage in repeated learning opportunities. Core motivational and teaching strategies include (1) use of reinforcers that are directly related to the child's goals and responses, (2) incorporating child choice into the teaching episodes, (3) interspersing previously acquired (or maintenance) tasks with acquisition tasks, (4) therapist reinforcement of child's attempts to perform the desired behavior at whatever level of accuracy the child can produce at the moment, (5) using activities that are highly motivating to the child, and (6) sharing control of the materials and interactions with the child. PRT is currently considered one of the empirically supported practices for building communication skills in children with autism, given its long history of published findings documenting enhanced child motivation, spontaneity, and social initiation; improved language, improved maintenance, and response generalization; and for concomitant reductions in unwanted behaviors. PRT strategies are incorporated into the teaching approaches used in the ESDM; their explicit incorporation represents one area of difference between the original Denver Model and the ESDM.

The approaches to autism just described have in common the view that early autism impedes an infant's early interpersonal experiences. In so doing, it creates barriers to social-communicative development, and these barriers result in a greater and greater impairment in the child over time due to the loss of social learning opportunities. The ESDM intervention seeks to stop this negative cascade of effects over time and increase child social learning in two ways: (1) by bringing the child into coordinated, interactive social relations for most of his or her waking hours, so that interpersonal and symbolic communication can be established and the transmission of social knowledge and social experience can occur; and (2) intensive teaching to "fill in" the learning deficits that have resulted from the child's past lack of access to the social world (Rogers et al., 2000). These goals are accomplished through teaching the ESDM curriculum using a specific set of teaching procedures.

THE ESDM CURRICULUM

In the ESDM, we understand autism as a disruption of development that affects virtually all developmental domains. This developmental orientation underlies our understanding of the impairments in the disorder, the curriculum that drives treatment goals and objectives, and the wide array of intervention techniques that are used. The ESDM curriculum is embodied in the ESDM Curriculum Checklist and Item Descriptions (see Appendix A). It lists specific skills sequenced developmentally within domains that include receptive communication, expressive communication, joint attention, imitation, social skills, play skills, cognitive skills, fine motor skills, gross motor skills, and self-care skills. Five of these domains carry particular weight in the ESDM: imitation, nonverbal communication (including joint attention), verbal communication, social development (including emotion sharing), and play.

On entry into the ESDM, children's current skill levels are evaluated using the ESDM Curriculum Checklist. Learning objectives are then written for the child, designed to be achieved within a 12-week period. At the end of 12 weeks, new learning objectives for the next 12-week period are written based on a new assessment with the Curriculum Checklist.

Language Development within a Social Context

The language intervention approach used in the ESDM comes from the science of communication development rather than behavior analysis and recognizes that verbal language develops from nonverbal social-communication behaviors as well as phonemic development (Bruner, 1975; Bates & Dick, 2002; Fergus, Menn, & Stoel-Gammon, 1992; Tomasello, 1992). Both verbal and nonverbal communication coordinate people's activities and allow partners to share their inner lives involving intentions, desires, interests, thoughts, and feelings. The ESDM intervention provides multiple and varied communicative opportunities and elicits many communicative behaviors, both verbal and nonverbal, from the child during each intervention session. The range of communicative, or pragmatic functions (Bates, 1976) is carefully developed so that a child not only requests an activity but also protests, greets familiar adults, shares attention, and comments or narrates during an activity. Spontaneous communication is carefully supported and children's communications exert much control over interactions and activities, thus demonstrating to children the power of communication and ensuring that communication is strongly reinforced. Consistent with the developmental emphasis, the adult's level of language is gauged and fitted to the child's language abilities, both in vocabulary and in the complexity of utterance used.

Building Up Complex Behaviors

The developmental skills that appear most affected in infants and toddlers with autism involve the more complex skills including joint attention, imitation, language, and symbolic play, which we assume require elaborated neural networks and significant brain connectivity to support. We further assume that the connectivity between brain regions required for complex activities needs to be stimulated through experience. Thus, we teach these behaviors by embedding them in highly preferred activities and we build them up from the simplest steps to the most complex. This is done by using a systematic breakdown of the skills based on developmental sequences in typical infancy as well as systematic procedures such as task analysis. These steps are described in detail in Chapter 4. However, we always target more than one skill domain during any teaching episode because we recognize that this is how skills typically develop. For example, in one teaching episode, we might target eye contact, expressive language, and motor behavior while the child is playing with building blocks, rather than teaching eye contact as an isolated behavior.

An Interdisciplinary Approach Underlies the Intervention

Autism is a disorder involving multiple deficits (Goodman, 1989; Happe, Ronald, & Plomin, 2006; Rogers, 1998). The curriculum items were extracted from research in early child development in multiple developmental domains: cognition, expressive and receptive language, social–emotional development, fine and gross motor development, self-care skills, play, and imitation. The curriculum was developed by a team of professionals from disciplines with particular expertise in these areas, including developmental and clinical psychology, ABA, early childhood special education, speech–language pathology (S-LP), and occupational therapy (OT).

Developmental and clinical psychologists contribute to the sequence of acquisition and the normative strategies for interaction, cognitive development, social–emotional development, play, and imitation. Applied behavior analysts contribute empirically derived strategies for effective teaching, and use functional assessment and analysis of behavior to develop approaches for unwanted behaviors and effective teaching practices. Early childhood special educators contribute expertise on early cognition and play, early education, and pre-academic development to develop teaching activities, peer interactions, and developmental sequences. Speech and language pathologists inform the sequence of speech development: oral–motor, phonemic, and word development, semantic development (vocabulary), morpho–syntactic development (grammar and word combinations), the varied pragmatic functions of communication, and use of augmentative and alternative communication approaches. Occupational therapists inform the sequence and content of motor skills, self-care skills, and personal independence, the use of functional activities to build developmental skills, and optimization of arousal and sensory responsivity to facilitate attention and engagement in learning. In addition, consultation with pediatrics contributes knowledge of the health-related concerns of individual children, such as seizures, sleep difficulties, nutrition, and allergies, that can interfere with children's ability to benefit from the intervention.

In the ESDM, this interdisciplinary team provides oversight and consultation regarding the intervention plan and progress for each child. When the ESDM is delivered mainly through parents or through 1:1 teaching, the direct delivery of the intervention is typically provided by one main professional, working with parents, and, often, therapy assistants. This generalist delivery model (Schopler, Mesibov, & Hearsey, 1995) is felt to keep the intervention approach consistent across treatment sessions and as economical as possible. It also models what parents need to do: address all of the child's needs. The full team is available as consultants to the primary therapist and family as needed. When the ESDM is delivered in a group preschool setting, the classroom teacher takes the generalist role with a consulting interdisciplinary team. The interdisciplinary team and its members are discussed in more detail in Chapter 3.

Systematic Individualization

There are four main methods of achieving individualization in the ESDM. First is the developmental curriculum, which targets the child's individual learning needs in each domain as described above. Second is the focus on children's preferences and interests, which individualizes materials and activities for each child. The third method is by incorporating family values, needs, and preferences into child objectives and parents' use of the ESDM at home and in other community settings. We discuss these three methods in the section that follows on teaching procedures. The fourth method is use of a decision tree that allows the therapist to make systematic changes in the teaching procedures when progress is too slow; we discuss this in Chapter 6.

ESDM TEACHING PROCEDURES

ESDM teaching is embedded inside play activities, addresses multiple objectives across developmental domains, and occurs at a very high rate. This allows for a great deal of teaching to occur in a typical play activity, and results in efficient use of the therapist's teaching time and the child's learning time. We emphasize efficient teaching because the children we serve have a great deal of learning to do to fill in the gaps and a very limited window of time in which to do so.

The ESDM uses teaching practices and procedures melded together from three intervention traditions: ABA, PRT, and the Denver Model. The core teaching practices to be used are those defined and assessed using the ESDM Teaching Fidelity Rating System, found in Appendix B.

Teaching Strategies from ABA

According to the basic principles of ABA, three components are necessary for learning. First, some stimulus must serve as a cue for the child to respond—and the child must attend to this stimulus event. Second, the child must emit a behavior immediately following the stimulus. Third, the child must experience some type of consequence or feedback that marks a correct performance (Lovaas, 2002). Over time, we want to see the child emit the new behavior more quickly, frequently, and easily in response to the stimulus, and to use the new skill or behavior in a widening range of appropriate contexts—generalization.

The science of learning goes back to the early 1900s, with psychological experiments and breakthroughs by Watson, Pavlov (classical conditioning), Thorndike (instrumental conditioning), and Skinner (operant conditioning; see Anderson, 2000, for an historical review). Research from the learning theory tradition is the foundation of ABA. Use of this research to help children and adults with developmental disorders began in earnest in the 1960s. It provided successful teaching approaches for persons who had previously been considered unable to learn (see Gardner, 2006, for a history of this development). The first publication describing the successful use of operant teaching procedures for a child with autism occurred in 1964 (Baer & Sherman, 1964), and the discrete trial teaching procedures (also referred to in this text as "massed trials" or the "Lovaas approach") so popular in autism intervention emanate from this period (Lovaas, 2002; Lovaas, Berberich, Perloff, & Schaeffer, 1966; Lovaas, Freitag, Gold, & Kassoria, 1965). (Note that the children involved were then often referred to as *schizophrenic* rather than *autistic*; the terms were essentially synonymous for a period of time when autism was seen as a type of schizophrenia.)

Basic practices of effective teaching used in ABA are summarized below. They include capturing attention, delivering teaching within an antecedent–behavior–consequence sequence, prompting, managing consequences, fading, shaping, chaining, and functional assessment. If more information is needed, consult excellent texts like Cooper, Heron, and Heward (2006); O'Neill et al. (1997); O'Neill, Horner, Albin, Storey, and Sprague (1990); and Pierce and Cheney (2008).

Capturing Attention

It is crucial to attain and maintain the child's attention until the instruction has been given or the action modeled, the action accomplished, and the reward delivered.

Antecedent–Behavior–Consequence (ABC)

An antecedent is a stimulus that occurs before a behavior. The consequence is an act that directly follows the behavior. Antecedent–behavior–consequence is what defines a three-term contingency and this sequence defines specific learning trials. Learning involves the formation of a new relationship between a stimulus event (the antecedent) and a behavior (or cognition). The nature of the consequence defines the nature of the relationship. Teaching involves manipulating the antecedent and the consequence to either strengthen or weaken the relation between the antecedent and the behavior. Consequences may involve reinforcement, punishment, or extinction (which is not actually a consequence—it is the absence or removal of a consequence that formerly was reinforcing). Increases and decreases in behavior due to the manipulation of the antecedent and consequence are the sine qua non of operant behavioral treatment.

Prompting Desired Behaviors

The learner must emit the behavior being taught in some fashion following the antecedent during the teaching episode so that it can be rewarded and its ties to the stimulus strengthened. Some behaviors are already in children's repertoires, but the children do not emit them under the appropriate stimulus conditions. Other behaviors are not in the child's repertoire at all, and the adult must build the behavior. The adult has to find a way to prompt the child to emit the behavior under specified stimulus conditions—the instructions, gestures, or materials that are to serve a stimulus function, or act as an antecedent, for the behavior.

Managing Consequences

Skillfully managing consequences allows children to attain rapid initial learning, to build strong habits that are not easily extinguished, to generalize the behavior appropriately, and to reduce unwanted behaviors. The strength, timing, and frequency of reinforcement delivery affect the quality, consistency, speed, and frequency of the behavior as well as the speed of learning. Different consequent strategies are needed for different learning goals.

Fading Prompts

While prompts are needed to assist a learner emit a new behavior in the presence of a certain stimulus, they have to be systematically faded so that the behavior is emitted in response to the discriminative stimulus rather than the prompt. Careful management of fading is crucial to avoid prompt dependence by children who do not initiate desired behaviors unless prompted by an adult. Fading prompts is one way to teach a child to generalize skills or demonstrate them with other people.

Shaping Behaviors

A child's performance of a new behavior is often only an approximation of the mature level of that behavior. Early speech of typical toddlers is an excellent example. Once children have learned to emit an immature version of a behavior, the adult must use careful prompting and reinforcement strategies to gradually shape the immature behavior into a more mature behavior.

Chaining Behaviors

Complex behaviors like speech, dressing, playing games, reading, writing, and so on are built up from individual actions that become linked together to form behavior sequences. Building up these sequences from the individual actions to produce fluent behavioral sequences is called *chaining*, and it requires careful prompting, fading, reinforcement, and task-analysis strategies.

Functional Assessment or Analysis of Behavior

A major tenet of behaviorism is that all behaviors are functional; that is, they are useful in achieving a particular goal and are in the behavioral repertoire because they lead to a reward. In order to replace undesired behaviors with more desirable behaviors, one must first understand what goal is achieved for the individual using that behavior. A functional assessment is a process of determining the functions of a behavior; that is, what goals it meets for the individual, and what reinforcement is maintaining that behavior. It is sometimes the case that functions of a behavior may be too difficult to identify during this type of assessment, and will require a full functional analysis. A functional analysis involves actively testing the effects of a variety of consequences that may be maintaining the behaviors in order to identify which variables are actually supporting it. A functional analysis is the only way to causally define the variables that underlie a behavior; however, it is a highly technical procedure, and requires a fair amount of expertise to design and carry out. There are also ethical implications at times, as when the unwanted behavior involves injury to self or others. Thus, we use functional assessment, rather than functional analysis, whenever possible. Behavioral analysts on the team are well positioned to determine the indicators that a functional analysis, rather than assessment, is needed.

Strategies from PRT

PRT is a treatment based on the principles of ABA and was first published in the 1980s by Robert and Lynn Koegel (Koegel & Williams, 1980; Koegel, O'Dell, & Koegel, 1987; Koegel & Koegel, 1988) and Laura Schreibman (Ingersoll & Schreibman, 2006; Schreibman & Koegel, 2005), who observed improved motivation, behavior, spontaneity, and generalization in children whose behavioral treatment was delivered in a more natural interactive framework rather than an adult-directed, massed trial format. They and their students and colleagues carried out a series of studies in which they demonstrated the efficacy of several additional teaching approaches to the basic principles of reinforcement, prompting, fading, shaping, and chaining discussed above (see Schreibman & Koegel, 2005, for a description of the supporting evidence).

PRT research suggests that two behaviors appear to be pivotal in improving a wide range of behaviors and in determining later adaptive capacities: *motivation* and *response to multiple cues* (Koegel, Koegel, Harrower, & Carter, 1999a; Koegel, Koegel, Shoshan,

& McNerney, 1999b). These behaviors are central to a wide area of functioning, so positive changes in these behaviors should have widespread effects on other behaviors (Koegel & Frea, 1993; Koegel et al., 1999b).

Compared to discrete trial teaching, PRT techniques result in children with more motivation to perform, better generalization of new skills, more spontaneous responding, and less problem behavior (Ingersoll & Schreibman, 2006; Losardo & Bricker, 1994). PRT works to increase motivation by including components such as child choice, turn taking, reinforcing attempts, and interspersing maintenance tasks. PRT builds the child's capacity to respond to multiple cues by varying the antecedents, purposefully setting up stimuli with multiple cues, and teaching children to emit the same behavior in response to varying related antecedents. PRT has been used successfully to target language skills, play skills, imitation, gesture, and social behaviors in children with autism (Koegel & Koegel, 1995; Schreibman & Koegel, 2005). However, PRT is an appropriate teaching method only when the skill to be taught has a direct relationship to a reinforcer (discussed in more depth in Chapter 5).

PRT Principles Used in the ESDM

1. *Reinforce child attempts.* Don't expect children to be able to deliver their best performance all the time. Rewarding attempts enhances motivation and perseverance and decreases frustration and unwanted behaviors.

2. *Alternate requests for new behaviors—acquisition skills—with requests for already learned maintenance skills.* This alternating of more difficult tasks with easy tasks also enhances motivation and decreases frustration. It also keeps learned skills under review, supporting their maintenance.

3. *Reinforcers have a direct relationship to the child's response or behavior.* The reinforcer flows from the child's initial choice and immediately follows the desired behavior. The child reaches for a car and ends up getting the car. The child reaches for your hands to play a game, and in the end you play that game. The child wants to be finished, and the target behavior results in the end of the activity. The reinforcer is a natural part of the activity, not extrinsic to it. This is also true of social or verbal rewards. When a child speaks, in the ESDM we do not respond by saying "good talking" (extrinsic reward). We respond by restating and expanding the child's words and giving the desired object or activity (e.g., child: "Car?"; adult: "Car. Here's the car.").

4. *Take turns in the activities.* Seek balanced interactions in which each partner has a chance to lead and follow—thus sharing control of the interaction. Taking turns makes the activity social, and it gives the adult access to the child's attention, the opportunity to model a behavior, and the opportunity to elicit a new child communication when it is time for the child's turn. It gives the child the opportunity to request, to imitate, and to see his or her actions mirrored by the adult.

5. *Instructions or other antecedents are delivered clearly.* The adult must have the child's attention and be sure that the antecedent, or stimulus, is appropriate to the task or activity and is present before the behavior is requested.

6. *Give children choices and follow their leads.* By using children's choices as an

opportunity to practice targeted skills, the adult builds child motivation, capitalizes on the strength of the reinforcer selected, and has the opportunity to reinforce children's self-initiated, or spontaneous, behavior.

These PRT principles are a fundamental aspect of the ESDM, and the explicit addition of these is one of the differences between the older version of the Denver Model, published and described before 2002, and the ESDM, developed and described since 2002.

Teaching Practices Developed in the Denver Model

The rest of the teaching practices in the ESDM come from the Denver Model. These focus on the affective and relationship-based aspects of the therapist's work with the child, the emphasis on development of play skills, and the use of communication intervention principles from the field of communication science (Rogers et al., 1986; Rogers & Lewis, 1989; Rogers et al., 2000).

1. *Adults modulate and optimize child affect, arousal, and attentional state.* The therapist skillfully modulates child affect and arousal through choice of activities, tone of voice, and level of adult activity so that the child can more optimally participate in learning. This practice targets affective characteristics as seen in a tired, lethargic, or underaroused child; a passive, perhaps avoidant child; a child who is whining, escaping, frustrated, hurt, crying, or otherwise upset; or an overactive, high-energy child who is not settling into an activity.

2. *Adult use of positive affect.* The adult displays clear, genuine, and natural positive affect throughout the episode matched by child positive affect. Positive affect permeates the episode, is well matched to child needs and capacities, does not overarouse the child, and serves teaching well.

3. *Turn taking and dyadic engagement occurs throughout.* The child is actively involved in adult turns, including giving toys, watching the adult, and showing awareness of both partners' acts. Reciprocity and social engagement between partners permeate the teaching activity.

4. *Adults respond sensitively and responsively to child communicative cues.* This refers to the adult's attunement to child states, motives, and feelings. A sensitive and responsive adult reads the child well and acknowledges communicative cues, whether verbal or gestural, by verbalizing or by acting contingently according to the child's communication so that the child seems to have been "heard." Or, in the face of an affective cue, the adult responds empathically to the child's emotional state by mirroring the emotion and communicating an understanding of it. The adult does not reinforce unwanted behavior, but acknowledges the child's cues and responds appropriately given the situation.

5. *Multiple and varied communicative opportunities occur.* The adult scaffolds multiple communications involving several different communicative functions during each play activity as specified in the child's objectives. Several different pragmatic functions are expressed, including opportunities to request, protest, comment, ask for help,

greet, name, expand, and so on. The range of pragmatic and communicative opportunities fits well with the child's language level. The adult uses a range of techniques including modeling, restatement, expansion of child utterances, and repetition of child utterances embedded in meaningful activities.

6. *Elaboration of activities.* The therapist encourages flexible, elaborated use of actions and materials by using multiple materials and varied schemas, theme, and variation, and/or narrative frames. The adult targets multiple objectives from different developmental domains in a single activity. Even if the child needs more adult-directed, mass trial teaching to learn, activities are still elaborated by having the child help take out, put away, and choose materials, or by interweaving social and communicative exchanges.

7. *Adult language is consistently appropriate developmentally and pragmatically for the child's verbal and nonverbal communicative intent and capacity.* Adults generally follow the one-up rule (i.e., the mean length of the adult's utterances is approximately one word longer than the mean length of the child's utterances), respond to child's communications with appropriate language, and use language to demonstrate a variety of pragmatic functions, semantic relations, and syntactic combinations.

8. *Transitions are effectively managed.* The adult scaffolds the child's shift of interest by closing down one activity and bringing up others, so that the child's interest flows smoothly from one activity to the next with minimal downtime. The timing of the transition is sensitive to the child's attention and motivation. Child independence is fostered and the child is attentive and quickly engaged in the new activity.

Using ESDM Teaching Strategies Together

When combined, the techniques outlined above are designed to engage the child in positive emotional experiences with another person, to draw the child's attention to social stimuli, to make such stimuli rewarding for the child, and to foster the child's motivation to continue such activities. Therapists use these techniques to elicit social and communicative behavior from the child that is as close to "normal" as we can create. We do this because we believe that these experiences are shaping brains as well as behaviors, and we want to stimulate and shape children's neural networks into patterns of greater sensitivity and responsivity to social partners than objects.

Use of Positive Affect

We focus closely on creating positive emotional states in children during social interactions, because we want to enhance the reward value of social interaction and recalibrate children's responsivity to voices, faces, and eyes. This includes the use of very pleasurable sensory social routines, focused on dyadic social experiences, and also on the use of highly preferred object routines that are accompanied and embedded in strongly social and communicative actions. Creating such positive routines also captures children's attention to support information processing of the social-communicative framework.

As mentioned in Chapter 1, research suggests that learning, especially language and social learning, is facilitated when it occurs in the context of an affectively rich and engaging interaction with another person. Thus, we use techniques in which social and language skills are taught within the context of playful, engaging experiences.

The ESDM's emphasis on positive affect and modulation of affective and arousal states to optimize social engagement and learning directly activates the social brain and its related neurotransmitters to foster the development of social and communicative behavior. The ESDM can improve the child's "social motivation" by stimulating two aspects of the social reward system: "liking" and "wanting," which are not the same thing. We can like things without having the incentive to attain them (want). Some children with autism appear to like social interaction, in that they respond positively to engagement, but they don't appear to seek it out. Others seem neither to like nor to want it. The ESDM addresses both liking and wanting by increasing the reward value of social engagement. During the first interactions, the adult partner focuses on "finding the smile"; in other words, finding sources of pleasure for the child. The goal is to make social engagement an intrinsic part of the reward. For children who do not "like" social engagement, this technique builds reward value through associative learning processes. In other words, social experiences are paired with nonsocial rewards, such as objects, to enhance the reward value of the social experience. We use both operant and classical learning paradigms to increase the reward value of social engagement and establish "liking," which also connotes proximity and attention to the liked stimulus.

The ESDM builds up the "want" by shaping children's self-initiated approach and requesting behaviors as they gain access to social and nonsocial rewards. But their access to desired social rewards needs to be controlled so that they are not satiated by the reward. This also ensures that to attain the reward, children need to intentionally use social and communicative acts.

The teaching approaches used in the ESDM do not only focus on simple stimulus–response associations that are required by a simple new habit. Rather, the approaches are designed to promote complex neural networks, involving a wider range of skills, by promoting skills that recruit neural activity from across brain regions. The types of teaching in the ESDM involve presenting one "theme" and then varying it; they target multiple domains during a teaching task, and involve affective engagement during the teaching of concepts. All of these practices result in increasingly complex neural networks and thus foster greater connectivity across multiple brain regions.

Play as the Frame for Intervention

Joint activity routines (Bruner, 1977) are play activities in which both partners have key roles and build on each other's contributions. The joint activities involve objects and activities that are typically found in natural environments for children of this age. In the ESDM, joint activities are the primary vehicles for teaching. Teaching is embedded in emotionally rich joint activity routines with and without objects. The play interactions are child centered, in that children's choices (i.e., their preferred activities and preferred materials), are featured throughout the activities. The adult shares control of the play by selecting what objects are available as choices for the child, what actions are modeled and reinforced, and how activities are sequenced. All developmental skills that can be taught through play are taught in this way: imitation, receptive and expressive communication, social and cognitive skills, constructive and symbolic play, and fine and gross motor development.

Intensive Teaching

We believe that one cause of the developmental delays in autism is due to a decreased number of learning opportunities, and we teach intensively in order to fill in the learning gaps. Teaching is woven into every social exchange, and accomplished ESDM therapists can deliver a learning opportunity as frequently as every 10 seconds. We expect that most young children with autism will learn quickly when appropriately taught, and intensive teaching is the means by which rapid learning is achieved.

This intensity is based on normal models of infant–toddler experiences. We know from the child development literature that infants and toddlers with a greater degree of interaction with sensitive and responsive caregivers who follow children's leads and use rich language to narrate the child's interests and activities have improved language development, more secure social relations with adults and peers, and have more positive social initiations and responses with others. We also know that infants and toddlers spend the majority of their waking hours (roughly 70 hours per week) in direct social interaction with caregivers. Further, we know that infants and toddlers who experience significant deprivation from this kind of social-communicative engagement with others experience lifelong changes in cognitive ability, language ability, social ties, symbolic play, and, in the most deprived children, increases in stereotypic and repetitive behavior. Finally, we know that a significant lack of this type of caregiving experience during the first 5 years of life affects ongoing development. While children never stop learning, the early childhood period is one of special sensitivity for social-communicative learning. If it takes this much social interaction to create "normal development" in typical infants and toddlers, then it is only logical to assume that infants and toddlers with ASD need at least as much of this kind of interactive experience as typically developing children if they are to progress as far as possible in social-communicative and cognitive areas.

Positive Behavior Approaches for Unwanted Behaviors

Unwanted behaviors—those that are aggressive, destructive, disruptive, or overly repetitive—are managed by following the principles of positive behavior approaches (Duda, Dunlap, Fox, Lentini, & Clark, 2004; Powell, Dunlap, & Fox, 2006). In positive behavior approaches, the focus is on replacement of unwanted behaviors with more conventional behaviors, rather than eliminating unwanted behaviors per se. Reinforcement strategies are used to teach alternative or incompatible behaviors, and the replacement behavior is very frequently an intentional communication or a more mature skill level. The overriding goal is to increase, rather than reduce, children's repertoire of skills in every area by using reinforcement strategies to develop, shape, and increase conventional and appropriate behaviors.

Family Involvement

Parent and family involvement is considered a best practice in early autism intervention (National Research Council, 2001) and it is an essential component of the ESDM intervention. If children with autism are to develop to their greatest capacity, they need to experience the same or more learning opportunities as do children who have no biological impairments that affect their learning. That means we must create social environments in which children with autism are in interaction with others throughout their waking hours. This can only happen if parents and other caregivers learn how to engage their child in ongoing interactions throughout the day. We, and many others (Schreibman & Koegel, 2005; Koegel, Bimbela, & Schreibman, 1996; Harris, Wolchik, & Weitz, 1981), believe that optimum outcomes for toddlers with autism require parent acquisition of interactive skills so that they can foster interaction throughout the child's waking hours. One major goal of the ESDM work is establishing this type of interactive environment at home and in other daily settings. A large part of the ESDM work with families involves coaching parents in the development and ongoing use of the interaction techniques described in this manual.

However, it is not a one-way street. Family styles, values, preferences, goals, and dreams influence their child's ESDM treatment plan. Parents are the primary teachers of all young children; parental teaching for young children with autism is crucial to child progress. However, autism is a complex disorder and parents typically need guidance, support, and help in order to embed treatment techniques into everyday life. Parents join in formulating priorities for intervention. Parents participate by implementing the teaching plan themselves and by identifying routines or opportunities throughout the day to implement (generalize) these new skills. Parents are co-therapists, both in teaching the developmental curriculum and when working on changing unwanted behaviors. They complete functional assessments of behavior, help generate a plan for teaching alternative behaviors, and implement these plans throughout the child's waking hours at home. The extent to which parents and other family members are involved in delivering the intervention at home varies considerably across families but is expected to involve at least 1–2 hours per day, embedded in natural family activities: mealtimes, play, outings, dressing, toileting, bathing, and bedtime.

The focus on parent–child intervention in the ESDM reflects research in typical child development that illustrates the powerful effect of certain parenting practices on children's communication, play, and social development (Tamis-LeMonda, Bornstein, & Baumwell, 2001). Parenting practices affect children's rate and quality of language development. They affect their school progress. Parenting practices affect children's emotional development and the quality of their important relationships—friendships, future romantic relationships, even parenting relationships with their own children. Parenting style affects children's development across children's lives and across generations (Steele & Steele, 1994).

For a long time we did not know if this would apply to children with autism, whose biological impairments involving social relations were expected to trump individual differences in parenting styles. However, evidence is now accumulating that indeed, the same relations exist for parents of children with autism as exist for children without autism. Children with autism demonstrate variability in their attachment security, and several different groups have found that, as in other groups of children, security was related to their parents' ways of sensitively responding to them (Rogers & Pennington, 1991; Rogers, Ozonoff, & Maslin-Cole, 1993; Sigman & Ungerer, 1984; Sigman & Mundy, 1989; Capps, Sigman, & Mundy, 1994; and see van IJzendoorn et al., 2007, for conflicting findings). There is some evidence that this pattern is also seen in older children with ASD (Orsmond, Seltzer, Greenberg, & Krauss, 2006; Bauminger et al., in review) and that attachment security with parents affects friendship patterns, as it does in typical development (Bauminger et al., 2008). Three studies have now demonstrated that parental communication styles involving following children's leads, as opposed to directing children's attention, positively contribute to language development for children with ASD over a very long period (Siller & Sigman, 2002; Mahoney, Wheeden, & Perales, 2004), as it does for children with typical development.

There is also new evidence that as parents become more attuned to their child's communications and interests and increase their sensitive responding, children's developmental rates accelerate in language, cognitive, and social development (Mahoney & Perales, 2005; Drew et al., 2002; Vismara & Rogers, 2008). Does this mean that parents of children with autism are less sensitive or responsive than others? No. Many studies have asked this question and all have found that parents of children with autism interact with their children very similarly to other parents (van IJzendoorn et al., 2007; Capps et al., 1994; Kasari, Sigman, & Yirmiya, 1993). However, children with autism as a group differ in their interactions with their parents compared to other children. Young children with autism typically do not initiate much interaction with their parents. They tend not to direct communications to them or share their emotions with them. They frequently do not express emotions clearly in their faces or bodies. They are often slow to develop speech and gesture, and even when they have these ways of communicating, they use them infrequently to share their own experiences with their parents (Kasari, Sigman, Yirmiya, & Mundy, 1994). Thus, while parents are doing their part to interact with their children, the children are not doing their part to initiate and sustain interactions with their parents, and so the number of interactions that occur between parents and children and the communicative content of those interactions is drastically reduced, limiting learning opportunities for children, limiting opportunities for parents to respond sensitively and responsively to child cues, and limiting positive feedback to parents (reinforcement!) that their interactions have been successful.

The ESDM style of intervention focuses on all of these issues. It drastically increases the number of child initiations and responses—child cues—that are occurring, and it shapes those cues into conventional communications that are more easily recognized. It also helps parents draw out and read the subtle cues that are present so that parents can respond sensitively and thus reinforce child communications. Finally, it helps parents detect the often subtle signs that their interactions have been successful, thus reinforcing parents for their interactive efforts.

EVIDENCE OF EFFECTIVENESS

Eight papers describing the effectiveness of the original Denver Model or the ESDM have been published or are in press in peer-reviewed journals at the time of this writing. The first four studies provided consistent evidence of developmental acceleration in a large group of children with ASD in Denver Model classrooms. Rogers and colleagues (Rogers et al., 1986) described the effects of the first iteration of the model, which highlighted a developmentally oriented, center-based, small-group preschool setting model with child:adult ratios of 1:2 and emphasized play, language, cognition, and social relations. Rogers and Lewis (1989) elaborated the above analyses on a larger group and demonstrated gains in symbolic play and social communication as well.

Rogers and DiLalla (1991) compared the effects of the Denver Model on the progress of a group of 49 children with ASD compared to a group of 27 children with other kinds of behavioral and/or developmental disorders but without symptoms of autism. The fourth study (Rogers, Lewis, & Reis, 1987) was a replication study of the Denver Model by five independent agencies, four in rural communities and one urban community in Colorado.

However, the within-group pre–post designs used in the above to evaluate the effectiveness of the Denver Model, while considered at that time to be an acceptable design for assessing effectiveness of early intervention (Fewell & Sandall, 1986) are no longer considered adequate for determining treatment efficacy (Kasari, 2002; Lord, Risi, & Pickles, 2005; Charman & Howlin, 2003). Current research designs in efficacy of early intervention suggest that preliminary positive data from pre–post designs need to be followed by methodologically rigorous controlled designs.

The next three studies published on the model used more rigorous quasi-experimental or experimental designs to examine treatment efficacy. Two recent papers have used single-subject designs to examine effects of the Denver Model or the ESDM on language acquisition of nonverbal young children with ASD (Rogers et al., 2006; Vismara, Colombi, & Rogers, 2009). Both studies involved 1:1 delivery of the model over a 12-week period in one individual therapy hour per week and parent training. Both studies revealed acquisition of single-word speech in most of the children treated in this low-intensity treatment. The 2006 study is the only paper to contrast the Denver Model treatment with another treatment. In this study, children were randomly assigned to either the Denver Model treatment or prompts for restructuring oral phonetic targets (PROMPT therapy) (Hayden, 2004) used to treat children with dyspraxia of speech. The majority of children (80%) in both approaches acquired intentional, spontaneous, communicative words during the course of the treatment, and the parent training component was assumed to play a pivotal role in the children's progress, given the minimal direct treatment provided. Furthermore, many of the children in this study had previously been involved in other language treatments, some for years, but did not acquire speech until this treatment.

The Vismara et al. (2009) paper tested the ESDM parent training content and process and examined its efficacy both in achieving parent implementation of the model and enhancing children's social-communicative development. Using a variety of measurement approaches and careful attention to threats to validity, Vismara and colleagues demonstrated significant gains in child spontaneous speech, social initiative, imitation skills, and parental acquisition of therapy skills in a 12-week period involving one therapy hour per week, focused on parent coaching. This study also demonstrated maintenance and generalization of the treatment effects in both parents and children. This was seen in continued child progress in both communication and social skills during a 12-week follow-up period after the end of treatment. Measurements were made during interactions with parents and also in interactions with an unfamiliar, untrained adult. Parents also demonstrated either stable or increasing skill at using the ESDM during the follow-up period.

The most recent outcome research is a National Institute of Mental Health (NIMH)–funded randomized controlled clinical trial of the ESDM, carried out at the University of Washington (Dawson, principal investigator). Dawson and colleagues (2010) recruited

48 toddlers with idiopathic autism between 18 and 30 months of age who were stratified on two levels of Full Scale IQ (below and above 55) and then randomly assigned to one of two groups: (1) an ESDM intervention group that received, on average, 25 hours of 1:1 delivered ESDM weekly from parents and trained home therapists, for 2 years (15 hours from therapists weekly, on average); and (2) a group provided with assessments and ongoing monitoring and referrals for standard community-based treatments, referred to below as the assessment and monitoring (AM) group. These two groups did not differ at baseline in severity of autism symptoms, gender, IQ, or socioeconomic status. Two-year follow-up data were obtained for 21 community-treated children and 23 ESDM-treated children.

At 2 years after the baseline assessment, the ESDM group showed significantly improved Mullen Early Learning Composite standard scores compared to the AM group. On average, the ESDM group improved 19.1 points compared to 7.0 points in the AM group. The bulk of this change appears due to improvements in both receptive and expressive language, which showed increases of 19.7 and 12.7 points, respectively, for the ESDM group, while the AM group improved 10.6 and 9.2 points, respectively. The ESDM group also showed a 10-point advantage on the Vineland Adaptive Behavior Composite standard scores relative to the AM group (see Figure 2.1). However, for these adaptive behavior scores, the ESDM group showed only 0.5-point improvement while the AM group showed a decline of 11.2 points. Thus, the ESDM group as a whole maintained a normative rate of growth in adaptive behavior compared to the normative sample of typically developing children. On average, they were no farther behind, nor any closer to same-age peers developmentally speaking. In contrast, over this 2-year span the AM group was on average increasingly more delayed in adaptive behavior

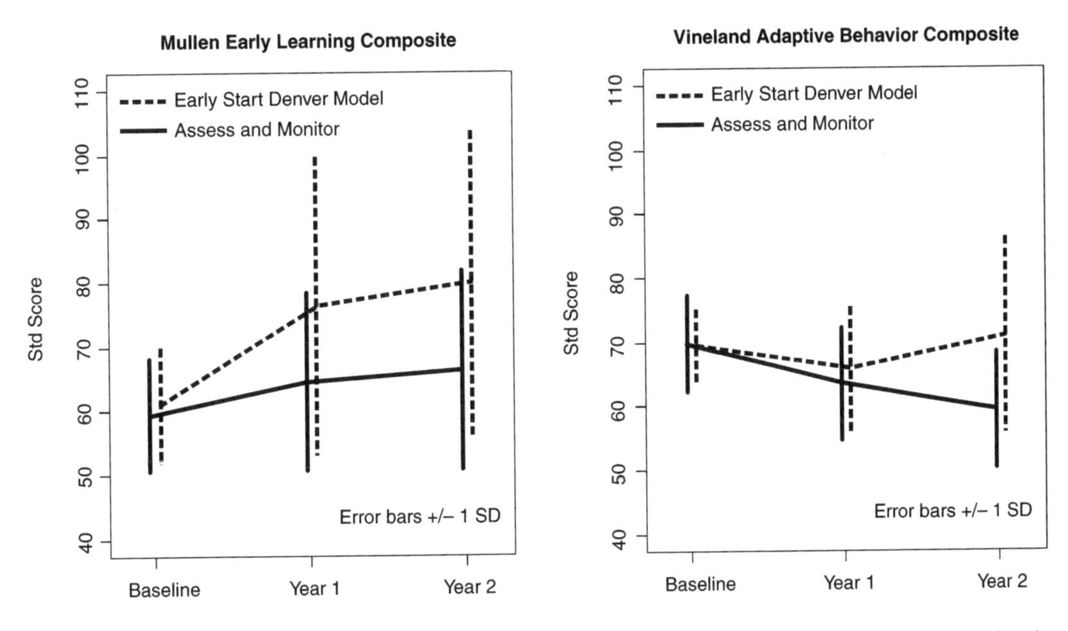

FIGURE 2.1. Comparative results of the ESDM and AM groups after 24 months on measures of development and adaptive behavior.

when compared to the normative sample. Closer examination of the Vineland subscales provides a more complicated picture. Children receiving the ESDM showed significantly better performance than the AM group on communication and motor subscales. Compared to their pretest scores, the ESDM group made substantial improvement in the communication domain but had declines in group means in socialization, daily living skills, and motor skills. The AM group showed no change in communication, but average declines in socialization, daily living skills, and motor skills well over twice that seen in the ESDM group.

Finally, in order to examine severity of autism at follow-up, we compared the clinically assigned diagnoses at both time points, which were made by experienced clinicians blind to group status using all available information to assign the appropriate DSM-IV diagnosis. All children in both groups continued to have some type of ASD diagnosis at Time 2. In terms of diagnostic stability, 15 (71.4%) children of the AM group received a diagnosis of autistic disorder both at baseline and at Time 2. In the ESDM group, 13 of the 23 (56.5%) children retained their diagnosis of autistic disorder from baseline to the 2-year outcome, and one (4.3%) child received a diagnosis of pervasive developmental disorder not otherwise specified (PDD-NOS) at both time points. In terms of increasing symptoms, five (23.8%) children in the AM group received a PDD-NOS diagnosis at baseline and then received a diagnosis of autistic disorder at Time 2. This same pattern was observed in only two (8.7%) children in the ESDM group. In terms of decreasing symptoms, one (4.8%) child in the AM group changed diagnoses from autistic disorder at baseline to PDD-NOS at Time 2 while seven (30.4%) children in the ESDM group experienced this change in diagnosis. This pattern of improvement in overall diagnosis in the ESDM group was assessed using Fisher's exact test on this 2 (treatment group) × 4 (diagnosis group; autistic/autistic, PDD/PDD, autistic/PDD, PDD/autistic) contingency table and found to be statistically significant ($p = .032$). Thus, children who received the ESDM were more likely to have an improved diagnostic status based on clinical assessment at the 2-year outcome compared to children in the AM group.

Thus, in this rigorous 2-year randomized controlled trial (RCT) that tested intensive delivery of the ESDM at home, we found significant IQ and language differences between groups that compare favorably with those published by Lovaas (1987), and larger and more widespread changes than those from the RCT of Lovaas's approach published by Smith, Groen, and Wynn (2000). We also found core symptoms of autism to be diminished, based on clinical diagnosis after 2 years of treatment, and these findings were achieved while delivering many fewer hours of treatment than the other two studies. While the ESDM needs to be independently replicated before it can be considered an empirically supported treatment for early ASD, these results are certainly consistent with earlier positive findings from the Denver Model studies.

Thus, a variety of studies, including an RCT, indicates that the ESDM is effective for increasing children's cognitive and language abilities, social interaction, and initiative, decreasing the severity of their ASD symptoms, and improving their overall behavior and adaptive skills. While longer-term follow-up studies and replications are necessary to determine the long-term benefits of this treatment approach, the consistency of the evidence across several different types of delivery (classroom, parent-delivered, and intensive at-home delivery) suggests that the ESDM is efficacious in addressing a wide range of early symptoms of ASD and improving child outcomes during the preschool period at least. Additional studies are ongoing.

SIMILARITIES AND DIFFERENCES BETWEEN THE ESDM AND OTHER INTERVENTION MODELS FOR TODDLERS WITH ASD

For those familiar with intervention models for early ASD, the similarities and differences between the ESDM and the other well-known models are likely becoming clear. The ESDM most closely resembles other intervention approaches with a strong emphasis on responsive interactions and a developmental orientation, like the responsive intervention work of Mahoney and Perales (Mahoney & Perales, 2003, 2005; Mahoney et al., 2004), DIR/Floortime (Wieder & Greenspan, 2005), Relationship Development Intervention/RDI (Gutstein, 2005), SCERTS (Prizant, Wetherby, Rubin, Laurent, & Rydell, 2006), and Hanen Centre programs (Coulter & Gallagher, 2001). All these intervention approaches are built on empirical evidence concerning patterns of typical social-communicative development. The ESDM uses a more explicit, behavioral teaching paradigm than is described by the other approaches, is more data driven, and it explicitly covers all developmental domains in its teaching practices, while most of the other models focus on social-communicative development.

The ESDM also has clear ties to the naturalistic behavioral interventions like PRT, incidental teaching (McGee, Morrier, & Daly, 1999), and milieu teaching (Yoder & Warren, 2001; Warren & Yoder, 2003; Kaiser, Yoder, & Keetz, 1992). Like the ESDM, these interventions use a child-centered, natural language frame delivered using careful behavioral teaching strategies. The ESDM differs from these interventions in the elaborated developmental curriculum used, the explicit emphasis is on affect and quality of relationships, and the comprehensive developmental framework.

Finally, the ESDM has in common with Lovaas's (1987) approach the use of a curriculum covering all domains of development, intensive teaching, use of behavioral teaching procedures, and a data-driven approach to decision making. It differs in the child- versus adult-centered teaching approach used, the focus on child positive affect, the focus on teaching communication embedded in ongoing social interaction and on nonverbal communication as a precursor of verbal communication, and in the empirical base for the curriculum and approach (i.e., developmental science rather than operant behavioral models).

Why might a person choose the ESDM over these other intervention approaches? First, it has a much stronger base in empirical evidence than do most of these other approaches. Only PRT and Lovaas's approach have as large a body of science behind them as does the ESDM. Second, it is the only autism intervention that focuses on all domains of development and is specifically constructed for toddlers both in curriculum and in interactional teaching styles. Third, it is transportable into every natural environment of toddlers. It does not require a small separate room for teaching, a specifically prepared special classroom, or special materials and visual systems. It uses the natural environment as the teaching environment. Finally, it is fun to do! Its focus on positive interactions provides plenty of reinforcement for parents, children, and therapists, and it uses a style of teaching that is quite familiar to parents and therapists from a number of different disciplines.

Is the ESDM better than other approaches? We have no comparative studies with which to answer that question. However, we assume that there is no one "best" approach for all children, families, and therapists. An intervention approach needs to fit the family's preferred way of interacting with children, a therapist's most successful way of interacting with others, and a child's own profile. The ESDM fills a current need in the field for a rigorous, empirically supported intervention that uses a developmental, relationship-based, and data-based approach to address the many developmental needs of very young children with ASD and the needs of their families.

CONCLUSION

The main principles of the ESDM result from a combination of empirical evidence from studies of early autism, studies of typical infant and child development, and studies of learning. The treatment is characterized by a set of principles and practices that underlie both the content and the delivery of the intervention. These involve interpersonal exchange and positive affect, shared engagement with real-life materials and activities, ongoing verbal and nonverbal communication, a developmentally based curriculum addressing all developmental domains, teaching practices based on learning theory and positive behavior approaches, a multidisciplinary perspective, and individualization of each child's program. The model has a long history, with ongoing changes and refinements as new data and new theories about early autism become available. The current model is the latest product of an interdisciplinary team of clinical experts and researchers in early autism at the University of California Davis and the University of Washington, who have been using and examining intervention models and carrying out research into the neuropsychological profile of early autism for a very long time. In the next chapter, we turn to the practicalities of delivering the ESDM.

Chapter 3

Using the Early Start Denver Model

DELIVERY SETTINGS

The ESDM's naturalistic teaching procedures allow it to be used in a variety of teaching environments: center-based preschools, inclusive preschools, parent-delivered interventions, and home-based interventions. The Denver Model, from which ESDM was developed, began as a daily, 25-hour-per-week group preschool program involving small groups of children taught both in small groups and individually, with a ratio of between 1:1 and 1:2 adults to children. The first efficacy studies, mentioned in Chapter 2, came from this preschool setting. This model was later used successfully in several inclusive preschools in the Denver, Colorado, area, which involved 15 or so children in a classroom, with 1–2 children having autism and the large majority of the other children with typical development. Activities included 1:1 teaching, small-group teaching, and large-group teaching. Techniques for delivering the ESDM in group settings, either specialized or inclusive, are detailed in Chapter 10.

The ESDM has been successful as an intensive, in-home, 20-hour-or-more-per week 1:1 treatment delivered by carefully supervised interventionists who could deliver the ESDM at high levels of fidelity (Dawson et al., 2010). This delivery modality does not exclude children attending group preschools or undergoing additional therapies. Techniques for delivering the ESDM intensively 1:1 in sessions typically running 2 hours each are detailed in the chapters that follow.

A version of parent delivery of the ESDM has also been used successfully (Vismara et al., 2009). In a clinical format, parent and child attend 1–2 therapy hours per week during which time the therapist both delivers the ESDM treatment directly *and* teaches the parent how to implement the ESDM at home during natural household routines and parent–child play activities. This delivery format requires that the clinician master the ESDM approach, develop the child's short-term objectives and daily teaching sheets, and pass on the skills and content to the parent in weekly sessions. A wide range of parents have learned to implement the ESDM model at high levels of fidelity and have made marked changes in their children's social and language abilities (Rogers et al., 2006; Vismara et al., 2009). Parent training and implementation have also been part of the treatment carried out in group settings and in intensive in-home delivery. It is important to remember that we do not have evidence that the ESDM approach is effective in 1–2 clinical therapy hours per week *unless* the ESDM parent-training component is used.

DELIVERY TO WHOM?

The ESDM has been developed for children with ASD starting at ages 1–3 years and continuing in treatment until ages 4–5. The curriculum addresses developmental skills from approximately 7–9 months to approximately 48 months of age. The curriculum content and the teaching procedures are derived from the studies of parent–child interaction in middle class Western cultures. Thus, the intervention is embedded in a particular cultural way of interacting with children. We have examined outcomes for a diverse group of American families ranging in both ethnicity and socioeconomic status (Rogers & Lewis, 1989; Vismara et al., 2009). Thus far we have not observed differences in child outcomes or parent usage related to ethnicity or socioeconomic status, but formal examination of this question has only begun. Families with non-Western cultural traditions may find some aspects of both content and procedures inappropriate as written; interventionists may need to adapt both content and procedures to fit inside family customs and values.

The ESDM is not meant to be used for children who are chronologically older than 60 months, even if their developmental skills are in the 12- to 60-month range. We do not consider it an appropriate curriculum or interactive style for older children. The focus of the curriculum on object use and nonverbal communication also makes the approach inappropriate for children developmentally younger than approximately 7–9 months. Importantly, we have observed that children need a minimum level of skill in object use to respond well to many of the teaching techniques and objectives of the ESDM. Therefore, as a rule of thumb, we recommend that the ESDM be used for children who are interested in objects and capable of carrying out some simple means–end actions, like putting in or taking out, and thus combining two objects in play. Children with ASD who are functioning beyond the 48-month level in all domains need a more advanced curriculum, though the teaching procedures may still be effective.

DELIVERY BY WHOM?

The ESDM was developed to be carried out and overseen by early childhood professionals in special education, educational, clinical or developmental psychology, speech and language pathology, OT, and ABA, and the people who are directly trained and supervised by these professionals. The curriculum and delivery draw directly from developmental and child clinical psychology, early childhood education, speech pathology, OT, and ABA. Any individual who is using the ESDM needs background in the knowledge base, concepts, and practices from these disciplines. This is mostly easily gained within a team of early interventionists who can cross train each other in the concepts and practices underlying the ESDM. Without access to this interdisciplinary input, it will be difficult for any single discipline to implement the ESDM model at high levels of accuracy. Fortunately, early intervention in the United States is typically organized in such teams, both in public schools and service delivery systems, and in autism and other health-related clinics. There is no good substitute for having colleagues from other disciplines observe your treatment sessions and review your treatment objectives as a way of gaining interdisciplinary expertise. This is how the ESDM was developed, and how it has been refined over the past 20 years. Later in this chapter we return to the topic of the interdisciplinary team and its members.

Therapists who learn the ESDM model generally approach it from one of two backgrounds. Some are very well trained in behavior analysis and have much experience in discrete trial teaching. These therapists have mastered the basic behavioral teaching strategies involving antecedent–behavior–consequence relations and the use of prompting, shaping, fading, and chaining to teach new skills and replace unwanted behaviors. The challenge for them in learning the ESDM model is the use of dyadic, play-based activities, induction of positive affect in the child, following children's leads, and fitting many different teaching objectives into child-chosen activities.

Therapists from special education, speech pathology, OT, and clinical or developmental psychology may come from a strong developmental background. They generally have well-developed skills in play-based intervention that follows child choice, and they typically find the affective aspects of the model easy to do. For them, the challenge in this model is the precision of the teaching approach that requires teaching very specific skills inside the play at a high rate, with careful application of reinforcement, prompting, fading, shaping, and chaining principles. Thus, interventionists from each tradition enter the ESDM approach with some very well-developed skills, but also some new teaching skills to learn.

ESDM PROCEDURES

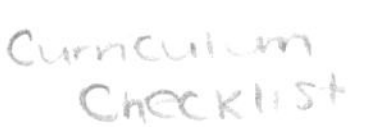

Formulating Teaching Objectives

Before the start of treatment every child receives an assessment using the Curriculum Checklist (see Appendix A). The team leader then develops two to three short-term teaching objectives in each of the Checklist's developmental domains. These objectives are designed to be met within 12 weeks and they define the skills that the child will be taught during that 12-week period. The teaching target is adjusted across the weeks based on data taken during sessions, and at the end of 12 weeks, the objectives are revised based on a new Curriculum Checklist assessment. New objectives are then developed or old ones revised. The process of formulating these short-term teaching objectives is explained in Chapter 4.

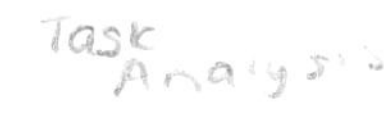

Task Analysis and Teaching Steps

At the time the objectives are developed, each one is broken down via a developmental task analysis into a sequence of steps. These steps serve as the intermediate teaching targets that lead to the full mastery of the objective. The steps guide what is taught in each session. Sessions focus on teaching every objective's "acquisition" step, which is the step the child currently needs to learn, and providing practice on the "maintenance" step, which is the immediately preceding step that the child has mastered. During the sessions, the interventionist pauses at regular intervals (e.g., every 15 minutes) to record the child's performance on a Daily Data Sheet (explained in more detail in Chapter 5).

The data sheet ties together the 12-week objectives, the teaching task analysis, and the child's individual performance. Hence it provides a way of tracking what was taught and what the child is learning.

The Treatment Notebook

The child's teaching plans are organized into a treatment notebook that includes: objectives, task analyses, and Daily Data Sheets as well as other relevant information. For example, it may include a schedule, so that the hours of treatment are easy to track; it may have space for different interventionists to write down notes about the session—important new steps or problems, questions to others, or skills that need special focus. Telephone numbers and names, such as for physicians, are often useful to keep as well. Additional teaching materials will also be included; these are described in the following chapters. The notebook typically stays where most of the treatment occurs. If the treatment is home based or involves mostly parent delivery, the notebook stays at home. If the treatment occurs at a center, the notebook stays there. Interventionists need to have the notebook accessible to them throughout treatment sessions.

Ethical Issues

For intensive home-based delivery, it is crucial that staff members are well trained in the ethics of care and professionalism before they begin to work in homes. Furthermore, it is crucial to provide ongoing supervision from a clinician with expertise in family dynamics to identify issues as they emerge, to help staff members be aware of their feelings and reactions, to review ethical standards, and to act accordingly.

As intervention progresses, parents and interventionists will come to know each other very well. Many ethical issues can arise as the relationships develop, and ongoing supervision is needed for staff members to be aware of these issues (Fuentes & Martin-Arribas, 2007). A staff member in the family home on a daily basis begins to be seen as one of the family. Parent–professional boundaries can be easily crossed, as parents share more and more and as the staff member sees the family in every aspect of home life. Parents may begin to ask for additional help, like child care, or they may suggest social contacts, inviting staff members to family events, birthday parties, and so on. Parents may want to give gifts to staff, and staff may want to give gifts to family members. Staff members may become emotionally involved in the family members' lives, pulled into marital disputes, and privy to private conversations and parental habits. Staff members may develop strong feelings about the family's ways of parenting, interacting, housekeeping, daily habits, and financial practices, and these feelings may affect the staff members' interactions with the family and the child, making it harder to maintain professional boundaries and distance.

Common ethical issues that arise and have to be carefully thought through and discussed in supervisory sessions include parental mental health, parenting adequacy and responsibility to report risk of child abuse and neglect, questions of spousal abuse, how much accommodation to provide to parents who request it, continuing to treat children who do not progress or who worsen, and other issues involved in referring families elsewhere, supporting parents' independence and initiative around decision making, lifestyle, cultural, and value differences, and many others.

USING THE GENERALIST MODEL TO DELIVER INTERVENTION

The interdisciplinary ESDM team uses a generalist model in the delivery of intervention to children and families (Schopler et al., 1995). This means that there is only one treatment plan in the ESDM that covers goals from all the disciplines (i.e., the teaching objectives with their developmental task analyses) and this plan focuses on the integrated functioning of the whole child. The child's treatment plan is delivered by parents at home, in individual speech–language pathology (S-LP) or OT sessions, in an intensive home delivery, or in preschool group-delivery settings. One professional person (the team leader) oversees the entire treatment plan, including developing the treatment objectives and the data collection system, guiding the treatment implementation, examining the progress data, and determining any changes in the plan. The ESDM treatment may occur in a single therapy model, like speech and language therapy, in which the therapist works with parent and child and the parent continues the interventions at home. However, even in that situation, we assume that the therapist has access to evaluations from other disciplines, has access to other professionals from different disciplines who know this child and could consult if needed, and has enough interdisciplinary training to carry out the ESDM. We have found the use of a generalist model to be important for the following reasons.

Children Develop in All Areas

Interventions in one area necessarily have impact on other areas. Any child learning activity affects multiple areas of development. For instance, in a motor activity, adults communicate with children. In a cognitive activity, the child's fine motor system is challenged to manipulate materials in specific ways. In a generalist model, the therapist working with a child knows the interventions to be delivered for that child in every domain and can tailor activities to target specific skills in multiple domains. This results in a very precise intervention in which each activity simultaneously addresses the child's developmental needs in multiple domains. This maximizes the amount of teaching in a given activity because multiple objectives and domains are being taught.

It Is Economical

The child's complete intervention plan can be carried out by parents and by any one staff member, thus avoiding the need for multiple expensive therapists involved with the child each week, with overlapping goals and treatments. In rural settings and others in which professional resources are scarce, it allows the professional staff to cover the maximum number of children while avoiding redundancy.

It Maximizes Teaching Consistency and Repetition

Multiple professionals, each working independently, cannot provide the kind of consistency in language, expectations, routines, and practice trials that we know enhance learning for children with autism. Conversely, children with autism have difficulty generalizing across settings and people and are unlikely to extract general learning principles across markedly different hourly interventions that occur once or twice each week

(Plaisted, 2001). Using one treatment plan across all adults and settings maximizes consistency and the number of teaching trials, thus maximizing child learning.

It Provides a Unified Intervention for Parents

Having a single team leader and a unified intervention plan prevents situations in which parents are given differing advice on what to do from every therapist they see. It focuses the parents' interactions on the team leader, and thus simplifies communications for the family. It also allows parents to see how one person can address all the child's developmental needs in play and typical daily activities, which is what we help parents learn to do, and it models for families how several different people can deliver the same intervention plan while each has a unique relationship with the child.

We next take a more detailed look at the interdisciplinary team, its organization, and members.

THE INTERDISCIPLINARY TREATMENT TEAM

Autism is technically defined by its three primary symptom areas—communication, social behavior, and a repetitive, restricted behavioral repertoire—however, many more areas are frequently affected including motor functioning, sensory responsivity, sensory processing, intellectual development, academic learning difficulties, attention problems, psychiatric problems like anxiety and mood disorders, behavioral problems like tantrums, and health-related problems involving food intake, sleep, and allergies (Hansen & Hagerman, 2003). Many of these associated difficulties are already present in the infant–toddler period (Zwaigenbaum et al., 2005), and there is frequently an increase in related problems during the preschool period. Thus, early interventionists working with young children with autism will face these difficulties in their work during the toddler and preschool periods.

Abnormalities in neural networks underlie many ASD symptoms, like those involving abnormal gait and movement patterns, sensory overreactivity, and difficulty producing intentional speech sounds. Interventions like the ESDM that seek to stimulate more typical developmental patterns in ASD must be built on a sophisticated understanding of the underlying neural, neuropsychological, and developmental foundations of various skills that will be targets of intervention. Delivering comprehensive intervention for young children with ASD thus requires expertise in early childhood development in the affected developmental domains, and this necessitates an interdisciplinary team.

Definition of the Team

The ESDM is an interdisciplinary model in which early childhood special education, child clinical and developmental psychology, S-LP, OT, pediatrics, and behavior analysis work together to build the intervention plan and guide its delivery. To be sure that the child's health needs are part of his or her plan, the child's physician needs to be seen as a part of this team; in some cases, this will be the developmental behavioral pediatrician who was part of the child's diagnostic assessment. For some children, child psychiatrists are also involved. Paraprofessionals often play major roles in the delivery of care in group programs and intensive home interventions. They also have an important role on the team. Regardless of the type of ESDM delivery being used (center based, inclusive preschool, parent coaching, or intensive home delivery), an interdisciplinary treatment team is necessary for developing and monitoring appropriate delivery of the ESDM.

Parents are also important members of the treatment team. Working with infants and toddlers means working within the context of the infant–parents triad (McCollum & Yates, 1994). Even more than with interventions for older children, infant–toddler treatment requires family work, a fact that has been well articulated by the infant mental health community (Gilkerson & Stott, 2005). People on an autism intervention team may lack formal training in infant mental health, but the concepts are crucial, and a family focus is considered fundamental to successful infant–toddler interventions (Shonkoff & Phillips, 2000). The necessity of a family focus is represented in the Individuals with Disabilities Act (IDEA, 1991), which requires of participating states that education for children under 3 years of age be organized and delivered according to an individualized family service plan (IFSP) which includes home visits, training, and counseling services to the family in addition to direct services for the child.

Organization of the Team

The team leader and parents are at the hub of the treatment team as illustrated in Figure 3.1. The other professional members of the team provide consultation, oversight, and

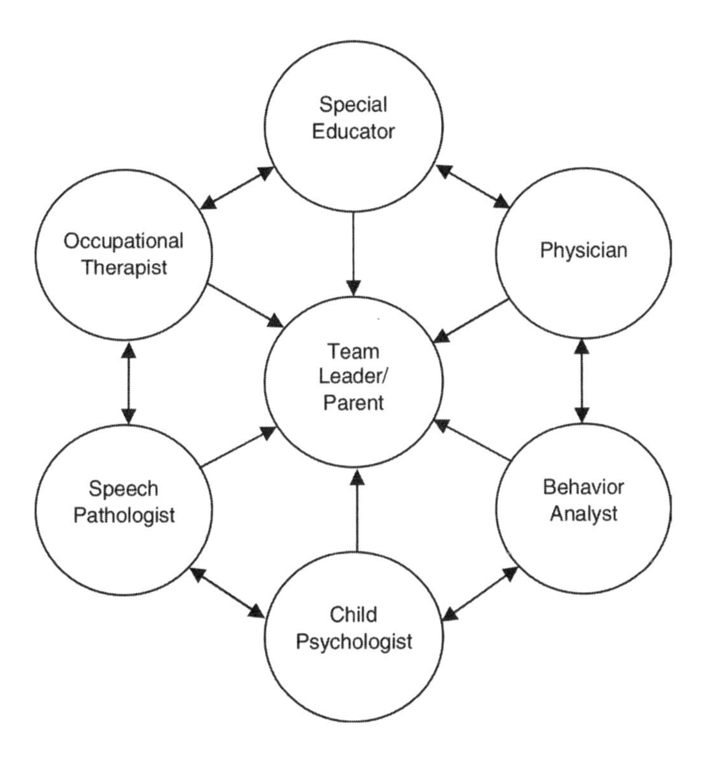

FIGURE 3.1. Organization of the interdisciplinary team.

support to the team leader and to the parents. Next we review the professional members of the team and their roles, followed by a discussion of issues for parents.

Team Leader

Professionals from a variety of disciplines may serve as team leaders depending on the setting and the child's needs. At the start of treatment, the team leader typically carries out an assessment using the Curriculum Checklist (see Appendix A). Based on the results of the assessment, the team leader develops the child's quarterly objectives, the developmental task analysis for each objective, the teaching activities and programs, and data collection systems, and sets these up in the treatment notebook. The team leader works directly with the parents to support them in delivering the intervention plan in natural care and play routines at home and in the community. The team leader also works with the child directly, during clinic visits in clinic-based models, during home visits with the parents or in the classroom, and works directly with paraprofessionals to implement the objectives. The team leader provides training as needed to paraprofessionals and monitors the child's progress through ongoing classroom contacts, or in biweekly visits in the center or the home with parents, child, and intervention providers. (Note: If this is a single-discipline therapy with parent implementation, the individual therapist is the team leader and carries out these steps.)

As treatment progresses, the team leader ensures that the intervention is proceeding successfully and the child is progressing as rapidly as possible. The team leader observes and fine-tunes the intervention being implemented, reviews data weekly, directs all changes in the teaching approach, develops and implements positive behavior support plans, and consults with other team members as needed to gain their disciplinary input. The team leader is the parents' main contact, sees the parents at least every 2 weeks, observes paraprofessionals who are teaching in the home or classroom regularly, evaluates their skills, and provides teaching as needed to ensure treatment fidelity.

Other Team Member Roles and Responsibilities

Other team members support the team leader with their disciplinary expertise. Each quarter, the other professional team members help the team leader update treatment objectives and the treatment plan and evaluate the course of treatment. The other members may act as consultants, evaluators, or occasionally, additional therapists for children with severe additional disabilities in their related areas of expertise. Remember that therapists of any discipline may be the team leader.

Early Childhood Special Educator

The early childhood special educator has particular expertise in curriculum development and individualization, physical organization of the classroom, management of the schedule and transition planning, and organization of the adults in the classroom. Early childhood special educators also have particular expertise in child development in multiple domains and in creating learning activities that address certain developmental areas. They tend to be excellent generalists, with training in all the developmental domains and with a deep understanding of how toddlers and young children learn. In many school-based settings, early childhood special educators assess children, determine the teaching goals, supervise the team, teach the parents the intervention, gather data, and update programs. In a preschool classroom-based delivery of the ESDM, the early childhood special educator is either the lead teacher for the entire group or provides consultation and support for the lead teacher. The early childhood special educator is typically responsible for the curriculum and supervision of teaching assistants in a classroom. In a home-based or parent-delivered implementation of the ESDM, the early childhood educator often takes a team leader position to develop the child's intervention plan, teach parents how to implement the ESDM, and supervise paraprofessionals and any others who are delivering the intervention plan. At the point when children are transitioning to new group programs, the early childhood special educator on the ESDM team may coordinate with the special educator in the new group setting to foster coordinated approaches to the child's intervention plan. In clinical settings, there may not be a special educator.

Clinical or Developmental Child Psychologist

The child clinical psychologist is a key member of the diagnostic team and is typically also responsible for ongoing monitoring of behavioral and mental health issues and consulting with other team members regarding family adjustment and family mental health concerns. The psychologist is typically responsible for conducting standardized assessments of the child's functioning, including assessments of intellectual and developmental abilities, behavior problems, and adaptive behavior. The psychologist will often contribute to the development of cognitive, social–emotional, and behavioral objectives for children. The psychologist may take a team leader role, particularly for children for whom there are significant family needs, those who need referrals for social or mental health services, or those for whom coordination with their ongoing mental health professionals needs to be part of the treatment plan. The psychologist may also provide regular (often weekly), ongoing clinical group supervision to team leaders and paraprofessionals regarding the various clinical issues and difficulties that arise in work with families. Finally, the psychologist will often provide help and support to staff members who have questions around the need to report possible child abuse or neglect. On some teams, the mental health roles described here are filled by licensed social workers.

Speech–Language Pathologist

Implementation of the ESDM requires ongoing input from the S-LP because of the intense focus on communication development in early ASD. In all ESDM delivery modalities, the S-LP is responsible for initial evaluation of children's speech and language, assessing the potential impact of difficulties in oral–motor function, and providing input to the communication objectives developed for each child. The S-LP consults and oversees the communication development of each child, assisting the treatment team to maximize language development and reassessing the child at regular intervals to monitor his or her communication progress. The S-LP has a major role in decisions to move to alternative communication systems for children. (This involves a specific decision-making process, discussed in detail in Chapter 9.) For children with a specific speech impairment that requires direct services, like a severe dyspraxia of speech, the

S-LP may provide direct treatment or refer children to others who can provide such treatment. It is extremely helpful to have S-LPs who are trained in a specific treatment approach to dyspraxia, like PROMPT (Hayden, 2004) treatment. PROMPT is very compatible with the orientation and practices of the ESDM, and we have found it essential for some children in order to develop speech.

The S-LP's other levels of involvement will depend on the delivery setting being used. In some settings, the S-LP may use the ESDM model to deliver individual, clinic-based therapy and to teach parents to deliver it at home (Rogers et al., 2006). In a group preschool setting, the S-LP may deliver regular weekly clinical speech and language therapy using the ESDM and following the child's quarterly objectives, but focusing on the communication and social objectives. In intensive home programs, the S-LP may head a treatment team, supervising the assistants and being the primary professional therapist, assuming that the S-LP has cross trained with the other team members and has developed expertise in ABA and the other disciplinary areas. In all these formats, the S-LP may have a consulting role rather than a direct role, assessing children, adding to the treatment objectives, monitoring progress, problem solving, and supporting the team leaders. For children who are receiving speech–language therapy from another professional, either privately or in a preschool setting, the ESDM S-LP maintains an open line of communication with this person to foster a coordinated approach to the child and family.

Occupational Therapist

The OT on the team, like the S-LP, has a critical role because of his or her expertise in motor and sensory development in early childhood and his or her knowledge of adaptive behavior development. The OT is a core member of the team whose input is essential for full realization of the model. For all children, the OT will support the team leader to ensure that motor objectives and treatment plans are appropriate and will follow the progress of those children with significant sensory and/or motor impairments and help the team make adaptations of the plan when needed.

The OT may play many roles depending on the type of ESDM delivery being used, from 1:1 clinical therapy and parent training to the evaluation and consultation role. The OT is responsible for initial screening, assessment if needed, review of objectives and implementation of treatment, and consultation regarding sensory and motor functioning for children who present with marked impairments in these domains. The OT may be a team leader for some children. For children whose severe motor impairments require direct treatment, the OT may provide care or refer children to others who can provide the needed treatment. For children who are receiving OT from another professional, either privately or in a preschool setting, the OT will communicate the child's current program and objectives in the ESDM and work with other therapists to foster a coordinated approach to the child and family.

Behavior Analyst

Expertise in behavior analysis is critical for the full realization of the model. The board-certified behavior analyst (BCBA) has particular expertise in the functional assessment of behavior, application of behavioral teaching principles, implementation of data collection strategies, and the use of data to monitor learning and change. Thus, the BCBA is a core team member and will often be in a team leader role, assessing children on the Curriculum Checklist, developing their individual objectives, and overseeing others to ensure correct implementation of the plan. For children with significant behavior problems, the BCBA will provide a functional assessment of the behaviors (O'Neill et al., 1990), develop a positive behavior support plan (Carr et al., 2002), teach parents and team members to implement the plan, and will examine efficacy data. The BCBA will also consult with other team members regarding application of learning theory principles. It is often the case that special educators, psychologists, and S-LPs have been thoroughly trained in the use of ABA within their discipline. However, given the complexity of ASD and the importance of accurate use of behavioral teaching strategies, functional assessments, development of positive behavior support plans, and the need for ongoing data collection and data-based decision making in the ESDM, the BCBA has a key role to fill on the team.

Physician

Another important member of the team is the child's pediatrician or primary care physician, and, in some cases, the pediatrician who was part of the child's diagnostic evaluation. Children with autism often experience a wide range of medical problems, including feeding problems, sleep difficulties, allergies, gastrointestinal problems, and seizures, among others. These conditions have a significant impact on the success of an intervention program. A child who is in pain, hungry, or tired will be irritable and have difficulty attending to the teaching that is occurring. Children newly diagnosed with ASD need a thorough medical examination to determine whether medical conditions are present, and if so, how they are to be treated. In addition, parents often have medical questions; for example, concerning a biomedical treatment they might have read about that the physician often is in the best position to address. Ideally, the child's primary physician is well-informed about ASD or has ties to other physicians who are expert in ASD, so that the bulk of the child's medical care can be provided by the primary physician with consultation from the medical specialist. With parental consent, the physician should be informed of the child's participation in the ESDM by the team leader, should have the team leader's name and phone number, and should be provided with a copy of the child's diagnostic and progress reports and intervention objectives.

Paraprofessionals

Paraprofessionals deliver much of the child's individual intervention when the ESDM is delivered intensively at home, as well as in group delivery in preschool classrooms. They deliver the plan as specified by the team leader, record progress data accurately, communicate changes in acquisition and mastered tasks to others on the child's teaching team, notify the team leader of any unexpected events or behaviors observed, and respect professional and ethical boundaries regarding their interactions with families. They meet regularly with the team leader and the clinical psychologist to discuss their interactions with children and family members and are regularly observed and provided with feedback about their treatment delivery.

Paraprofessionals are often in the complex role of having the most contact with parents, spending the most time delivering the treatment, but having less authority over treatment design than the professional team members. In homes, paraprofessionals enter the family's space and life, and they face many ethical issues concerning professional boundaries, family privacy, parental concerns about the child, and the dynamic relationships that play out in the day-to-day life of families. They are engaged in interactions with child and family throughout their workdays in a treatment model that requires emotional engagement during each therapy hour; it is an intense, demanding role. Furthermore, in the ESDM, the activities are not scripted, and instead, successful intervention relies on the interventionist's knowledge of the treatment plan, the child, and their own creativity as they create learning activities out of everyday materials and events.

Paraprofessionals need ongoing professional supervision and support in order to manage this set of expectations in a responsible and ethical way, and they also need ongoing emotional support and guidance from the professional team members. Weekly supervision from the team leader is crucial for supporting the paraprofessionals in their work with the children and their interactions with parents and other family members. This needs to involve both observation of their teaching and discussion about their work with each assigned child. Regular supervision by the clinical psychologist has been quite helpful for us when the ESDM is being used for intensive 1:1 home delivery of the model. All disciplines should provide ongoing training and consultation to the paraprofessional staff, who carry the lion's share of the child's intervention in some settings and thus need considerable knowledge and skill if the ESDM is to be fully realized.

Other Professionals

Other professionals who may be a part of an individual child's team include those in nutrition, physical therapy, music therapy, audiology, and medicine including specialists in allergies, ophthalmology, gastroenterology, psychiatry, and neurology, among many others. When other disciplines are involved in treating the child, the same communication procedures apply. These include obtaining parental consent, sharing teaching objectives and teaching plans, and working to establish consistency in intervention approaches.

While we focus on a generalist model, there are certainly some children whose profile of disabilities requires some individual discipline-specific therapy within the ESDM. This occurs for children who are progressing in all other skills but still do not imitate consonants and syllables after the first 3–6 months of intensive treatment. We have typically added 1 hour of speech–language therapy from the S-LP using the PROMPT approach for such children. (Note: With this addition in our intensive home-based approach at the University of Washington, over 90% of children developed meaningful speech in 2 years.) Another use of disciplinary therapy from the S-LP that comes up from time to time involves children with significant oral–motor problems affecting eating as well as speech.

Disciplinary consult and treatment is also sometimes needed from the OT, especially for children who have very poor muscle tone or other motor problems and need significant accommodation regarding seating, other positioning, postural control and stability, and efforts to normalize tone. In these situations in which additional individual therapy is added, the ESDM intervention plan is still followed, and the specialized therapists consult with the other treatment givers on the team, joining their therapy sessions and teaching them the techniques and accommodations needed for an individual child.

It has seemed much more helpful for the ESDM professional staff to provide these additional therapy hours than to refer children to professionals outside of the ESDM, both because of the common approach and common objectives that the ESDM staff uses, and because the ESDM professional can pass on additional treatment techniques to other ESDM staff members' treatment sessions (e.g., paraprofessionals). However, when children need additional health-related interventions that cannot be provided by the ESDM staff, then appropriate referrals need to be made and a bidirectional flow of communication and information needs to be established.

Fostering Communication across the Team

Given all the people in the team and the many roles involved, communication systems and procedures need to be designed thoughtfully to ensure that each person with an area of responsibility for a child and family has knowledge of child progress and input into the direct delivery system. Two important ways to ensure communication are the treatment notebook, described earlier in this chapter, and team meetings.

The child's treatment notebook becomes a primary communication vehicle when multiple persons are delivering the child's treatment. Each person needs to leave their daily data sheet and progress notes for the next person so that all the child's objectives are addressed across the child's treatment day and any particular accommodations or other nonroutine events can be noted. This also allows the team to coordinate maximum teaching of the more difficult aspects of the child's program. The notebook should be reviewed weekly by team leaders to examine and update the child's program for the following week.

Conducting a weekly or biweekly team meeting or group supervision with the paraprofessionals is necessary to maintain consistency of treatment across the various members, as well as in sharing discussions about difficult situations with family members and managing the ethical dilemmas that inevitably arise. The team leader should lead these discussions, and the clinical psychologist may be involved as well, in order to supervise the work going on in the homes from a clinical perspective. These meetings may be conducted in the field, in the center, or in a phone conference call; they are necessary for optimal child progress.

Some settings have established teams involving one team leader and several paraprofessionals who care for a specified number of children and families and thus can review all their shared cases together at one time. In this situation, the reviews can be scheduled with the team leader and paraprofessionals, and the other team members can attend these standing meetings for children who require their disciplinary input. For children in group delivery, this allows for multiple children to be reviewed simultaneously by different teams. When teams are more flexibly assigned in terms of team leaders and paraprofessionals, phone conference calls around a specific child can be a more efficient way to proceed, allowing for people out in the field to call in. We have found that 15–20 minutes is enough to review and update programs weekly or biweekly for one child, assuming treatment is progressing smoothly.

A general meeting of treatment team professionals is also necessary at regular intervals to ensure that the consulting team members have updates about child progress and concerns. Holding quarterly progress review meetings for each child at the time of their quarterly assessments allows for ongoing interdisciplinary input to children's programs.

Staff Training

The ESDM Teaching Fidelity Rating System (see Appendix B) was developed to assess an adult's mastery of the teaching practices that are core to the ESDM. The fidelity tool allows one to score the quality with which each of the core practices is used in a particular play activity. A Likert-based scale allows one to rate each practice on a 5-point scale, with 1 being very poor usage to 5 being an optimal example of the practice. We define competence in the use of the ESDM teaching practices as (1) achieving 85% or greater of the number of possible points in each play activity, *and* (2) consistent scores of 4 or 5 on each practice, *and* (3) no scores lower than a 3.

Professionals and paraprofessionals need both didactic and apprenticeship training with an experienced professional to master the skill sets involved in using the ESDM. At the end of training, each professional staff member should demonstrate competence in delivering an intervention session at 80–85% fidelity, using the Curriculum Checklist in its entirety, writing objectives, task analyzing them, and setting up and using a data system, so that they are fully trained in the model and can knowledgeably supervise others.

Team leaders need additional training to learn the intricacies of the assessment and treatment design procedures—using the curriculum, writing and analyzing the objectives, developing and using the data and program sheets, monitoring and updating progress, and working with the paraprofessionals to ensure high-quality delivery. This is done through apprenticeship with experienced team leaders.

Paraprofessionals need to acquire considerable understanding of child development in the areas targeted by this intervention: imitation, joint attention, verbal and nonverbal communication, play, social development, and ABA. They need to learn about family styles and the family issues that often arise in this kind of work. They also need to learn to deliver the model at high levels of fidelity, and to manage the paperwork systems with a high level of accuracy.

For those who wish to learn the ESDM, use of the fidelity rating system is an excellent way to examine one's own skills and areas in need of improvement. While the teaching practices may seem simple, even experienced teachers and therapists of young children with autism may not have mastered each teaching technique listed above so that the skill is automatic and consistent.

It is extremely helpful to examine one's own teaching skills and identify teaching behaviors that could be more consistent or precise. We recommend videotaping yourself teaching children and then take a look at your videos to watch for these or other teaching inaccuracies using the ESDM Teaching Fidelity Rating System. As you see teaching problems, stop the video and think through what you wish you had done instead. Analyze the problem, focusing on the concepts targeted above. Imagine the teaching carried out more optimally. The next time you are in therapy and that difficulty occurs, fix it on the spot. Carry out this process with other team members or colleagues as well, watching each other's tapes or therapy sessions and using the fidelity tool to critique the teaching. Over time, considerable growth will occur in your facility with the ESDM practices.

The most common teaching problems are these:

1. Antecedents are unclear.
2. Reinforcers do not follow quickly enough.
3. Behaviors other than the target behavior are reinforced; both accidental behaviors and unwanted or maladaptive behaviors.
4. Reinforcers lack reinforcement value or strength.
5. Appropriate behavior is not reinforced.
6. Minimal levels of a skill are not shaped into mature, independent, and spontaneous levels of the skill.
7. Reinforcer schedules are not systematically reduced or shifted to intrinsic reinforcers.
8. Too much time is spent on mastered skills; too little time spent on new skills.
9. Too much time is spent on new skills, with resulting problems of child attention and motivation.
10. Prompts are not quickly faded and children are prompt dependent, or prompts are confused with antecedents.
11. When behavioral sequences are being taught, the child is not being taught all the steps.
12. Verbal antecedents or other social behaviors are used to instruct intermediate steps in behavior chains that do not involve language (dressing, handwashing) rather than teaching the skill in such a way that each behavior becomes the antecedent for the next.
13. Very few actual teaching trials (A–B–C chains) occur inside an activity. The therapist may be entertaining the child with pleasurable activities, but little teaching is occurring.
14. A skill taught in a very artificial or highly structured and adult-directed setting is not generalized to natural settings and developed as a spontaneous behavior.
15. Data are not collected, or if collected are not used to plan the approach for the next therapy session.
16. Teaching opportunities are missed because the therapist is not attending to what the child is playing with or how the child uses the materials in play.

We have developed a curriculum for training in the ESDM model that consists of readings, discussions, video training materials, and observation and practice during teaching sessions. When new staff members enter the model, they begin to learn through a written and video curriculum that includes the materials here and much more. It is taught in a 1.5-hour weekly seminar, with weekly pre- and posttests on the content, and apprenticeship with a highly experienced staff member. The weekly training topics consist of the following:

Ethics and family dynamics
Introduction to autism
Typical toddler social and communicative development

Cognition, imitation, and play
Motor and adaptive behavior self-help skills
The Denver Model, joint activity routines and sensory social routines
Principles of ABA and behavior problems
Naturalistic ABA and PRT

In addition to the didactic curriculum, this training period also involves an apprenticeship with one of the most senior and competent staff members for observation and supervised experience with teaching. New staff members accompany the most experienced staff members to therapy sessions and also observe team leaders running clinic sessions. Through these apprenticeship experiences, new staff members are gradually introduced to the ESDM methods of working with children with autism.

As a new person begins to work with children under supervision, the team leader rates his or her work using the Fidelity Rating System. Beginning therapists are expected to achieve an overall score of 80–85% for three or more consecutive administrations of these measures before they use the ESDM independently with children. In addition, staff members are required to use the child's data collection form during several treatment sessions and must obtain 80% reliability or higher with a team leader for at least three training probes.

For those already experienced in teaching young children with ASD, this training typically takes 4–6 weeks. (Note: The full syllabus for training, including written and video materials, is available from the authors for the cost of copying and shipping.)

PARTNERING WITH FAMILIES

A primary goal in the ESDM is to help the child become more socially engaged with others and to do so not only with a therapist but especially with family members and important others; there is no better way to promote such abilities than to involve the parents in delivering the treatment. However, the only common element among families with autism is that there is a person with autism in the family. On all other characteristics, they are as different from one another as any other group of families randomly selected from a community. Finding a way to partner with each family who enters the ESDM treatment requires open dialogue with families, excellent listening skills, cultural awareness, flexibility, creativity, and self-awareness from staff. Sensitivity to cultural differences among families is crucial for forming strong alliances with them and designing an intervention approach that recognizes and respects their cultural practices and values (Lynch & Hanson, 1992). The greater the cultural differences between a target family and the interventionist's own family, the more challenged the interventionist will be to see the strengths and needs of the family. However, just as in individual therapy, the quality of the relationship between therapist and patient is crucial in determining the success of the treatment (Zeanah & McDonough, 1989). The parents must feel unconditional positive regard from the interventionist, both for themselves as parents and for their relationship with their child, in order to trust the interventionist and commit to the treatment. This is why parental goals are included in the 12-week objectives; it reflects the importance of the family's ideas and goals and the family's power to determine what their child should learn.

The Effects of Autism on Families

Families of toddlers with autism are stressed when they enter treatment, and the stressors grow over time (Dale, Johoda, & Knott, 2006). Autism stresses families to a greater degree than do many other developmental disorders (Schieve, Blumberg, Rice, Visser, & Boyle, 2007). Stressors include the slow and often inconsistent diagnostic process, the uneven and unusual development course that children show, the resulting ebbs and flows of parental hope and pessimism, the tendency to interpret child inconsistencies as refusal rather than inability, the lack of communication and affection shared by children, the contrast between the children's typical appearance and their very atypical behaviors, the children's embarrassing public behavioral displays, increased rates of parental mental health concerns, the number of professionals that parents must maintain relations with, the constant barrage of new and fad treatments, and the pressure from other parents to try yet another therapy (Marcus, Kunce, & Schopler, 2005).

The very poor outcomes that are associated with autism and the public stereotypes involving high levels of aggression and self-injury cause parents much worry about the future with their child. Books that report child recoveries after hundreds of thousands of dollars of care foster guilt and feelings of inadequacy in parents who cannot access or afford such treatments. Guilt and pressure arise from the amount of time that parenting a child with autism requires and its depletion of the finite amount of time available to parents to care for each other, other children in the family, and themselves. Child food refusals, poor sleep habits, and lack of personal care skills add further work and strain on parents. Other families of children with autism can add guilt as well, with their ongoing encouragement to other families to try whatever treatment appeared to help their own child, and the unspoken message that if parents don't try every single intervention, they may be denying their child the hope of recovery or great improvement.

According to Seligman and Darling (1997), mothers tended to be more severely affected by having a child with autism than fathers, and affection between partners can be weakened. On the positive side, Baron-Cohen and Bolton (1994) note that statistically, parents of children with autism are no more likely to separate and divorce than parents of nonhandicapped children. However, early intervention can affect the structure of many families as one or both parents become highly involved with the child with autism; the parents need to be supported to tend to their marital relationship and their relationships with the other children. Families of children with autism report greater difficulties in family functioning than do those of children with other disorders or children with severe chronic health problems. Families of children with autism experience a greater loss of income than families of children with other disorders related to the need for a parent to provide more care at home (Montes & Halterman, 2008). Family activities outside the home are more restricted by autism than by other disorders, and support networks for families are fewer (Higgins, Bailey, & Pearce, 2005). Families of children with autism tend to use more coping strategies associated with distancing and escape from their stresses than do families with other disorders that tend to use a greater number of coping strategies associated with social support and problem solving (Sivberg, 2002).

Siblings are also affected by the presence of a child with autism in the family, and, as with parents, there are both positive and negative effects on sibling development. In some ways, having a sibling with ASD enhances a child's psychosocial and emotional development. Siblings' self-concepts have been found to be enhanced as they evaluate their own intelligence, school abilities, and personal traits (Macks & Reeve, 2007). This may reflect their comparisons of themselves with their sibling with autism; however, it may also reflect their increased maturity (Gray, 1998). Interestingly, parents in this study did not share this positive view of the sibling, and in fact were somewhat more negative about the sibling's adjustment than were the comparison parents. Importantly, however, sibling well-being in these families with a child with autism was significantly affected by the socioeconomic status of the family. Autism in a sibling is likely a stress factor for children, and the more stressors that accumulate, like lower income, less parental education, and other family stressors, the poorer the sibling does (Macks & Reeve, 2007). Other studies have also found some increases in behavioral and social difficulties as well, though these are likely both genetic contributions and social contributions, respectively (Orsmond & Seltzer, 2007). The effects on relationships persist across the lifetime. Adult siblings of persons with autism report less involvement and more pessimism about their affected sibling than do adult siblings of persons with Down syndrome (Orsmond & Seltzer, 2007; Hodapp & Urbano, 2007).

The Effects of Treatment on Families

Families are resilient, and ongoing parent education as part of ASD diagnosis and intervention leads to improvement of parental mental health (Tonge et al., 2006). Involving families in successful work with their children has beneficial effects on parents as well as the children involved. As reviewed by Marcus et al. (2005), parents in such interventions report greater feelings of competence and self-efficacy, children maintain their gains for a longer period, and other children in the family also demonstrate positive effects. The ESDM family focus and involvement can thus be expected to benefit all family members.

However, for reasons that are poorly understood, there is extremely wide variability in the outcome of children who received even high-quality, intensive early intervention (Sallows & Graupner, 2005). Research has shown that differences in brain development measurable during the preschool period partially account for the tremendous variability in autism outcome (Elder, Dawson, Toth, Fein, & Munson, 2007; Courchesne, Redcay, & Kennedy, 2004). Some children respond quickly and make rapid progress. Others make steady gains but at a slower rate. Other children may struggle to make the smallest improvement in their behavior, despite the fact that parents and professionals are providing the best intervention possible. It is important, therefore, that parents not take on the burden of guilt when their child's progress is slower than expected. Importantly, even for a child making slower-than-expected progress, high-quality interventions will undoubtedly have a significant effect on the child's quality of life and outcome ((Eldevik & Gardner, 2006; Smith, Eikeseth, Klevstrand, & Lovaas, 1997). Early intensive interventions have improved outcomes for virtually all children with ASD. For example, whereas previously, autism was associated with mental retardation in the large majority of cases and only 50% of children learned to speak, today we find that many more individuals with autism do not have mental retardation and the majority of individuals with autism develop at least some spoken language (Chakrabarti & Fombonne, 2005).

The concepts from family systems theory provide an important lens through which to understand family functioning (Mashal, Feldman, & Sigal, 1989). Because each family system exerts efforts to maintain an emotional equilibrium among the members, changing the nature of behaviors and expectancies between a parent and a child with autism will affect every member of that family. The family system may respond in ways that do not reinforce the changes that are occurring, because the family equilibrium is upset and other family roles and access to reinforcement are also challenged. For example, a parent who begins to spend some periods of concentrated time each day working with a toddler with ASD during playtime, meals, and bath time may begin to hear from older children that the parent is now spending too much time with the child with autism, even though the parent has been careful not to reduce time with the older children. The older children's complaints reflect their awareness that the child with autism is now getting more attention—more family resources—than before. The closeness that develops between the parent and the child with autism during intensive treatment can result in feelings of exclusion from other family members (i.e., spouses, siblings), resulting in structural changes that have lifelong implications for family functioning.

Interventionists can help family members to predict and/or recognize changes in the family system that may occur as intervention proceeds and roles and expectations are changed vis-à-vis the child with autism. In the same vein, interventionists need to consider the effect of treatment on various family members, and be sure that each member has a way of experiencing some "gain" from efforts to support the child with autism (e.g., through their own contributions, from increased family playtime or other activities, more fun with the sibling, or perhaps some alone time with a parent). Understanding and reflecting on behavioral changes in family members from a family systems perspective may allow a new equilibrium to emerge. An ESDM staff member with clinical training in family dynamics should provide consultation and support to other members regarding this aspect of the ESDM treatment.

Interventionists who work closely with families learn about each family's stressors, as well as their hopes and dreams for their child. The intervention team can help each family identify the strengths they bring to their own child's life and thus alleviate some parental guilt. Strengths are not only finances, teaching skills, number of toys, and space for play, but also the amount of time a family can spend in 1:1 interaction. Strengths also include the number of other siblings for play and modeling, a large and supportive extended family, parental interactive or creative talents, parental enjoyment of their children and vice versa, well-established family routines, or, conversely, a relaxed and accepting parenting style and the parents' ability to be in the moment, the parents' strong faith, the parents' strong work ethic, and their determination to provide well for their child and family. Interventionists can help families accept, at a deep level, that they did not cause their child's autism, and that they are an ongoing source of help for their child. Finally, interventionists are a source of social support for families and can help families find other support among parent groups. Connecting with other parents of children with autism can help families identify ways to manage their children successfully in the community and thus allow for more participation in community activities. All these add to the families' networks of support, increase quality of life and well-being, and reduce stress.

Parents as Powerful Advocates for Their Child

The needs of children with autism are many, the resources are few, and the expenses are large. There are neither enough services nor enough funds to meet the needs of all children with autism. Nor is there enough expertise in many public systems to understand and meet each child's needs. Parents must learn to become strong advocates for their children in order to access needed resources available for their children. In order to advocate fully,

1. Parents must learn to understand their child's needs in many domains.
2. They must be able to articulate these needs to a variety of other people.
3. They must understand the public and private systems of care and know where to find resources to meet their child's needs.
4. They have to understand their child's legal rights and routes of recourse.
5. Finally, parents have to make informed decisions about choosing from the many different types of services and care that are available in a community and in the nation.

ESDM treatment is often the first service delivery system that families in the ESDM experience, and it has a responsibility to prepare families well for a lifetime of advocacy for their child. Parents will need to take on the team leader role for their child for a very long time, often a lifetime. Thus, in the ESDM there is a partnership of parents and team leaders that allows for an apprenticeship learning opportunity for parents. The ESDM emphasizes partnership, collaboration, and shared responsibility with parents so that parents can learn the elements needed to carry out the role of advocate. The ESDM team leader does not take an authoritative role. Rather, the collaborative nature of the team leader–parent relationship also gives parents opportunities to practice advocacy within a family-friendly intervention approach and prepares them for the next systems of care that they will encounter.

Preparation for IFSP/IEP Meetings

Individualized education plan (IEP) meetings can be very painful and difficult experiences for families. However, the ESDM staff members can help parents prepare for these meetings and take some control and ownership of the process, fostering their sense of competence in their advocacy role. Parental preparation for the IEP process includes the following:

- Knowledge of requirements and assurances stated in the IDEA.
- Understanding of the purpose, goals, and steps of the IEP process.
- Meeting the members of the IEP team before the meeting.
- Gathering and understanding the assessment data that will be discussed in the meeting (and meeting ahead of time with each assessor to hear the results, if possible).
- Considering which people to invite to be part of the parents' and child's "team."
- Thinking through the parents' goals and objectives for the child so that parents can contribute to developing the annual IEP objectives.

- Parents' statements about strengths, needs, and necessary supports, and accommodations for their child.
- Concepts regarding least restrictive environments.
- The concepts of decision making based on child needs rather than existing settings and services.

There are excellent publications to recommend to parents that explain the laws and requirements of the IEP process (Siegel, 2007). Some parents may want to write a parental report concerning their child's strengths, needs, characteristics, and their own goals for their child. Some parents will benefit from role playing the IEP or walking through each part of the process together so they can visualize the process. Finally, parents should use the IEP process to establish ongoing progress meetings with the next intervention team, so that the parents have formalized ways to monitor progress and maintain close involvement with the new program staff.

It is common for an ESDM team leader to attend IFSP/IEP meetings and to provide a report of the child's current curriculum and supports in the ESDM. One of the most important things that an ESDM team leader can do is to facilitate the parents' active role in the meeting and support the parents' advocacy for their child. The first IEP meeting becomes a template for all others and the parents may face a lifetime of such meetings ahead of them; hence the importance of parental advocacy, preparation, knowledge, and confidence in their understanding of their child's educational rights and needs, and the safety net of supports available to ensure that the child's needs will be met.

When Parents Are Not Comfortable with the ESDM Philosophy or Procedures

For some parents, the types of interaction core to the ESDM seem unnatural or inappropriate. They may feel that their child will gain more benefit from a more structured and adult-directed learning environment. If this is the case, those families should be referred to a different intervention that uses a more adult-directed approach, such as traditional discrete trial teaching. There are no comparative studies demonstrating that a more child-centered approach is better for overall outcomes than a more adult-directed approach. There are pros and cons to both, and parents should be encouraged to choose empirically supported interventions that they believe will be most effective for their child and family. Belief in the efficacy of a treatment is an important part of treatment response (Beecher, 1955).

TRANSITIONING OUT OF THE ESDM INTERVENTION

Over time, parents should become quite knowledgeable about the ESDM intervention processes and procedures, and the relationship between the team leader and parents may change. Parents may become much more active about the objectives they want to see worked on, the staff members they want working with their child, and activities that they find helpful or not helpful. This is evidence of the parents' expertise in their child's needs, style, and learning responses, and it demonstrates that they are prepared to be advocates for their child in future settings. For team leaders and staff members who are used to having a great deal of authority over the child's program, this may be somewhat uncomfortable, and the staff member may feel that his or her knowledge, skill, or role is being challenged. However, this level of parental involvement will likely serve the child well in other settings. If parents are belittling staff members, complaining, or asking for more control than can be shared (like staff assignments), then the issues must be processed to determine the nature of the conflicts and the best resolutions to them. Again, the presence of clinical supervision should help the staff members have the needed dialogue with families.

There are also points at which children and families have gained all they can from their current interventions, and it is time to move on. Ongoing challenges from parents may signal that the time has come to transition. Other signals that a program transition is needed include children approaching kindergarten age, or children who are not progressing and thus are not benefitting from the intervention. Discussions about program transitions signal the last phase of the ESDM intervention. As with all other ESDM decisions, the decision that a transition is needed should come from the team, and the team includes the parents. Parents may become anxious about a transition because of losing their relationship with the staff or the services they have provided. They may not want to transition because the child has done well and they worry that progress will not be sustained. Or the child may not have done well and they feel that a move will further jeopardize the child. Allowing ample time for the transition will help the parents and the child come to know new staff members and allow enough transfer of information that the new setting can benefit from all that has been learned and can support the child's current skill set and continue progress.

Sometimes, parents want to transition their child before the staff thinks it is beneficial for the child, and this can result in negative feelings all around. It is quite important to listen carefully to the parents' reasoning and to support their goals for the child, since the parents are the experts on their child and how he or she will be raised. Staff members may well need help managing their feelings about an unexpected termination, since staff members can become deeply attached to children in their care, and a parent decision to leave can feel like rejection and failure as well as loss to some staff members. Clinical supervision is often quite helpful in managing these feelings so that when the parents do terminate, no bridges are burned.

Preparation for transition includes programmatic preparation, involving IEP meetings, transition plans, transition activities, and interface with the new staff members. It can be helpful to parents to remember all their child has learned in the ESDM setting and to see how the child is ready for the next setting. Children's developmental gains reflect good parenting, and the child's readiness should be credited to the parents' success. It is a bittersweet experience for most parents to see their child through a life transition that leads to greater independence, and it may be helpful to highlight the normalcy of this parental response for parents of a child with autism. Parents may be quite anxious about the transition, and concerned about the loss of support and expertise. Helping them think through which support systems will continue to be available to them can help. If parents do not have any providers for their child other than the ESDM staff, other community providers can be developed who will continue to serve the child and family after the transition. If parents have not joined any community family support or advocacy groups, this should be encouraged, because these are relationships that can continue after the transition. Hopefully, the ESDM staff can continue to be available to the parents and child as consultants for a set period of time after the transition, to help the new setting and to reassure parents that there will be support through the initial transition period.

CONCLUSION

The ESDM incorporates interdisciplinary expertise into the intervention model because of the multiple domains that are affected in autism: motor functioning, sensory functioning, communication development, intellectual development and learning difficulties, behavioral functioning, health-related problems, and effects on family members. The interdisciplinary team provides disciplinary training to those from other disciplines and provides disciplinary expertise for children with specific problems in addition to their autism. However, the use of a generalist model supported by the interdisciplinary team results in an integrated approach to the child's therapy across his or her multiple domains of need, provides a single line of communication for the family, and ensures that one professional has the "big" picture of an individual child's and family's needs and progress. It is an economical and efficient approach to providing professional care for young children with autism and their families. However, it requires significant interdisciplinary training across the team and disciplinary "role release" in order to realize the potential of this aspect of the ESDM. When done well, it creates an exciting environment for staff members and families alike, an environment of continual learning from the other team members, and sharing and support across the team that fosters team cohesion and solidarity in the face of work that is often both physically and emotionally demanding.

Parents and families are central members of the interdisciplinary team. The work with children in the ESDM is work within a family system. Success can be measured by the quality of parent–child relationships, parental satisfaction with child progress and the ESDM services received, quality of the working alliance between parents and the ESDM staff, parental knowledge of child needs and service systems, and parental advocacy skills. Termination of ESDM direct services should be a celebration of all that has been accomplished by staff, parents, and child, with optimism joined with careful planning for the next stage in the child's development.

The next chapter begins a more detailed discussion of how to teach children using the ESDM. The process begins with the development of short-term learning objectives.

Chapter 4

Developing Short-Term Learning Objectives

One of the most important parts of the intervention process in the ESDM is the construction of short-term (12-week) learning objectives for the child. The objectives guide the intervention like a road map guides a traveler, directing the course of all the teaching. There are so many things to teach a young child with autism that it is easy to lose track of teaching targets during a play-based treatment session. The objectives help interventionists, whether new or highly experienced, to stay focused on specific skills and behaviors so they can provide sufficient learning opportunities for the child to master targeted skills.

The construction of the short-term objectives begins with an assessment of the child's current skill level using the ESDM Curriculum Checklist (see Appendix A). Two to three target skills in each relevant developmental domain are then formulated and taught over the next 12 weeks. Each skill is defined as a measurable learning objective in terms of the antecedent event (discriminative stimulus), behavioral response, and generalized mastery-level criteria. This chapter describes this process of assessment and the development of measurable 12-week learning objectives.

ASSESSMENT USING THE ESDM CURRICULUM CHECKLIST

The ESDM Curriculum Checklist is a criterion-referenced tool that provides developmental sequences of skills in a variety of developmental domains: receptive communication, expressive communication, social skills, play skills, cognitive skills, fine motor skills, gross motor skills, and adaptive behavior skills. The Checklist is organized into four skill levels, which roughly correspond to the developmental age periods 12–18 months, 18–24 months, 24–36 months, and 36–48 months. However, the Curriculum Checklist was developed specifically for young children with ASD and reflects their typical developmental profile. This involves relatively more advanced visual motor skills and relatively less advanced social and communication skills than other children of the same developmental age. Thus, in each level, the communication and social items are developmentally more immature than the fine and gross motor items, if one uses a standard of typical development as a point of comparison. The skills within a domain come from wide-ranging reviews of the literature on typical child development. The placement of the items in a specific level reflects both typical child development research and also the clinical experience of several different expert ESDM interdisciplinary teams working with hundreds of young children with ASD over the past 25 years.

The Evaluator

The Curriculum Checklist is developed to be administered by early intervention professionals. It can be administered in several different formats, depending on the organization of the team and the intervention program. It can be used by a single early intervention professional who has cross-disciplinary knowledge of development in the various domains and has practiced the tool and its scoring. This evaluation format would be used when the ESDM is delivered as a single-discipline therapy, or in an intensive 1:1 delivery format using a generalist model, with the team leader administering the Checklist. If a single disciplinarian is going to use it, that person will need cross training in other disciplines on the items that are outside of that person's knowledge base. In group programs involving a multidisciplinary team, different domains can be administered by the various professional team members, with each disciplinarian administering the sections most relevant to his or her skill set.

Administration

As with other assessment tools that cover a wide range of skills, the goal is to assess the child's current levels of ability rather than to administer the entire tool. At the end of the assessment, the assessor should have identified the skills in each domain that define the child's most mature skills, those skills that are currently emerging, and those skills that are currently not in the child's repertoire. Most children's skills will cluster in one of the four levels for each domain. However, for children whose skills fall in the earlier items in a level, be sure to review the final items in the previous level to identify any critical skills that the child is failing in the level below. Similarly, if a child has mostly passes in one level and only a few fails, you will need to move into the next level and assess at least the first half of the items in that domain to be sure you have good information about what the child's real repertoire is at this particular time. As with other developmental tests, your goal is to determine the child's basal and ceiling levels, and particularly to identify the range in which passes turn to failures in each domain. This will be the target area for teaching.

The Curriculum Checklist is administered in the same way that intervention occurs—in a play-based interactive style using a joint activity frame. Using play activities allows for a variety of domains to be assessed within a single activity; this is because most toy-based interactions between a child and adult involve motor skills, cognitive skills, communicative skills, and social skills. A play-based assessment also allows one to examine social and communication components inside typical social interaction patterns for young children. The assessor organizes a play session that includes the materials needed to complete the items and develops play activities with the child. The assessor should engage the child in a play activity that interests the child, carry out the activity with the child until a natural ending point or until no new behaviors are being elicited, and then pause and note the items on the Curriculum Checklist that were observed, as well as those that were tried but were not elicited. The assessor then begins another play activity and proceeds as before. After each play activity, one should pause, take notes, check the items, and determine what items still have to be administered. Then, the assessor chooses materials and play activities that elicit the remaining items. For those items that cannot be observed (e.g., bath time), the parent is interviewed. If there are other therapists' reports, incorporate that information as well. There are columns for each of these information sources: direct observation, parent report, and other therapist or teacher report. The parent should be present throughout the assessment, and the level of parent participation is up to the assessor.

The Curriculum Checklist can generally be administered within one play session of 1–1.5 hours. The best setting is a therapy room, with a small table and chairs, beanbag, floor area, comfortable chair for the parent, and materials that will be needed to elicit the skills on the Curriculum Checklist. A list of necessary materials is presented in the beginning of the Curriculum Checklist. It is very helpful to remove materials from the room that will not be used for the assessment, so that time is not lost and children's attention is not focused on materials that cannot provide useful information for the assessment. Video recording of the assessment is not necessary but is helpful as a source of information later, and also as a documentation of the starting point of treatment.

Scoring

Three scoring conventions are used with the Checklist: P (for pass) or + (for consistent performance or mastery), P/F (pass–fail) or ± (to capture inconsistent performance), and F (fail) or – (to use when no examples are seen or the behavior is difficult to elicit).

The Curriculum Checklist Item Descriptions specify what level of response is needed to pass an item. The assessor records the parent report and the direct assessment scores in the appropriate columns, along with information provided by other team members if it is available. For both passed and failed items, one needs to know whether the child displays this behavior at home and/or in other settings, and if so, how consistently. There will also be behaviors that cannot be observed in the assessment setting, like self-care skills, and the parent will provide information on these skills. After the assessment is complete, the assessor integrates the information into a final code for each item, indicating the child's mastery level of each item in a domain within the particular level that contains both passes and fails. (*Note:* Items that are considered mastered or passed will not be targets for any teaching objectives, so it is quite important to not optimize child performance. Passes should be reserved for skills that are consistently and reliably used as described in the item description and well generalized, if appropriate, across different settings, people, and materials.) When the assessor has a good sense of the child's working repertoire of skills and the Curriculum Checklist clearly reflects the child's current level of skills with a group of Ps, P/Fs, and Fs in each domain, the assessment is complete. The following is a narrative description of the administration of the ESDM Curriculum Checklist.

Case Example: Isaac's ESDM Evaluation

Isaac is a 26-month-old boy of Hispanic origin diagnosed the previous week with autistic disorder. He is the third child of young parents with high school educations. This assessment takes place in a clinic setting and is scheduled to last 75 minutes. The assessor is an

ESDM therapist who will provide intervention via parent coaching in the ESDM. The setting is a therapy room, as described above, with toys needed for the assessment in closed cabinets and on high shelves. The description below occurs in roughly 5-minute intervals, which represents the length of time this particular child tended to spend in an activity. The therapist will carry out an activity, and then fill out the Curriculum Checklist at the end of the activity, before starting a new one.

Minutes 0–5: Entry

Isaac is "jumped" into the room by the assessor, in response to great resistance at walking with the family from the waiting room into the assessment room. As he enters, he looks around and approaches the open toy shelf. While the assessor describes the coming activities to the mother and aunt, he looks at the toys, selects a clear box with two trucks, puts the box on the floor, and removes both trucks. He returns to the shelf and operates a pop-up toy, using a different hand movement to open each of five little boxes, and then puts all the lids back down. He removes a box with art supplies, places it on the floor, removes a marker, takes the top off, looks around for a piece of paper, and begins to scribble in large circular scribbles using a right-handed radial grasp. Another ESDM staff member enters the room to observe, and he looks up at her entry but does not respond to her greeting. He finds a pinwheel on the shelf, picks it up, holds it by the stick, waves it to make it spin, and then spins it with his hand.

ESDM Curriculum Checklist Level 1 Item Observations

Refusal to walk cooperatively with hand held, understands container-contained relationships. Means–end understanding of tools involving marker, crayon, push-button toy, and pinwheel. Operates a number of different push-button-type actions. Conventional play with pinwheel and art materials. Radial grasp, circular scribbles, lack of response to greeting. Independent play is very brief—60 seconds or less. Fairly organized during exploration.

Minutes 5–15: Mother–Child Play

(*Note:* It is important to observe some parent–child play and interaction during the hour. When it occurs at the beginning, it allows one to begin to sample the child's skill level, and it helps children become comfortable in the new setting. Some parents will be pleased to be asked to play with their child, and others will be quite hesitant to begin this way and will be more comfortable later.) His mother joins him on the floor, selects a container of small magnetic train pieces, and offers him the box, asking, "Isaac, do you want to play with trains?" He takes one and they both sit down. She demonstrates driving a train piece back and forth on the carpet, and he imitates her. He reaches to a toy phone in front of him in the cabinet, his mother helps him get it and dials it, and Isaac dials, picks up the receiver, and babbles into the phone. She says, "Hello, Isaac," and he responds with a long string of variegated babble with melodic contour, and then he hangs up the phone. Mother repeats this activity of dialing, and Isaac carries out the sequence of dialing, lifting the receiver, vocalizing, and hanging up one more time before he is finished and returns to the pinwheel.

Mother finds a box of play dough material and turns to him. He is watching her and she says, "Sit down," and points to the floor, where he sits and they both begin to remove materials. He sits on his knees, facing 90 degrees away from her, and they maintain this position for the rest of this play episode. He has trouble with the lids, pulling at them and using his teeth, but he cannot open them. He does not offer them to her or request her help in any way, and when she tries to help and reaches for the cans, he turns away. She opens the cans for him, and he ignores her "give me" request conveyed by language and gesture. They engage in a shared game of taking out the play dough and putting pieces on top of the train cars. They begin to take turns putting pieces on top of one car, and they repeat this turn taking through three rounds. He imitates her moving the cars with the play dough. She makes some sound effects, "beep beep," and he imitates her with a rough approximation and then offers some more jargon. His vocalizations appear intentional, but he does not direct them to her with gaze or orientation. He reaches to take one of her pieces and she pulls it away. He protests angrily by saying, "No no no," and bounces on his knees, and she says, "You have to share," and directs him to his own play dough. She shows him how to use the play dough press, and he watches and then copies her actions, and the two together fill the press before turning back to the trains with the flat pieces from the press. As she drives her train, he adds a sound effect. She demonstrates the magnet on the train and shows him how the cars will stick together. He offers his piece to her for the magnet effect. Then they return to the parallel train play, and he smiles and laughs and provides a long string of variegated jargon as he shares his enjoyment of the activity with eye contact. Another person in the room speaks, and he turns to look, and then connects his train pieces and drives the whole line of cars.

ESDM Curriculum Checklist Level 1 Item Observations

Vocal imitation of sound effect, word "no no," variegated babble with intonation, intentional vocalizations, no gaze accompanying vocalizations. He followed gesture and instruction to sit down, imitated several actions on objects, including a novel action, and demonstrated functional play with the phone, train, and play dough. He showed sequenced play with the phone. He demonstrated some nonverbal requests through gesture and a verbal protest, but no means of requesting help. He shared enjoyment with gaze alternation. He did not give objects in response to a gestural request. He looked to a voice and watched a play partner's actions. Turn taking occurs repeatedly, for short rounds.

Minutes 15–20

Assessor now joins the train activity on the floor and the mother gradually moves to the side. Assessor says, "Put on," while modeling placing play dough on the train and he then does so. She then models and offers a coloring activity, but he refuses by turning away. She says, "Time to clean up," and begins to put the play dough in the cans. She offers him a can, says, "Clean up," and points to it, and he places his piece of play dough into it. She thanks him, puts more away, repeats the request, and he ignores two more requests, so she assists him to put it away, again thanking him, and then quickly cleans up all the play dough props. He wanders away.

Skills Observed

Occasionally followed simple instructions plus gesture. He helped with clean-up. He followed the proximal point and imitated actions on objects.

Minutes 20–25

He goes to the toy cabinet and reaches for the pop-bead bag. The assessor opens it and assembles three different beads together and then wiggles them. He tries to put them in but cannot and throws it down. She hands him hers, and he takes each out and throws them on the floor. Then he reaches for a slinky. She picks it up, labels it and offers it to him, and he says, "No no no," with an angry whine while reaching for it. He takes one end while she holds the other and he walks away. She begins to wiggle her end and he turns to look, then he wiggles his end as well and smiles at her. He releases his end; she gathers it up fast and offers it to him with the words, "Want slinky?" He approaches her, she says, "More slinky?" and he gestures with reach to the slinky in response. She gives one end, as before, and he walks away, turns to her, and repeats the wiggle game from before with directed smiles before wandering away.

ESDM Curriculum Checklist Level 1 Item Observations

Lack of appropriate verbal request, shared pleasure with eye contact, imitated a novel action, gestured to request, and enjoyed the dyadic game.

Minutes 25–30

Assessor demonstrates a party horn, blowing it out to the side. He smiles, looks, flaps hands excitedly, and then waits expectantly. She repeats and he smiles, takes it, approaches Mother, and hands it to her. Mother blows it for him and he looks, smiles, and laughs, and then takes it to his aunt and offers. She repeats and then puts it to his mouth. He blows but cannot operate it and he hands it back for her to blow, again with smiles and laughter.

Minutes 30–35

He wanders away and pats a big ball as he passes it. The assessor pats the ball as well, then models kicking the ball into the wall. He watches but does not imitate when she offers the ball. She repeats, and he again does not respond to her model or imitation, so she picks him up and sits him on the ball, and bounces him while counting, "1, 2, 3, stop." She repeats this twice. He smiles but averts face and leaves. She follows him and offers another game, a jumping game similar to the one that was used to bring him into the room. She jumps him up and down while counting to 5. He again smiles, averts his face, and leaves when she stops. He wanders over to the beanbag and picks up the picture book lying there. He turns pages one at a time, looking at the pictures. She points to the chicks, saying, "See the chicks—peep peep peep," and he looks and says, "Peep peep." He turns the pages and they repeat this with the cow. She then says, "Take the book to Mommy," and points to his mother. He does not follow her point and ignores her request. She repeats once more, with no response.

ESDM Curriculum Checklist Level 1 Item Observations

Uses gaze and gives objects to request others' actions, differentially prefers parent and grandparent to assessor, shares pleasure with directed smiles and laughter, imitates blowing. He turns pages in a book, looks at pictures, follows proximal point to pictures, and imitates an animal sound. He is much quieter with the assessor than with the parent. His play is less organized and less mature than in the first 15 minutes. He does not follow an instruction involving an object and does not look to Mother when her name is mentioned.

Minutes 35–45

He dumps a container of "sensory social toys" (balloons, balls, bubbles, noisemakers), and she offers the nerf balls and bucket to him. She tosses a ball in the bucket and offers him a ball and encourages him to do the same. He tosses the ball toward the bucket. She praises this and gives him another, this time aiming the basket to catch his ball. He throws and succeeds, and everyone claps. He looks around at the applauding people while smiling. She rolls a ball to him, but he ignores both that one and the next one she rolls. She then offers bubbles. He smiles and says, "No no no," while reaching for them, so she operates the bubble gun, saying, "1, 2, 3, go," and he imitates "One, go!" He smiles to her, flaps his hands, and watches the bubbles but does not request more and wanders away. She operates a balloon and he reapproaches her, moving in a well-coordinated fashion through the materials on the floor, smiling and reaching for the balloon, flapping hands while she blows it, and when she gently deflates it, he takes the other balloon to his mother and gives it to her. When his mother asks, "More?" he whines and says, "No no no," angrily while waiting for her to blow the balloon.

ESDM Curriculum Checklist Level 1 Item Observations

Verbal imitation of "one, go." Requests are confusing because he uses "give" gestures combined with angry whining and "no no no" to request. He flaps hands when excited. There is a lack of sustained engagement in activities with assessor. He has good balance, walks around objects instead of on top of them or tripping over them, is aware of the environment, and his muscle tone looks good when he sits and stands (straight back, good posture, no lordosis or rounded shoulders, no splayed legs when sitting).

Minutes 45–55

Assessor puts a box of drawing materials on a small table and takes him by the hand to a small chair, asks him to sit, and he does so. She holds up two markers for him to choose from, and he reaches to one, which she hands to him, takes her own, and they both make marks. She models circular scribbles ("circle, circle, circle") and he imitates. She shifts to lines ("line, line, line") and he copies. She shifts to fast movements, back and forth, and he copies, mirroring her movements in both hands. He gets out of the chair to get new markers that he opens with his mouth. He ignores his mother's "no" and when Mother retrieves the marker lid from his mouth, he is very angry, yelling and protesting, but he returns to the markers and colors with a marker in each hand, using ulnar grasp and wrist rotation during circles. The assessor begins to sing a song with hand movements—"Eensy Weensy Spider." He looks up at her, smiles and listens, then returns to coloring. When she stops, he looks up and waits. She begins singing again and encourages him to bring his hands together for the "spider." He says, "No no no," and leaves the table. He vocalizes a little, with variegated jargon, walks back to the toy cabinet and stands a minute, vocalizing while making small hand and body movements, moving his hands rhythmically up and down like a drummer, bending and straightening his knees, and vocalizing as if copying a little dance routine. The therapist joins and copies his movements, and he watches her and repeats them, as if the two of them are dancing.

The therapist then takes two tinkertoy sticks, puts knobs on the ends, and drums on one of the boxes on the floor, handing a stick to Isaac. He imitates her drumming. She drums on the side and he imitates. She bangs two sticks together and he imitates. She adds a word, "Bang bang bang," and he imitates. She models clapping her hands together—he does not imitate. He then gets two sticks and bangs on the box, facing her and smiling as she joins in. He shifts his gaze from the banging sticks to share smiles. She models how to make the drumstick and hands him two pieces, which he assembles. She begins to make a star out of the tinkertoy piece, with sticks jutting out and offers it to him. He adds sticks in the right places.

ESDM Curriculum Checklist Level 1 Item Observations

He imitates actions on objects, imitates block construction, imitates familiar body movements, imitates new words, and imitates lines, scribbles, and circular scribbles. He copies both actions and differing tempos of actions. He gets angry very quickly, ignores "no," is aware of being imitated, and enjoys it. He likes the imitation game, and he shifts gaze from the object to smile at his partner in a display of affect sharing. He likes being sung to but does not join in. He makes a choice from two offered objects by reaching.

Minutes 50–60

He picks up a 12-piece inset puzzle frame, and she provides the box with the puzzle pieces and instructs him to sit down—he says, "No no no," so she helps him sit and provides a piece, which he places. She provides another, which he misses, and she points to the correct place, and he places it. She provides a third, and he places it and then gets up, to which she says, "All done," and he imitates "all done" and goes to the door. She offers a bag with a small round pegboard and six 1" × 6" pegs, and he takes them with interest. His mother says, "Sit down," and he plops to the floor, opens the bag, takes out the pieces, and begins to assemble the pegboard. Instead of placing all the pegs, he stacks some on others and even gets them to balance, but he does not finish and tosses it away. A third shape sorter interests him, and he tries to place the pieces but needs help on all but the circle and square. He does not finish this either. He is now vocalizing freely.

ESDM Curriculum Checklist Level 1 Item Observations

He does not complete toy routines, but rather places two to three pieces and then turns to something else. He does simple shape matching, varies schemas. He is curious and interested in novel objects.

Minutes 65–75

The assessment ends with a brief interview with the family members. They are extremely worried about him because of his lack of language and his very difficult behavior. Biting, sleep, and tantrums are huge problems. He bites everyone and is not safe around smaller children. His aunt, who keeps him during the day, showed his bite marks up and down her arms. When angry, he screams, throws himself on the floor, and bangs his head. He attempts to bite multiple times per day and has tantrums every hour. He does not go to bed, does not stay in bed, and is up several times every night. He eats well, however, with good use of spoon, fork, and open cup. He eats a wide variety of food and eats the family meals, though he does not stay in his chair but rather climbs up, eats a few bites, leaves, and comes back. He does not wander the house with food and is not allowed to take anything except his water cup away from the table. He can use a straw, will eat new foods, and is not spoon fed by others. He is not on a bottle. He helps pull off his clothes for undressing and helps pull his shirt back on. Diapering is not a problem because he does not like to be wet. He likes water and enjoys hand-washing routines and his bath. He will rub a washcloth and towel on his body and will put his toothbrush in his mouth, although he will not let anyone else brush his teeth. His hair is cut very short so hair washing and combing is not a problem. He does not reliably follow any instructions at home and does not do any chores like putting his clothes in the hamper or putting his cup on a shelf. He does not help clean up toys. Very few demands are placed on him because of his severe temper tantrums. In terms of strengths, they see Isaac as a smart little boy who can figure out how to operate objects and how to get his way. They see him as athletic and fearless, able to climb up and down tall playground equipment, and run, jump, and roughhouse with bigger kids. They describe him as coordinated on his tricycle, when throwing balls, and when climbing on equipment, and also in his ability to stack blocks, color, and use a spoon and fork. His parents are very young, of Hispanic origin, and both work long hours. English is their primary language, but they mix in a significant amount of Spanish with each other and with Isaac. He stays with his aunt and uncle during the day, and Spanish is their primary language with him and with others.

Isaac now clearly wants to leave. He gets up and goes to the door. It is time to go, so the examiner tells him, "Yes, it's time to go." She kneels to his level and directs a very clear "bye-bye" and wave to him. He imitates both back to her, and she takes him out of the room while his mother and aunt gather their things and leave. The family members feel that he has done extremely well during this session and are pleased at the words he has spoken, his good cooperation, and his lack of behavior problems.

Isaac's ESDM Assessment Profile

Isaac has significant strengths in fine and gross motor skills. His interest in objects and knowledge of how objects work will be very useful in therapy. He is motivated to act on materials, and he seems to enjoy social play with a mirroring partner. He is able to attend for a reasonable period of time, does not avoid others, and has some reciprocal play. He imitates actions on objects easily and occasionally imitates words. His speech contains many consonants, speech-like intonation, and phonemic structure. He imitates some words and initiates at least one. His play involves short sequences of related acts and some conventional play. His curiosity and enthusiasm for objects will be a great help in treatment. His skills fall within Level 1 in all domains except gross motor, in which he passes all but one item—kicking the big ball—and he is ready for Level 2 items.

Receptive Communication

He scores passes or pass–fails on the first six items, involving looking toward sounds and voices and following a proximal point. He responds consistently to an instruction, "sit down," with and without gestures.

Expressive Communication

His expressive communication strengths involve his developing phonemes and intentional vocalizations. He does not use conventional gestures consistently for any pragmatic functions, nor does he appear to understand others' communicative gestures.

Social Skills

In terms of social skills, he watches his play partner when engaged in parallel play, and he will imitate his partner and do a few turns in a reciprocal exchange. He allows touch, but he only occasionally shares smiles and uses eye contact communicatively. He demonstrates imitation of some novel actions involving actions on objects, oral imitations, and vocal imitations, although only actions on objects are consistently imitated. We would expect to see imitation develop quickly given his current skill level. He did not demonstrate any matching skills, though he groups like objects in his play (trains, drawing materials), and we expect to see this area progress rapidly as well. Several beginning play items are passed, including 1, 2, 4, 5, and 7. He has a nice range of play schemas, but he does not sustain them and does not yet seem to have a goal of task completion. This will be a primary target area for his objectives. Thus, building play sequences with more materials and more steps will be a main focus of play activities, including the clean-up sequence.

Fine Motor Skills

His fine motor skills are well developed, and most of his failures are actually "no opportunity" scores because they were not probed, like the ring stacker, lego stacks, and scooping. We did not observe a pincer grasp and need to probe for it in a snack routine with Cheerios.

Gross Motor Skills

His only fail in the gross motor domain was kicking the big ball; the rest of the items were completed by parent report.

Eating, Dressing, Grooming, Chores

His self-care skills are developing well, though he needs to learn to stay at the table throughout a meal. Bedtime needs to be dealt with, but his severe tantrums, self-abuse, and aggression are preventing his family members from knowing how to teach him. It will be crucial to complete a functional assessment of his problem behaviors and get positive support plans going quickly, so that both his developmental and his behavioral difficulties can be addressed.

CONSTRUCTING THE LEARNING OBJECTIVES

The child's team leader and the child's parents formulate the objectives to be learned by the child over the next 12 weeks. The objectives are constructed using the parents' goals, data from the ESDM Curriculum Checklist, and input from any other professionals who support the child and family. We write objectives that we fully expect an individual child to master in 3 months, but that are sufficiently challenging so that it will take 2 or 3 months to teach them, given the intensity of teaching that will be provided.

BALANCING OBJECTIVES ACROSS DOMAINS

The ESDM advocates choosing a balanced number of objectives in each of the domains, rather than emphasizing one domain at the expense of the others. The reason for this is twofold. First, we wish to counteract the natural tendency to emphasize those domains in which the child has weaknesses. Building a set of objectives on the most affected areas can result in frustration for the therapist, parents, and child because progress is liable to be slowest and teaching most difficult in the most affected areas. Second, we do not want to focus only on strengths. After all, it is exhilarating to see a child easily succeed in his or her area of strength. The problem with focusing on strengths is that the core domains that are affected in autism, such as the domain of social reciprocity, are neglected at the expense of the areas of strength. Such unbalanced teaching only accentuates the uneven pattern of strengths and weaknesses that is so characteristic of autism. In the ESDM, we write objectives in all domains, the strongest as well as the weakest domains, so that we are supporting the development of areas of talent as well as weakness. This tends to ensure highly motivating activities for the child and therapist.

HOW MANY OBJECTIVES?

Write two to three objectives for each domain. This translates into more than 20 objectives but we find it provides a manageable set for intensive treatment over a 12-week period. What if there are not two to three Curriculum Checklist items in a domain that you feel relatively confident that the child can pass in 12 weeks? You can either write fewer objectives in that area, or you can break a particular item into two smaller steps. Having more objectives helps the interventionists think of teaching targets within activities. Be aware when the same underlying skills will logically affect development in two different domains; you can then write related objectives for both domains. For instance, if you write an objective that specifies that the child will use 10 different specific verbs for expressive language development, it only makes sense to also write a receptive communication objective that targets those same 10 verbs.

SELECTING SKILL CONTENT

The task, then, is to identify two to three skills in each domain to be taught over the next 12 weeks. The assessment information from the Curriculum Checklist is used in two different ways to construct objectives. First, one identifies the skills in each domain that represent the child's first P/Fs and Fs. We expect that these skills will be learned in 12 weeks. Second, the team leader must project the child's learning rate ahead over the next 3 months and think about what the child can reasonably accomplish given consistent daily teaching from parents and/or staff. Some children learn rapidly, and these are typically the children with ASD who have more skills relative to their ages in the language, cognitive, and fine motor domains on the objectives. For these children, you would not necessarily highlight the first skills failed as the targets, but rather later skills in the same level sequence that also address those first failed skills.

For example, on 24-month-old Nathan's initial evaluation, he failed Level 2 Receptive Communication item 2, "Follows eight to 10 one-step verbal instructions involving body actions and actions on objects." He only followed six of them at the time: give me, come here, sit down, looks to name, high five, and bye-bye. However, for a 24 month old with autism who has not yet received treatment, this is an impressive receptive language repertoire, and it seems clear that it will not take him 12 more weeks of daily teaching to acquire another two instructions. Using this item as it is written in the Curriculum Checklist for his 12-week objective is not appropriate. It is better to set the bar higher by writing receptive communication objectives that target the items toward the end of Level 2. These are skills involving placing items in locations, pointing to live examples and pictures of various people and objects, and following several different action words with objects. With these as learning objectives, the therapist will have taught virtually all the receptive language skills in Level 2 by the end of 12 weeks.

Other children learn more slowly in certain areas. Joshua has the same level of performance on item 2 as Nathan. However, Joshua is 38 months old, has been in the ESDM intervention for 12 months, and has received intensive daily teaching. Communication is extremely difficult for him; over the past 12 months he has mastered all of Level 1 receptive communication and he follows six instructions. Given Joshua's rate of progress, the objectives written for him will differ from those written for Nathan. For Joshua, it would be more appropriate to target item 2, mastery of 10 instructions, for his Level 2 Receptive Communication 12-week objectives. It will likely take him 12 weeks to learn four more instructions.

Thus, knowledge of the child's learning rate gained from the assessment is used to decide what skills can reasonably be expected to be mastered in 12 weeks of teaching. Keeping objectives challenging but accomplishable is crucial for motivating the child, the team, and the parents, and for giving the therapists enough to do in their sessions.

In summary, to identify the skills to be taught, look at the pattern of skills passed and failed in a specific developmental domain. Identify the Curriculum Checklist level in the domain that contains the most advanced consistent passes for this child. Your objectives should focus on completing this level. You can assume that every child can master his or her P/F items in a level within 12 weeks of good, consistent, daily teaching; those skills should definitely be targeted in the objectives. Then, look beyond the first P/Fs to the first few Fs. You have to use your own knowledge of the child, gleaned from your assessment, to gauge how far into unlearned areas to venture with your objectives. When in doubt, be conservative! Why? It builds confidence for everyone, child included, when the child masters objectives, and it is discouraging for everyone when the child does not master most of the 12-week objectives. Child mastery keeps motivation for teaching and learning high for child, interventionists, and parents, and child mastery requires choosing appropriate learning objectives and teaching approaches, and then ensuring their daily delivery.

ELEMENTS OF THE OBJECTIVE

Every professional person who reads this book has likely written educational or treatment objectives previously. However, we use a very specific format for objectives in the ESDM that supports adult teaching and child learning in very helpful ways. After the target skills are selected from the Curriculum Checklist, as explained above, each skill is then described in measurable, behavioral terms. Thus each ESDM objective has four main characteristics: (1) a statement of the antecedent stimulus or event that precedes and will elicit the behavior (skill); (2) specification of an observable, measurable behavior (the skill to be taught); (3) the criterion that defines mastery of the objective; and (4) a criterion that involves functional, generalized performance of the target behavior. We offer guidelines for writing these four elements below.

Statement of the Antecedent Stimulus

Skills and behaviors occur in response to something, and that something is the antecedent stimulus, or the discriminative stimulus (Sd) for the behavior. Some behaviors are performed in response to another person's behavior (e.g., approaching an adult who calls your name, taking a toy when another child hands it to you). Other behaviors are responses to an environmental cue (e.g., many preschool transitions are cued through lights, bells, songs, and so on in addition to verbal instruction). Some behaviors occur in response to an internal cue (e.g., getting a drink of water when thirsty, choosing a toy and playing with it in free play activities, requesting something to eat when hungry). Finally, some behaviors are part of a chain or sequence and are cued by the preceding behavior (e.g., turning off the water when you have finished washing hands, turning off the light when you leave the bathroom, hanging up your coat after you have removed it).

The reasons for specifying the antecedent or stimulus condition in the objective are twofold: First, it helps us teach children with autism to respond to the same stimuli that also cue behavior in other children. Second, it tells the interventionist what antecedent stimuli must be used to teach the objective, which should improve the consistency of teaching and the rapidity of child learning. We believe that using consistent antecedents in teaching improves child learning rates. This is why we stress them.

How do you choose what antecedent, or Sd, to specify? There are several points to consider. First and foremost, think about the Sds in natural environments—home, preschool, day care—that elicit this behavior in typically developing children of the same age. This is the best Sd to use. If that does not seem appropriate for this child, then think about how adults would typically *instruct* a child of this age to do this behavior in a natural setting. What language and gestures would they use? Those are the Sds to target. (*Note:* The child does not have to understand the antecedent or Sd in order for you to specify it. That is what will be taught.)

The following are examples of stated antecedents: "When an adult establishes eye contact, waves, and says 'bye-bye'" (she will imitate the wave ...); "When another child approaches, extends his or her hand to an object the child is holding, and asks for a turn, to share, or to give," (the child will extend the toy ...); "When the child approaches the toilet and stands within 12–18 inches in front of it" (he will spontaneously unfasten pants ...). (*Note*: This last antecedent phrase is written for a spontaneous behavior. Spontaneous behaviors also have Sds; either environmental, internal, or preceding behaviors occurring in a chain.)

When the target behavior is a spontaneous social behavior, the antecedent may be harder to specify. What is the antecedent for a spontaneous greeting? Is it seeing a familiar person for the first time that day, hour, and so on? The familiar person is likely also looking at you and smiling at you. Here is an antecedent phrase for a spontaneous greeting: "When Jason first enters the therapy room and the therapist approaches him with eye contact and a smile, Jason will say 'hi' or wave." Here is an antecedent phrase for a spontaneous request: "When Jason enters the kitchen and approaches a drink container that is prominent but out of reach, he will look at the adult and ask, 'Drink, please.' " In both these situations, there is an environmental stimulus that precedes the request and that is incorporated into the objective as an antecedent, or Sd, for spontaneous speech.

Beware!

People often mistakenly treat a setting as an antecedent. A setting is a situation or environment in which a behavior occurs. Examples are "In the classroom," "during 1:1 treatment," and "during circle time." These are settings, not antecedents. They can be helpful in specifying situations in which the behavior should occur, but they are not antecedents—they do not elicit a certain behavior.

A behavior may occur under more than one stimulus condition. In this case, the objective could specify several appropriate conditions (e.g., "Sara will establish eye contact and say, 'Help me,' to her partner while offering the object in three conditions: when presented with a container she cannot open; when she cannot complete a fastener on her clothing; and when she cannot locate the correct position for a puzzle piece.").

Statement of the Behavior to Be Demonstrated

Our only real evidence of child learning is observable child behavior. We cannot observe knowledge of color concepts, but we can observe children matching and sorting by color, naming colors, and selecting colors by name. Because we often think in more abstract terms about child development, it can be difficult to translate a developmental concept, like "knowledge of" or "has the concepts" or "engages in," into a clearly observable behavior.

Each objective should describe specific child behaviors. Children give, point to, say, kick, match, sort, pedal, name, and jump. They demonstrate joint attention behaviors by giving, showing, looking, pointing, and following points. They respond to others with observable behaviors as well—they orient their heads and bodies, make eye contact, speak, and gesture. Visualize the child performing the objective that you are writing. What is the child actually doing? What muscles have moved? What action has occurred? Those actions are the behaviors that your objective is targeting.

A single objective may involve more than one behavior. This happens for two reasons. First, it may happen because the behaviors are generally combined in a motor sequence. For example, cleaning up involves placing or sorting things (matching) into containers, and putting containers away, on shelves or in drawers. Advanced-level joint attention skills involve pointing, following points, or showing, combined with eye contact and gaze shifts from object to person, and are often accompanied by vocalizations as well. Dressing and toileting involve long chains of behaviors. Behaviors like these that occur in a sequence are often taught together, so objectives concerning such sequences of behavior will specify the multiple behaviors involved in one objective. For example, the following objective targets two joint attention behaviors, gaze shifts, and following points:

In response to an adult saying, "Johnny, look!" while looking at and pointing to the object on the shelf or floor from a distance of up to 10 feet, Johnny will visually follow the point, look at the object, and then make eye contact with the adult at first opportunity, three times in a 20-minute period, in three consecutive sessions, and for two or more different adults.

In this objective, there are three behaviors that Johnny will have to demonstrate, in a sequence: following the point with eyes and head, looking at an object, and then looking back and making eye contact. These will occur in response to a stimulus involving adult behaviors, including turning, pointing, and speaking. The child will have to exhibit this combination of behaviors three separate times in 20 minutes, and he will have to do it at the very first stimulus presentation each time to pass this objective.

The second situation in which there are multiple behaviors in one objective involves using the same class of behaviors, like naming, pointing, or imitating, for multiple exemplars. Verb use is a good example: In response to the partner's example or to spontaneously narrate her own activity, Shannon will use 10 different action words (verbs) appropriately to describe acts of self, other, or object during a 1-hour dyadic play period.

This objective is measurable without listing the specific verbs to be used. As written, the child's display of any 10 verbs would pass this objective. However, if it matters which verbs the child is to use, which might occur because there are certain verbs that are really difficult for this child or are quite necessary for communication, then you would name them in the objective. For example: Shannon will use the following five verbs: give, help, up, down, and finished, in two-word utterances during snack routines, either imitatively or spontaneously, to request, daily for 3 consecutive days.

Specification of the Criterion That Defines Mastery

Each written objective needs to specify the criterion for judging successful learning and mastery of the objective. This serves two very utilitarian purposes. First, it helps to focus the teaching on a certain level of achievement, and second, it allows one to be quite clear about whether the child has succeeded or failed and thus provides clear feedback about whether the child is learning what you are trying to teach.

Setting the criteria for mastery at an appropriate level of difficulty is dependent on the team's knowledge of the child's developmental rate. As stated earlier, we write criteria that represent mastery of a skill, but also with the expectation that the child will achieve that mastery in 12 weeks. Setting the criteria involves a good sense of the child's learning rate, the amount of teaching that will occur, and a healthy dose of optimism. As mentioned earlier, when it is not clear what the child can reasonably be expected to learn in 12 weeks, be conservative. It is better to err by being too easy than too hard because everyone—child, parents, teaching staff, and team—is negatively affected by failure. It is better for everyone to be pleased at the level of mastery attained.

A criterion for success may specify the number of skills learned (e.g., naming eight colors), or the latency of the response (e.g., the child will return a friend's greeting by orienting, looking, and saying "Hi" within 1 second). The criterion may involve a specific level of independence in a sequence of skills (e.g., the child will complete 70% of the steps involved in hand washing independently, without any prompts). It could involve a temporal duration (e.g., plays independently and appropriately with toys, with no adult prompts, for 10 minutes). The nature of the behavior in the objective will indicate the appropriate measurement dimension.

Beware of Percentage Statements!

A common mistake is to overuse a percentage statement as the criterion for mastery. Percentages don't characterize mastery of many behaviors very well. Percentages work best when the objective involves a number of behaviors over a percentage of time, like naming 10 action words in response to adult questions in an hour of interactive play. For example, the objective could be written in this way: During a 15-minute dramatic play activity involving vehicles, action figures, and props, Max will use 10 different action words either in response to his partner's questions and comments or to narrate his own play, in 80% of play sessions, for five consecutive sessions.

As written above, Max will need to produce 10 different action words 4 days out of 5 in a row. However, for many important skills, like eye contact, coordinating gaze with language, and so on, a percentage is not a good criterion. Eye contact does not happen continuously and so specifying that Max will make eye contact 80% of the time in a 1-hour speech therapy session is not a good criterion statement. It would also require that one monitor eye contact over the whole session to measure success, which is very difficult to do. Eye contact happens at certain times in interactions; for example, when initiating a new exchange. Thus, the following mastery criterion better captures how eye contact is used in typical exchanges: "Max will make eye contact combined with speech or gesture during at least three of five requests."

Also avoid percentages in mastery criteria for spontaneous or independent behaviors in a sequence. If the target behavior involves cleaning up after a play activity, setting the criterion at 85% (i.e., Johnny will clean up after free play 85% of the time) requires that the child complete the entire clean-up in 85% of the opportunities measured. For small children, completely independent clean-up is not typically expected. For a child who is learning to clean up, it would be more helpful for teaching and for measuring progress to specify what we would expect from other children. For example: At the end of an activity, when the adult says, "Let's clean up," Johnny will participate by picking up four or more pieces and putting them in a container spontaneously or in response to adult modeling, for four or more play activities during an intervention hour, across four consecutive sessions.

Another way to gauge children's current skill repertoire involves their first response to the antecedent. First response can be considered a good indicator of the stability of a behavior. If the child performs a skill the first time the antecedent occurs in a session, for several days or sessions in a row, it is likely that the skill is a stable one for the child. Thus, one might use response on a first trial as a mastery criterion. For example: Becci will respond to a peer who approaches, looks, and says "Hi" to her by answering hi with eye contact in less than 1 second at the first opportunity, daily for 5 consecutive days.

In addition to specifying the quantity, accuracy, fluency, or latency of performance, the criterion should specify the level of independence the child is expected to demonstrate. For many skills, it is not appropriate to expect completely independent performance from young children. Typically developing preschoolers receive prompts, assistance, and repeated reminders in many situations. Thus, many objectives should contain a phrase that defines the level of adult support: playing with toys for 10 minutes with no more than two redirections; completing all the steps to hand washing without more than two motor or verbal prompts; responds at first request (that means no adult repetitions or coaching) to point to 10 or more different pictures of familiar objects in a book during book reading; responds without prompts to greetings from a familiar adult at preschool with eye contact and says "Hi" in 80% of opportunities over 3 days.

(*Note:* To help identify the level of support to specify, gauging the criteria in terms of typical behavior of peers ensures age-appropriate teaching. When in doubt, observe some typically developing children of the same age as the target child.)

The definition of mastery, however, is not complete without specification of generalized performance of the skill. This is the fourth and final element of the child's learning objectives.

Specification of the Criterion That Indicates Generalization

We want to be sure that a new skill becomes a stable part of a child's repertoire, rather than performance on a really great day or with one favorite person or in one setting only. Generalization usually involves performance of the skill in more than one natural environment, performance using several different objects or materials, and/or performance with multiple people. A measurable generalization criterion helps us know that what we are seeing represents a true picture of the child's current responding rate to the antecedent. For a behavior that doesn't occur very often in a single day, like returning people's greetings, you might want to see the behavior demonstrated in most opportunities over 3 or 4 consecutive days to be sure that it is mastered. For a complex behavior that occurs frequently, like washing hands, you would be more likely to get a representative sample of the child's behavior in a single day or 2 consecutive days. For example, setting a generalization criterion like the following would give you a good sample: "Performs 90% of the steps of hand washing without assistance or prompts in each opportunity over a 2-day period."

Finally, we know that behaviors are generalized when they occur across different settings, materials, and people. Unless the behavior or skill is itself specific to an environment, object, or person, each 12-week objective should include in the criterion statement that the behavior will occur in two or more environments, with two or more materials, and with two or more different people.

There are both strengths and weaknesses to requiring this. The strengths are that the interventionists and child will have to practice this skill in multiple environments and with multiple people in order to pass the objective, and this will lead to a much more stable and permanent set of behaviors. It will also require people in various environments to be working on the skill, which extends teaching across various people and across the child's life settings, another strength. The weakness is that it becomes more difficult to measure. You will need data or reliable reports from other settings. It will also take longer to get to mastery, since the objective will take more teaching to accomplish. However, the strengths will generally outweigh the weaknesses, and in so doing, you will prevent the frustrating situation that we see too often in which the child has a repertoire of skills that never occur outside the therapy room and are not used functionally.

WRITING FUNCTIONAL OBJECTIVES

It takes child and adult time to teach skills, and we want to be sure the time is well spent and that children are learning adaptive skills that will serve them in multiple environments. The antecedent statement can and should target functional, adaptive use of the behavior.

Let's use expressive vocabulary development as an example here. Children don't usually walk around naming objects in the room. We use language to request the things we want, give people what they ask for, protest, begin and end interactions, share our interests, experiences, feelings, and thoughts with others, and identify our own needs and ask for help with them. Children should learn to use their skills in adaptive and typical situations. Objectives that specify this help keep the teaching functional. Writing an objective that involves naming 25 pictures on flashcards in a therapy room is not a very functional use of early language. A more functional and expressive language objective would target naming pictures in several storybooks during book reading, or requesting several different preferred foods by name during a meal, or requesting their favorite play themes during thematic play hour, or asking for favorite toys from other children during free play. These much more functional objectives help ensure that the teaching and learning will serve the child well in real-life settings. They also help ensure that teaching will occur within real-life experiences and interactions at home, in preschool, and in community settings, and with parents, friends, and teachers.

How might one check the functionality of an objective? Imagine a typically developing child you know of the same age carrying out this objective. Is it something the child would typically do or be expected to do? Where, with whom, with what materials, and in response to what stimuli would you expect the behavior? If agemates carry it out in a similar way and in the specified settings, it is likely to be functional for a child with ASD as well.

With practice, writing objectives becomes faster and easier. It helps to write the objectives as soon as possible after you have administered the Curriculum Checklist. The target behaviors will be much clearer in your mind and the objectives will flow

TABLE 4.1. Guidelines for Writing Learning Objectives

Select the skills to be learned.
- Include the current P/F items
- Focus on completing the domain level that contains the most advanced consistent passes
- Look beyond the P/Fs to the first few Fs and gauge the child's learning rate
- When in doubt, be conservative

Select the antecedent.
- Use natural cues for the behavior (another behavior, environmental cues, internal cues, preceding behaviors)
- If appropriate, more than one antecedent can be specified for the behavior
- Beware of using setting events as antecedents

Specify the behavior—the target skill to be learned.
- It must be specific, observable, and measurable
- It can be more than one behavior

Specify the mastery criterion.
- Quantity
- Accuracy
- Fluency
- Latency of performance
- First response
- Level of independence
- Time duration

Specify the generalization criterion.
- Across different settings and/or
- With different objects or materials and/or
- With different people

more easily. Check each objective for the four elements: antecedent, behavior, criterion, and generalization. Table 4.1 summarizes the guidelines for writing objectives covered in this chapter. More detailed information about developing and writing educational objectives can be found in a variety of texts for educators. Cipani and Spooner (1994) is one such useful text.

ISAAC'S 12-WEEK LEARNING OBJECTIVES

Earlier in this chapter we described 26-month-old Isaac's evaluation and the ESDM assessment profile. The following lists the set of 12-week learning objectives written for Isaac. All of these are in Level 1 and cover six out of seven domains: expressive communication, receptive communication, social interaction, imitation, cognitive skills, and play skills. Because this was a brief intervention carried out completely by families, and because he had no motor delays, we did not write motor objectives. However, Isaac had a behavior plan for his tantrums and biting in addition to the objectives listed below. The initials of the Level 1 domains along with the Curriculum Checklist item numbers are noted in parentheses at the end of each objective. For the first three objectives, we have labeled each of their four elements.

Expressive Communication

1. [*Antecedent*:] During vocal games or in intentional vocalizations at home and in the clinic, [*Behavior*:] Isaac will spontaneously use two to three different vowel-consonant combinations and will vocalize five or more times [*Mastery criterion*:] in a 10-minute period [*Generalization*:] over three consecutive periods. (Expressive Communication [EC] item 12)

2. [*Antecedent*:] When desired activities or objects are offered to him, [*Behavior*:] Isaac will request them from his partner by using directed gestures, vocalizations, and/or eye contact [*Mastery criterion*:] in 90% of opportunities [*Generalization*:] across three consecutive 10-minute periods, across at least two environments and three or more people. (EC items 1, 2, 3, 10)

3. [*Antecedent*:] During social interactions at home and in the clinic when the adult offers desired materials, unwanted materials, and materials for which he needs help, [*Behavior*:] Isaac will communicate protest, negation, requests, and requests for help using gestures combined with gaze by pushing objects away (protest, negation), directed reaching for request, and handing objects to people (help), [*Mastery Criterion*:] three or more times in 45 minutes of play over 3 consecutive days [*Generalization*] across two or more people and settings. (EC items 5, 7, 8, 9)

Receptive Communication

4. When an adult calls Isaac by name from across the room and out of his line of sight, he will look to the adult with eye contact and orientation three times in a 20-minute period over three consecutive sessions, at home and in the clinic. (Receptive Communication [RC] items 3, 7)

5. When an adult points to a location, picture, or object more than three feet away, Isaac will follow the point and respond appropriately with the associated action, three or more opportunities in three consecutive 10-minute periods at home and in the clinic. (RC items 5, 8, 9)

6. In response to a direct adult verbal request with or without gesture, Isaac will perform five different instructions involving body actions: sit down, stand up, clean up, get the (object), give me (object) in 90% of opportunities across two different 1-hour sessions in the clinic and across two different play periods with parent or grandmother at home. (RC items 13, 14, 15)

Social Interaction

7. During song, book, or sensory social routines in the clinic and at home, when an adult offers a routine or stops a routine, Isaac will use eye contact and gesture consistently to request or continue five different routines (e.g., songs, physical games) with three or more different people. (Social Interaction [SI] items 2, 3, 4, 5, 6; RC items 10, 11; EC items 1, 9)

8. In multiple environments, when greeted by an adult in close proximity with a wave and hi or bye, Isaac will return the greeting by waving back in 90% of opportuni-

ties over 2 consecutive days, including two different people and settings. (SI items 8, 9; Imitation [IM] item 2)

Imitation

9. During object play at the clinic and home when the adult engages in various actions on objects, Isaac will spontaneously imitate in 80% or more of 10 or more actions, both familiar and novel, during three consecutive sessions. (IM items 1, 2; SI item 7)

10. During songs, finger plays, and sensory social routines at home, in speech therapy, and at the clinic, Isaac will spontaneously imitate five or more different body movements not involving objects within 1 second of the model, over three consecutive sessions (these can be approximations rather than perfect imitations). (IM items 2, 3; SI item 7)

11. When Isaac vocalizes using consonant–vowel–consonant–vowel (CVCV) combinations and an adult imitates his vocalizations, Isaac will repeat the CVCV vocalization in 80% of opportunities across three 10-minute periods, at home, in the clinic, and in speech therapy. (IM item 4; Level 2 IM item 1)

Cognitive Skills

12. During clean-up, blocks, and other appropriate activities at day care, home, and in the clinic, Isaac will follow an adult model and match, group, or sort a set of up to eight materials by identity 90% correctly, over three consecutive opportunities. (Cognitive [CG] item 1; IM item 1; RC items 10, 14; Play [PL] item 8)

Play Skills

13. During ball and beanbag-type activities, in response to partner verbal or gestural requests and initiations, Isaac will throw or roll objects back and forth with a partner for three to five rounds or more, over three consecutive opportunities, in two or more environments and with two or more people. (PL item 1; IM item 1; SI items 3, 5, 7; RC items 10, 14; GM items 7, 8)

14. During play activities using five or more realistic objects from well-established routines like mealtime, bath time, toothbrushing, or bedtime, Isaac will imitate and initiate five or more appropriate actions on self and partner in three consecutive sessions at home and in the clinic. (PL items 1, 4, 7; IM item 1)

15. In day care, in the clinic, and at home, during play with construction or art materials, Isaac will carry out five or more reciprocal acts during a 5-minute activity involving taking turns, co-construction, or imitating and being imitated in a shared activity, twice each session for three consecutive sessions (PL Items 1, 4; IM items 1, 12; SI items 3, 5, 7, 11)

Isaac and his family participated in our once weekly parent–toddler sessions for 12 weeks and then went on to a public preschool program. He progressed well in the parent–toddler clinic, acquiring very consistent single-word speech and some two-word combinations, with excellent behavioral progress and nice social, play, and imitation development. He is now 4 years old, with consistent, elaborated speech, excellent social skills with peers, and no significant behavior problems. He has a loving, playful relationship with his new baby brother. He does well in Head Start preschool and does not display the social problems that one expects to see in a child with ASD.

CONCLUSION

Well-written objectives define the content of the teaching and allow one to gauge teaching effectiveness. It takes time to write these well, and the time that is put into this is time well spent. Teaching will move along much more rapidly and carefully when the objectives lay out what the child is to learn and under what conditions the teaching should occur. The ESDM Curriculum Checklist provides a comprehensive set of targets for the teaching objectives, and the objectives are the cornerstone of teaching in the ESDM.

Share the objectives with everyone who spends time with the child. The more practice children receive, the more quickly they will learn. In an ideal situation, the objectives not only serve the intervention team, but also everyone else who interacts with the child. Parents can integrate them into their daily interactions with their child during typical life routines. Other interventionists as well—preschool teacher, speech therapist, OT, music therapist, Sunday school teacher, day-care provider—can help the child by incorporating relevant objectives into their own interactions. The more the ESDM interventionist can share what he or she is doing with others and help others incorporate teaching into their interactions, the more rapidly the child will progress.

Chapter 5

Formulating Daily Teaching Targets and Tracking Progress

In the last chapter, we described the ESDM approach for constructing the child's short-term learning objectives. These objectives define the child's curriculum over a 12-week period. This chapter focuses on turning each of those objectives into small teachable steps that build toward mastery of the full objective. The process involves carrying out a task analysis of each objective beginning with the child's current baseline level and ending with the fully mastered and generalized objective as written. These learning steps from the task analysis then guide daily teaching and target behaviors for daily data collection within the session. Session data allow close tracking of each child's progress.

MAPPING OUT LEARNING STEPS FOR EACH OBJECTIVE

The process for mapping out the steps for teaching each objective requires one to combine knowledge of developmental sequences in the various domains with the process of task analysis. Most early intervention professionals reading this will be familiar with task analyzing a skill. A task analysis of a motor skill such as putting on a shirt or stringing beads involves breaking it down into separate motor actions. Each of the actions is then taught in sequential order ("chaining"). Prompts are faded between the acts so that each action in the sequence serves as the antecedent for the next act. Once learned, the chain of behaviors occurs independently as a motor sequence that begins with the antecedent and ends at the completion of the entire chain. If you need to review the process of task analysis, read further in texts for special educators or behavior analysis (Cipani & Spooner, 1994; Cooper et al., 2006).

Basic task analysis can be done by watching someone perform the steps and describing each action. However, task analysis of an ESDM learning objective is a somewhat expanded process. When you task analyze a learning objective, you have to *imagine* or anticipate how that skill will develop over the teaching period, based on previous experiences with children and your own knowledge of development. These are *developmental* task analyses, and they incorporate knowledge from typical development of various abilities as well as learning theory. Carrying out a developmental task analysis of an objective lays out the steps of the child's learning; these steps might involve stepwise gains in independent performance, increasingly refined approximations of the modeled behavior, performance of a skill on an increasingly wide range of exemplars, or increasing generalization across people and environments, among other things. Let's use the skill of *initiating joint attention to share affect* as an example. Twenty-eight-month-old Joshua currently makes occasional eye contact to request objects and social interactions and to share interest. He has the following expressive communication objective that has been task analyzed into the learning steps below.

> **Expressive communication objective:** During social games with objects (e.g., bubbles, noisemakers), Joshua will make joint attention bids to share affect involving eye contact with his partner via alternating gaze and smiling three or more times in a 10-minute period, across three consecutive periods, for two or more partners and objects.

(Note that there is no specified social antecedent provided by the partner, because we are targeting a spontaneous and independent social behavior.) This objective was task analyzed into the following six steps:

Learning Steps

1. Makes eye contact occasionally to continue interaction
2. Makes eye contact repeatedly and consistently to continue interaction
3. Occasionally directs smile with eye contact to continue interaction
4. Consistently directs smile with eye contact to continue interaction
5. Alternates gaze and smile between partner and object three or more times during activity
6. Alternates gaze and smile with two or more partners, for two or three object games, three or more times during activity

The first step describes Joshua's current baseline skill, an item that he passed on the ESDM Curriculum Checklist. The final step represents the fully accomplished, generalized objective. Mapping out the learning steps means charting the stepwise progression of this skill from baseline to mastery. There is no set number of steps involved, though typically we write four to six steps. We want enough steps so that progress can be documented from week to week, assuming the skill is being taught consistently.

Beginning at the Ends

A favorite approach for task analyzing an objective in the Sacramento ESDM site is to work "from the ends to the middle." Begin with the child's current baseline performance. The first step describes the behavior the child exhibits in relation to the stimulus at the present moment in time. If the child only rarely emits the behavior, then the step will describe the act occurring rarely, or infrequently. If the child never demonstrates the action in relation to the stimulus unless fully prompted, then the baseline-level step will include that full prompt in the description. The first step has to be a behavior that the child currently performs, in some way, in the presence of the stimulus, and that is related to the target behavior. Joshua's current behavioral skill related to the objective is to make "occasional eye contact to request social interactions," and that is the first step in the task analysis.

Next, we write the last step, which is the fully mastered objective, at the criterion specified in the objective. This final step usually involves the generalized description in the objective, involving multiple materials, environs, and people. In Joshua's case the last step, 6, describes the generalization criterion of the objective. The step that precedes this last one often describes the ungeneralized skill performed at the numerical criterion level, as shown in the example for Joshua. This penultimate step may also specify the consistency of the performance (e.g., 85% of opportunities in three consecutive sessions), or the frequency of the behavior (e.g., two to three times in 15 minutes), or it may involve increasing consistency of the response to the antecedent (e.g., one out of three, two out of three, three out of three opportunities). However, it will reflect the quantitative criterion for mastery as specified in the objective.

The Middle Learning Steps

The nature of the middle steps depends on the skill involved. Most child objectives fall into one of four types: those that involve (1) developmental sequences, (2) behavior chains and behavior "bundles," (3) increasing behavioral frequencies and adding content, or (4) linking existing behaviors to new antecedents. We discuss each in turn.

Developmental Sequences

Some aspects of child learning follow a sequence seen in virtually all typically developing children. Young children with autism tend to follow many of these same sequences—even in their most challenged areas, like language and in symbolic play (Tager-Flusberg et al., 1990; Lifter, Sulzer-Azaroff, Anderson, Coyle, & Cowdery, 1993; McCleery, Tully, Slevc, & Schreibman, 2006). The interdisciplinary members of the team will often be excellent resources for these developmental steps as seen in typical development. S-LPs are experts in the steps of typical language development. Pediatric OTs are quite knowledgeable about the development of fine motor control. Early childhood special educators have expertise in many developmental areas, as do many developmental psychologists. Thus, we can turn to the team's disciplinary expertise for ideas.

A second source for developmental sequences is the ESDM Curriculum Checklist. It lays out these sequences, within and across levels. Other early childhood curricula are often developmentally sequenced, and those can also be aids.

Behavior Chains and Behavior "Bundles"

Many skills represent a chain of behaviors linked together, with each behavior serving as the stimulus for the next. When the objective involves a behavior chain, like a self-care skill, the learning steps involve mastery of the individual behaviors and their performance in a sequence or chain. In this type of skill, the middle steps of the analysis may follow the order in which you plan to teach the skill (e.g., removes shirt from head, from neck, from last arm, from both arms, from belly). Alternatively, the steps may represent the number of steps completed independently, which often works well for a chain in which the actions are not necessarily related (e.g., table setting: completes one step independently, completes two steps independently ... five steps independently). The following is an example of an objective and set of learning steps that involve backward chaining to teach the skill of removing an open jacket.

Personal independence objective: When Joshua's jacket is opened and he is told to take off his jacket while standing near his cubby and coat hook at preschool, he will remove it and put it on the hook, 90% of opportunities.

Learning Steps

1. Independently hangs jacket on hook
2. Removes jacket from second wrist and hangs on hook
3. Independently removes jacket from second arm and hangs on hook
4. Removes jacket from second shoulder and hangs on hook
5. Removes jacket from first wrist and hangs on hook
6. Removes jacket from first elbow and hangs on hook
7. Removes jacket from first shoulder and hangs on hook
8. Removes unfastened jacket and hangs on hook following instruction 90% of opportunities
9. Removes unfastened jacket and hangs on hook in more than one setting 90% of opportunities

The alternative way of writing this would look like this

Learning Steps

1. Completes one to two steps with partial prompts only
2. Completes one to two steps independently
3. Completes three to four steps with partial physical prompts
4. Completes three to four steps independently
5. Completes five to six steps with partial prompts
6. Completes five to six steps independently
7. Completes entire task with no more than one to two partial prompts
8. Completes task independently 90% of opportunities, one setting
9. Completes task independently 90% of opportunities, two or more settings

A related skill involves performance of multiple behaviors that typically co-occur in a given situation—"behavior bundles." In typical development, these bundles are easily seen in early communicative behavior when eye contact, gesture, and vocalizations or speech are generally integrated into a single communicative act. Picture a toddler who wants the juice from the pitcher that is out of reach. He or she will point or reach with his or her hand to the pitcher while looking back at you and making little whining noises that convey his or her desire very clearly! Several communicative behaviors are *bundled* into a package. The following is an example of a developmental task analysis for bundled behaviors.

Twenty-eight-month-old Joshua currently gestures by reaching for objects he desires, and only occasionally looks or vocalizes. He does not currently integrate gesturing, looking to adults and vocalizing.

Expressive communication objective: When desired activities or objects are offered to him, Joshua will request them from several partners by combining directed gestures, vocalizations, and eye contact in 80% of requests made in a 10-minute period across three consecutive periods.

Learning Steps

1. Directs reach or point gesture consistently
2. Occasionally adds vocalization to gesture
3. Consistently combines vocalization with gesture to request
4. Occasionally combines gaze with voice or gesture to request
5. Consistently combines gaze with vocalization or gesture to request
6. Combines all three inconsistently
7. Combines all three 80% of requests
8. Combines all three 80% of requests, with two or more partners

(*Note:* "Directs" means that the gaze and the vocalization are directed to the adult, but the gesture is directed to the desired object.)

Increasing Behavior Frequencies and Adding Content

Objectives of this sort involve increasing the frequency of an existing behavior or elaborating the child's knowledge base and/or the size of his or her behavioral repertoire involving a certain skill (e.g., names nine colors, identifies 10 body parts, draws five geometric shapes). Both the language and cognitive domains of the Curriculum Checklist contain many items like this. For these objectives, the child already has the underlying behavior needed—he or she names objects, gives items on request, and can copy a block design or a simple line drawing. What he or she lacks is the content or the number of exemplars.

When writing out the learning steps for objectives like these, it is sometimes efficient to break down the steps quantitatively. For example, if the full criterion is to name eight or more colors, the steps might be broken down into: names one to two, three to four, five to six, and seven to eight colors. This is preferable to naming each new color addition in a different step (e.g., red, blue, green, yellow, white, black, brown, purple). Naming each color addition can lead to directive teaching rather than the more flexible teaching style that we espouse in the ESDM. However, there is no right or wrong way; the decision should be based on what will help the child most easily and quickly. Somewhere the content of teaching has to be specified, either in the objective, in the learning steps, or on a data sheet or program sheet. Choose the approach that will work best for your teaching.

For an example of learning steps focused on increasing frequency of a specific behavior, we turn again to 28-month-old Joshua. We want to increase his vocalizations. His currently vocalizes using vowels only, and these occur every 10 minutes or less.

> **Expressive communication objective:** During sensory social routines, Joshua will spontaneously vocalize five or more times using vowels and several consonants in a 10-minute period across three consecutive sessions, with multiple partners and in multiple settings.
>
> *Learning Steps*
>
> 1. Produces vowel vocalization one time every 10 minutes
> 2. Produces vowel vocalization two to three times every 10 minutes
> 3. Two to three vocalizations with one to two consonants every 10 minutes
> 4. Two to three vocalizations with three or more consonants every 10 minutes
> 5. Five vocalizations with three or more consonants every 10 minutes
> 6. Five vocalizations with three or more consonants every 10 minutes, with two or more partners and settings

Linking Existing Behaviors to New Antecedents

In this teaching situation, the target behavior is already in the child's repertoire—he or she sits, reaches, looks, smiles, laughs, vocalizes, grasps and handles objects, and so on. However, the behavior does not consistently occur in the presence of the specified antecedent (the discriminative stimulus, or Sd). (Many of the Level 1 skills fall into this category.) The learning steps will involve eliciting the existing behavior through prompting in response to the desired antecedent stimulus, and then fading prompts as the behavior comes under stimulus control. The teaching techniques will largely involve prompting and fading. However, the child's learning steps, or benchmarks, will focus on independence. We tend not to write steps that involve prompt levels because we want prompts faded as soon as possible. When teaching, we need to stay at the same step until that step is mastered and demonstrated on several consecutive days. Thus, if prompts are used as steps, we cannot fade prompts as fast as possible, given the rule about staying on a step until mastery is achieved. By focusing on the degree of independence achieved, we can withdraw prompts as fast as possible.

In the following example, Joshua is capable of picking up a fork or spoon, loading it with food, and putting it into his mouth, but he seldom does this; instead he either eats with his hands or is fed.

> **Self-care objective:** During mealtimes, Joshua will use utensils to feed himself independently for most of his meal, across three consecutive meals, both at day care and at home. (Note that the criterion was not set at 100%, since it is not unusual for 28 month olds to put their hands in their food occasionally or to be given a bite or two by a parent.)
>
> *Learning Steps*
>
> 1. Uses both spoon and/or fork (utensils) with assistance for five to ten bites
> 2. Uses utensils spontaneously independently for five to ten bites

3. Spontaneously independently uses utensils 25% of meal
4. Spontaneously independently uses utensils 50% of meal
5. Spontaneously independently uses utensils 75% of meal
6. Spontaneously independently uses utensils 90% of meal, with two or more people or settings

In the above objective and plan, the specific utensil is not named because this child uses both spoon or fork without difficulty, though seldom. For a child who is struggling to manage both a spoon and a fork, the objective might target one or the other rather than both.

Building a Completely New Skill

Teaching a brand new skill—kicking a ball, pointing to request, imitating motions in songs—involves a variety of teaching strategies including prompting, fading, shaping, and chaining. The learning steps you write will likely involve increasing accuracy of the behavior and decreasing prompts and other supports.

Twenty-eight-month-old Joshua has the following play objective involving the spontaneous production of functional play actions with familiar objects. He currently has no spontaneous functional play, and he only occasionally imitates familiar actions with objects. We build up functional play from imitation skills, which are covered in a separate objective with its own learning steps.

Play objective: During pretend play activities involving mealtime, bath time, or bedtime props, Joshua will carry out three or more functional play acts on self, partner, or doll spontaneously using three or more of the props appropriately (tissues, necklace, sunglasses, hairbrush, hat, cup, spoon, bowl, etc.) in three consecutive sessions.

Learning Steps

1. Imitates functional play act on one object inconsistently
2. Imitates one to two play acts on one object consistently
3. Imitates one to two functional play acts on two to three objects consistently
4. Initiates one to two functional play acts on one object spontaneously
5. Initiates one to two functional play acts on two objects
6. Initiates one to two functional play acts on three to four objects

(*Hint:* If you feel very unsure of what the steps should be for a particular skill, don't struggle too hard. Do the best you can and begin to teach it. If the steps aren't right, you will learn this as you start to teach. Then, revise the steps as needed based on your teaching experience. It's the nature of teaching that we learn a great deal about the learner's learning processes as we try to teach.)

Following the above steps for breaking down each objective into small teaching targets provides the lead therapist or team leader with a very specific plan that will cover all of the teaching that needs to occur in the next 12 weeks to accomplish the objectives. There is a full set of examples at the end of this chapter to illustrate the process further.

TRACKING PROGRESS

We can track the child's progress on the learning steps by adding two columns to the list of steps: date started and date passed, as shown in Figure 5.1. This figure lists one of the learning objectives with its learning steps for Isaac, the child discussed in Chapter 4. A complete list of Isaac's learning objectives and their respecting learning steps can be found in Appendix 5.1 at the end of this chapter. We have found it helpful in the Sacramento ESDM site to use this date-started/date-passed format as a summary sheet to track child progress through the steps. "Date started" refers to the date of the first session in which we begin to teach that step of a skill. "Date passed" refers to the date at which the child first performed the skill specified at that step at the criterion specified in the objective. Using these columns provides a simple chronological record of learning progress. For more detailed session-by-session tracking of child progress, the Daily Data Sheet is used.

The Daily Data Sheet

The Daily Data Sheet (see Figure 5.2) is used in the intervention session to conduct interval recordings of child performance and also to cue the interventionist as to the skills and steps to be taught to an individual child. The Daily Data Sheet is essentially a telegraphically written version of the objectives with their learning steps. It can usually fit onto two sides of a single sheet of paper, which makes it easy to use and quick to scan. It can be brought into the session on a clipboard with a pen.

Figure 5.2 shows a Daily Data Sheet set-up for teaching Brittany on March 8, 2007. Each objective appears in a telegraphic form of three to five words. Each objective is followed by a telegraphic description of each of the learning steps, with columns in which to record data (P1, P2, etc.). The number of columns reflects the number of coding periods (P) planned for a given session. In Brittany's case, data will be collected every 15 minutes for an hour session. The data sheet ties together the 12-week objectives, the teaching task

EXPRESSIVE COMMUNICATION

1. During vocal games or intentional vocalizations at home and in the clinic, Isaac will spontaneously use two to three different vowel–consonant (VC) combinations and will vocalize five or more times in a 10-minute period over three consecutive periods.

Date Started	Date Passed	Steps
		1. Produces several Vs in spontaneous vocalizations in 30 minutes.
		2. Produces several Cs in spontaneous vocalizations in 30 minutes.
		3. Produces two to three different VC combinations in 30 minutes.
		4. Produces two to three different VC combinations in 15 minutes.
		5. Produces four to five VC combinations in 10 minutes.

FIGURE 5.1. Example of data-started/date-passed format for learning steps.

Daily Data Sheet for: Brittany Date: 3/8/07 Provider: ____________

Behavior Coding

15 min	30 min	45 min	1 hr	FINAL CODE

1	Severe behavior (e.g., aggression, self-injurious behavior, frequent and intense tantrums)
2	Mild behavior (e.g., noncompliance, some tantrums but able to participate in activity)
3	Some behavior (e.g., fussy, whiny,, some noncompliance but able to participate in most of activity)
4	No problem behavior but difficulty staying on task
5	Compliant, on task, working at ability level
6	Above average performance for that child; pleasant, excited about activity

1. Uses five consonants intentionally (main gist of objective)

P1	P2	P3	P4	Steps
				1. Uses one to two consonants, self-directed
				2. Uses one to two consonants responsively
				3. Uses one to two consonants in 10-minute period
				4. Uses three to four consonants responsively
				5. Uses three consonants in 10-minute period
				6. Uses five consonants responsively

2. Uses gaze for spontaneous requests

P1	P2	P3	P4	Steps
				1. Reaches without eye contact
				2. Uses gaze three times fully prompted in 20 minutes
				3. Uses gaze to request, partially prompted
				4. Uses gaze to request after vocal prompt
				5. Uses gaze to request spontaneously, object out of reach
				6. Uses gaze to request spontaneously, three times in one activity

3. Communicates intentionally with voice

P1	P2	P3	P4	Steps
				1. Vocalizations are undirected and unintentional
				2. Intentional vocalization occurs occasionally
				3. Intentional vocalization occurs in several activities
				4. Intentional vocalization occurs in majority of activities
				5. Intentional vocalization occurs in each activity

4. Uses three or more conventional gestures

P1	P2	P3	P4	Steps
				1. Reaches to grasp object
				2. Uses two different gestures
				3. Uses one gesture combined with gaze
				4. Uses three different gestures
				5. Uses two different gestures combined with gaze
				6. Uses three different common gestures with gaze in 20 minutes

5. Consistently looks to human sounds

P1	P2	P3	P4	Steps
				1. Looks to object noises inconsistently
				2. Looks to human sounds occasionally, within 3 feet
				3. Looks to human sounds frequently, within 3 feet
				4. Looks to human sounds, occasionally, from within 10 feet
				5. Looks to human sounds, frequently, within 10 feet
				6. Consistently looks to human sounds, once per minute

6. Consistently looks to name

P1	P2	P3	P4	Steps
				1. Looks to name rarely
				2. Looks to name occasionally, within 3 feet
				3. Looks to name frequently, within 3 feet
				4. Looks to name occasionally, from within 10 feet
				5. Looks to name frequently, within 10 feet
				6. Consistently looks to name, once per minute

7. Responds to several instructions, verbal plus gesture

P1	P2	P3	P4	Steps
				1. Responds rarely to instruction
				2. Responds to one instruction, partial prompt
				3. Responds to two to three instructions, partial prompt
				4. Responds to one instruction, 80% unprompted
				5. Responds to three to four instructions, partial prompt
				6. Responds to two to three instructions, 80% unprompted

8. Follows proximal point

P1	P2	P3	P4	Steps
				1. Follows proximal point rarely
				2. Follows proximal point once per 30 minutes
				3. Follows proximal point two times per 30 minutes
				4. Follows proximal point three times per 30 minutes
				5. Follows distal 4-inch point one to two times per 30 minutes
				6. Follows distal 4-inch point three times per 30 minutes

9. Responds to greetings with gaze plus gesture or voice

P1	P2	P3	P4	Steps
				1. Responds to greeting with gaze occasionally
				2. Responds with gaze, gesture, or voice 50% of opportunities
				3. Responds with gaze, gesture, or voice 70% of opportunities
				4. Responds with gaze plus gesture or voice occasionally
				5. Responds with gaze plus gesture or voice 50% of opportunities
				6. Responds to greeting with gaze plus other 70% of opportunities

10. Responds to social and object routines with gaze plus gesture or voice

P1	P2	P3	P4	Steps
				1. Responds with gaze to social routines only
				2. Responds with gaze to social and object routines
				3. Responds with gaze plus gesture or voice to either social or object routines
				4. Responds with gaze plus gesture or voice for one to two social and object routines
				5. Responds with gaze plus gesture or voice for three social and object routines
				6. Responds with gaze plus gesture or voice for 10 routines

11. Imitates 10 different familiar actions on objects

P1	P2	P3	P4	Steps
				1. Imitates one to two familiar actions
				2. Imitates three to four familiar actions
				3. Imitates five to six familiar actions
				4. Imitates seven to eight familiar actions
				5. Imitates nine to ten familiar actions

12. Imitates three different body actions in social routines

P1	P2	P3	P4	Steps
				1. Watches body actions on sensory social routines
				2. Imitates one body action, partial prompt
				3. Imitates one body action, no prompts
				4. Imitates two body actions, partial prompts
				5. Imitates two body actions, no prompts
				6. Imitates three body actions, partial prompts

(cont.)

FIGURE 5.2. Example of Daily Data Sheet for Brittany.

13. Imitates three to five different sound patterns

P1	P2	P3	P4	Steps
				1. Imitates vocal contours
				2. Imitates one to two open vowels
				3. Imitates one familiar consonant
				4. Imitates two consonants
				5. Imitates one to two animal sounds
				6. Imitates three to five different sounds

14. Imitates three different facial movements

P1	P2	P3	P4	Steps
				1. Watches self wiggle tongue in mirror
				2. Imitates partner imitating his or her tongue wiggle
				3. Imitates partner's tongue wiggle
				4. Occasionally imitates second facial action
				5. Occasionally imitates third facial action
				6. Imitates three different facial movements in 30 minutes

15. Uses several props appropriately

P1	P2	P3	P4	Steps
				1. Uses one prop infrequently
				2. Uses one prop consistently, partial prompts
				3. Uses two to three props, partial prompts
				4. Uses two to three props, independently
				5. Uses four or more props on self and other, partial prompts
				6. Uses four or more props on self and other, unprompted

16. Repeats action to complete toy

P1	P2	P3	P4	Steps
				1. Completes two pieces independently, one to two toys
				2. Completes two pieces independently, three to four toys
				3. Completes three to four pieces independently, one to two toys
				4. Completes three to four pieces independently, three to four toys
				5. Completes five to six pieces independently, three to four toys
				6. Completes five to six pieces independently, five to six toys

17. Combines play actions in a sequence

P1	P2	P3	P4	Steps
				1. Uses one play action on objects
				2. Uses two play actions on several objects
				3. Uses two play actions routines
				4. Combines three or more play actions occasionally
				5. Combines three or more play actions consistently on one to two toys
				6. Combines three or more play actions on three to five different toys

18. Following model, matches objects

P1	P2	P3	P4	Steps
				1. Matches two identical objects, full physical prompts
				2. Matches two objects, partial prompts
				3. Matches one set of identical objects, independently
				4. Sorts two sets of identical objects, some errors
				5. Sorts three to five sets of identical objects, few errors

FIGURE 5.2 *(cont.)*

analysis, and the child's individual performance. It also provides a way of tracking what was taught during each intervention session, and how the child performed.

When to Take Data

ESDM therapy requires too much ongoing interaction with the child to allow for trial-by-trial recording. Instead, the ESDM uses a time interval recording system. Therapists record data every 15 minutes during a session, resulting in four recordings over a 1-hour session. This requires that therapists keep track of time by using a watch, timer, or a very visible clock in the therapy room. As each 15-minute interval comes to a close, the therapist needs to be sure that the child has attractive toys that he or she can play with alone for a couple of minutes. If the therapist is in the middle of a joint activity with objects, the therapist finds a natural point in the play to stop taking turns, pick up the clipboard, and record data. If the therapist is in the midst of a sensory social routine, then at its ending, the therapist gives the child a toy with which to occupy him- or herself for a few minutes—a puzzle, some cars or blocks, and so on—and picks up the clipboard to record. Data recording takes only a couple of minutes.

How to Take Data

It helps to prepare the Daily Data Sheet before the session by highlighting the current acquisition step for each objective in some bright color. This allows the therapist to see very quickly what is to be taught and what behavior data should be recorded. The therapist will record data on the highlighted step (the acquisition step) and the step just before it (the maintenance step) for each objective. The current acquisition steps for each of Brittany's objectives can be readily seen highlighted in gray on Figure 5.2. Taking data involves recording child performance on at least two specific learning steps for each objective addressed during the past 15 minutes. One is the acquisition step that is the current teaching target; the second is the preceding step, the child's most recent mastery, or maintenance step. You may also take data on other steps, but it is not necessary. The therapist reviews every objective on the data sheet and marks the level of performance for the acquisition and maintenance steps as follows. If the child performed the step consistently when presented with the opportunity during the past 15 minutes, the therapist marks "+" or "P." If he or she tried to elicit the response and the child did not perform it or performed it very inconsistently, he or she will mark "–" or "F." If the behavior is a high-frequency behavior and the child performed the skill inconsistently, use "±" or "P/F." If the behavior was only probed once, score that performance as "+" or "–." If behaviors for more advanced steps have been observed, these are also recorded. If the maintenance level skill has been failed, then the therapist records behaviors observed from steps that preceded the current maintenance step. (Note that not all objectives will have data from a specific coding period. It's hard to teach 20 objectives in a 15-minute time period!) If an objective has not been addressed in a 15-minute period, the therapist will just leave the space blank or code it "N/O" (no opportunity) or "N/A" (not addressed). As the session progresses, the therapist should be sure to address and code performance on all the current objectives.

Sometimes an objective relies on the mastery of a previous one that provides foundation skills. For example, Isaac's play objectives (mentioned earlier and in Appendix

5.1), cannot be mastered until he has learned object imitation skills, Objective 9. The steps for Objective 13, functional play, also involve object imitation. The therapist can easily design activities that will allow him or her to target both skills and thus can record data on both the imitation skill and the functional play skill from the same activity. It is not until the last steps of functional play that it becomes somewhat differentiated from object imitation. At the beginning of a new 12-week teaching period, when there are many new objectives, one often will not begin to teach all objectives at once, but rather start a few, and then add additional ones. These are choices that therapists make in order to meet the individual child's learning needs and styles.

Rating Child Behavior

The final portion of the Daily Data Sheet contains a section labeled "Behavior Coding." It allows you to quantify the child's behavior for each 15-minute period as well as for the session as a whole. A numeric score of 1 to 6 is used to characterize the child's behavior. A section for recording additional information may also be provided at the end of the sheet.

Using the Data to Inform Your Activities during the Session

The therapy session should provide for a probe of each maintenance step and multiple opportunities to teach each acquisition step. Reviewing the Daily Data Sheet and the objectives every 15 minutes helps the therapist see what has and has not yet been done. Unscored objectives indicate what objectives have not yet been targeted in the session. It also allows for adjustments in the session given the child's performance. If a child fails a maintenance step, it needs to be probed again during the current session. If any maintenance steps are performed inconsistently, they should be carefully probed at the next session as well. If the child continues to be inconsistent on these steps in the next session, these skills should be reclassified as acquisition skills and retaught. Finally, notice acquisition steps that were failed. If the child did not receive five to 10 opportunities to practice them, add additional opportunities to the current session. As the therapist reviews the data sheet each 15 minutes, he or she should make notes to help remember what objectives still need to be addressed in the current hour.

Data at the End of the Session

By the end of the session, the therapist should have data on child performance of the maintenance and acquisition step of every objective taught in the session. If not, be sure that the objectives that were not covered in this session are covered first in the next session. Write them into a plan for the next session or circle them on the next data sheet to be sure that they are covered first next time. Once the whole Daily Data Sheet has been completed for a single treatment session, it is time to summarize the performance onto the Data Summary Sheet. This sheet contains data on one objective over multiple sessions. It allows one to examine the data on acquisition and decide when to move to the next acquisition step.

Figure 5.3 shows the Data Summary Sheet for one of 30-month-old Daniel's expressive language learning objectives over four sessions. Each column represents one therapy session. The form can be adapted to contain columns for all the sessions over the 12-week period. At the top of each column is a row labeled Acquisition Step #, the acquisition step

Expressive Language
Child: Daniel
Asks "What's that?" (three or more times)

Acquisition steps	Date started	Date mastered
1. "What's that" once		
2. Twice + gesture		
3. Three times + gesture		

Objective: When an adult shows Daniel a novel attractive object, he will request information by asking "What's that?" and gesturing toward the object at least three times per session spontaneously for four of five consecutive sessions across two or more settings and people.

Materials/activity ideas:
Opaque bag with cookies inside, gift box with toy inside, activate a toy under a small blanket, activate a noisemaker out of sight

Acquisition Step #	3	3	3	3					
Notes	Attempted seven times, refused to imitate prompt four times	Attempted six times, performed after minimal verbal prompt four times	Attempted three times, refused to imitate after prompt all three times	Seven trials, four at P3, three at P2					
Goal Code	R	P3	R	P3					
Date	2/17	2/18	2/22	2/24					
Initials	SR	MR	mom	SR					

Acquisition Step #									
Notes									
Goal Code									
Date									
Initials									

Summary Performance Codes: Reflect the majority of the codes for this objective scored during this session for five or more trials.
R = refused P1 = fully prompted P2 = partially prompted P3 = minimally prompted A = acquired: performed consistently (80% of opportunities)

FIGURE 5.3. Example of Data Summary Sheet for Daniel.

for that day. The next row provides a place for notes. The third row involves the rating of the child's performance according to the Daily Data Sheet using the goal codes at the bottom of the page for the acquisition step. There are five codes: Refused (R), Acquired (A; correctly performed on 80% of trials), P1 (fully prompted), P2 (partially prompted), and P3 (minimally prompted). Refused means that for most opportunities that day, the child would not perform the acquisition step even when the therapist attempted to prompt the child. Acquired means the child performed the acquisition step as written consistently, either 80% of times it was elicited, or at the first trial (for a low-frequency behavior, like saying goodbye at the end of the session). There are three prompt levels coded P1, P2, and P3. These indicate what level of prompt was needed to achieve the acquisition step. At the end of a specific teaching session, the therapist rates the child's overall performance on each objective for that session according to the goal code that reflects the majority of coded responses. If there is no majority code because the child performed at two different levels an equal number of times, then use both codes: P2/P3. The Data Summary Sheet provides a rapid visual summary of child progress on a particular objective over sessions, and it allows the therapist to quickly spot objectives that are not progressing well.

The general rule for deciding when an acquisition step is acquired and needs to become a maintenance step, is when three consecutive sessions receive an A code. Once this happens, the next learning step becomes the acquisition step, and the Daily Data Sheet for the next session is highlighted accordingly.

SUMMARY

The ESDM takes a very structured and practical approach to building a daily teaching plan from the child's quarterly objectives. Through a developmental task analysis, learning steps are delineated for each objective and these steps are then used to construct a Daily Data Sheet. The Daily Data Sheet guides the therapist on what to teach and serves as a data-gathering device on how the child responds to the teaching. The therapist's teaching efforts and data-recording focus on (1) the "acquisition step" of each objective, and (2) the "maintenance step" the child has already mastered. The data are summarized to allow for easy examination of progress so that the team leader knows when progress is not optimal and the teaching plan needs adjusting. If the child is not progressing quickly, the teaching approaches need to be adapted; the process for this is discussed in the next chapter.

The ESDM approach to developing a child's teaching plan allows for maximum individualization, beginning with the use of the ESDM Curriculum Checklist and parent input to create objectives that target an individual learning profile. The profile uses a child's preferred materials and activities to teach the objectives, and a systematic plan to vary the teaching approach to improve progress when the initial teaching approach is not resulting in sufficient progress. The ESDM as a whole allows us to teach to individual learning styles, developmental strengths and needs, and personal preferences, as well as family values and priorities. It is not a one-size-fits-all approach, but rather an approach that is deeply individualized both for children and for families. This chapter and Chapter 4 have focused on setting treatment objectives for the child and tracking the child's progress on those objectives. In the next chapters, we describe the actual teaching strategies to be used, beginning with joint activity routines

Appendix 5.1

Learning Objectives and Learning Steps for Isaac

EXPRESSIVE COMMUNICATION

1. During vocal games or intentional vocalizations at home and in the clinic, Isaac will spontaneously use two to three different vowel–consonant combinations and will vocalize five or more times in a 10-minute period over three consecutive periods.

Date Started	Date Passed	Steps
		1. Produces several Vs in spontaneous vocalizations in 30 minutes.
		2. Produces several Cs in spontaneous vocalizations in 30 minutes.
		3. Produces two to three different CV combinations in 30 minutes.
		4. Produces two to three different CV combinations in 15 minutes
		5. Produces five or more CV combinations in 10 minutes.

2. When desired activities or objects are offered to him, Isaac will request them from his partner by using directed gestures, vocalizations, and/or eye contact in 90% of opportunities across three consecutive 10-minute periods, across at least two environments and three or more people.

Date Started	Date Passed	Steps
		1. Uses gestures to request.
		2. Uses eye contact to request.
		3. Produces vocalizations for intentional request.
		4. Combines two (eye contact, gestures, vocalizations).
		5. Combines eye contact, gestures, and vocalizations.

3. During social interactions at home and in the clinic, when the adult offers desired materials, unwanted materials, and materials for which he needs help, Isaac will communicate protest,

negation, requests, and requests for help using gestures combined with gaze: by pushing objects away (protest, negation), directed reaching for request, and handing objects to people (help) three or more times in 45 minutes of play over three consecutive days.

Date Started	Date Passed	Steps
		1. Gives for help to open hand.
		2. Pushes away to protest, negate.
		3. Gives for help, no open hand.
		4. Pushes away to protest, no fuss.
		5. Gives for help plus gaze, no open hand.

RECEPTIVE COMMUNICATION

4. When an adult calls Isaac by name from across the room and out of his line of sight, he will look to the adult with eye contact and orientation three times in a 20-minute period over three consecutive sessions, at home and in the clinic.

Date Started	Date Passed	Steps
		1. Looks with eye contact to name—no distractions—partner close.
		2. Turns and looks to name—no distractions.
		3. Looks to name while playing.
		4. Turns and looks to name while playing.
		5. Turns and looks to name while playing from 5 feet.
		6. Turns and looks to name while playing from across room.

5. When an adult points to a location, picture, or object more than 3 feet away, Isaac will follow the point and respond appropriately with the associated action, three or more opportunities in three consecutive 10-minute periods at home and in the clinic.

Date Started	Date Passed	Steps
		1. Follows proximal point (less than 3 feet) to indicate object.
		2. Follows proximal point to indicate picture.
		3. Follows distal point (more than 3 feet) to indicate object.
		4. Follows distal point to indicate location.

6. In response to direct adult verbal requests with natural gestures, Isaac will perform five different instructions involving body actions: sit down, stand up, clean up, get the (object), and give me (object) in 90% of opportunities across two different 1-hour sessions in the clinic and across two different play periods with parent or grandparent at home.

Date Started	Date Passed	Steps
		1. Follows one to two instructions: full physical prompt.
		2. Follows one to two instructions: partial physical prompt.
		3. Follows three to four instructions: partial physical prompt.
		4. Follows one to two instructions: only gestural prompt.
		5. Follows three to four instructions: gestural prompt only.
		6. Follows five to six instructions: gestural prompts only.

SOCIAL INTERACTION

7. During song, book, or sensory social routines in the clinic and at home, when an adult offers a routine or stops a routine, Isaac will use eye contact and gesture consistently to request or continue five different routines (e.g., songs, bubbles, physical games) with three or more different people.

Date Started	Date Passed	Steps
		1. Eye contact to request/continue.
		2. Gesture to request/continue.
		3. Combines eye contact and gesture to request one to two times in 15 minutes.
		4. Combines gaze and gesture three to four times in 15 minutes.
		5. Combines gaze and gesture consistently to request.

8. In multiple environments, when greeted by an adult in close proximity with a wave and "hi" or "bye," Isaac will return the greeting by waving back with gaze, in 90% of opportunities over two consecutive days, including two different people and settings.

Date Started	Date Passed	Steps
		1. Eye contact when adult waves and greets.
		2. Imitates wave when greeted, partial prompt.

		3. Imitates wave when greeted, close proximity.
		4. Imitates wave with gaze when greeted, close proximity.
		5. Waves back with gaze from 5–8 feet, spontaneous.

IMITATION

9. During object play at the clinic and home, when the adult engages in various actions on objects, Isaac will spontaneously imitate 80% or more of 10 or more actions, both familiar and novel, during three consecutive sessions.

Date Started	Date Passed	Steps
		1. Imitates one to two actions, partial prompt.
		2. Imitates one to two actions, spontaneous.
		3. Imitates three to four actions, spontaneous.
		4. Imitates five to six actions, spontaneous.
		5. Imitates seven to eight actions, spontaneous.
		6. Imitates 9–10 actions, spontaneous.

10. During songs, finger plays, and sensory social routines at home, in speech therapy, and in the clinic, Isaac will spontaneously imitate five or more different body movements not involving objects within 1 second of the model, over three consecutive sessions (these can be approximations rather than perfect imitations).

Date Started	Date Passed	Steps
		1. Imitates one movement, partial prompt
		2. Imitates one movement, spontaneous.
		3. Imitates two movements, spontaneous.
		4. Imitates three movements, spontaneous.
		5. Imitates four movements, spontaneous.
		6. Imitates five movements, spontaneous.

11. When Isaac vocalizes using CVCV combinations and an adult imitates his vocalizations, Isaac will repeat the CVCV vocalization, in 80% of opportunities across three 10-minute periods at home, in the clinic, and in speech therapy.

Date Started	Date Passed	Steps
		1. Repeats V occasionally.
		2. Repeats V consistently.
		3. Repeats C occasionally.
		4. Repeats C consistently.
		5. Repeats CVCV occasionally.
		6. Repeats CVCV consistently.

COGNITIVE SKILLS

12. During clean up, blocks, and other appropriate activities at day care, home, and the clinic, Isaac will follow an adult model and match, group, or sort a set of up to eight materials by identifying 90% correctly, over three consecutive opportunities.

Date Started	Date Passed	Steps
		1. Match/sort one to two identical objects after model.
		2. Match/sort three to four identical objects after model.
		3. Match/sort five to six identical objects after model.
		4. Match/sort seven to eight identical objects after model.

PLAY SKILLS

13. During ball and beanbag-type activities, in response to partner verbal and gestural requests and initiations, Isaac will throw or roll objects back and forth with a partner for three to five rounds or more across three consecutive opportunities, in two or more environments and with two or more people.

Date Started	Date Passed	Steps
		1. Responds with one turn.
		2. Maintains two rounds.
		3. Maintains three rounds.
		4. Maintains four rounds.
		5. Maintains five rounds.

14. During play activities using five or more realistic objects from well-established routines like mealtime, bath time, toothbrushing, or bedtime, Isaac will imitate and initiate five or more appropriate actions on self and partner in three consecutive sessions at home and in the clinic.

Date Started	Date Passed	Steps
		1. Imitates one to two actions, spontaneous to self or partner.
		2. Imitates three to four actions, spontaneous to self or partner.
		3. Imitates five actions, spontaneous to self or partner.
		4. Initiates one to two actions, to self or partner.
		5. Initiates three to four actions, to self or partner.
		6. Initiates five actions, to self and to partner.

15. In day care, the clinic, and at home, during play with construction or art materials, Isaac will carry out five or more reciprocal acts during a 5-minute activity involving taking turns, co-construction, or imitating and being imitated in a shared activity, twice each session for three consecutive sessions.

Date Started	Date Passed	Steps
		1. One to two reciprocal acts, one activity.
		2. Three to four reciprocal acts, one activity.
		3. Five or more reciprocal acts, one activity.
		4. Five or more reciprocal acts, two activities

Chapter 6

Developing Plans and Frames for Teaching

Two-year-old Dominique and her father, James, are playing on the floor with toys. Parent and child have a bag of blocks in front of them. They are building a tower with the blocks, crashing them down by running a toy truck into the tower, and then building the tower again. James and Dominique each add blocks to the structure, and James cues her to crash them by saying, "Where's the truck? Can you crash it?" while demonstrating by rolling the truck toward the blocks. Then, James rolls the truck to her, counts "1, 2, 3," and Dominique crashes down the tower. Both say, "Crash!" in a big voice, sharing looks, smiles, and laughter. Dominique begins to build the tower again and the game repeats. As the play goes on, James elaborates the play by turning the towers into a bridge, so that he and Dominique can drive the truck "under" the bridge. She begins to line up the blocks and James calls it a road, and each drives a car along the "road," alternating between driving "fast" and "slow," with a few more crashes just for fun. As Dominique's interest wanes and turns to other objects, James follows her gaze to an animal book on the floor and asks whether she wants to read the book. Dominique stands up and goes to the book and brings it back to her father, turning to sit on his lap. He hands her the book to open and comments on the picture of a horse on the cover. Dominique points to the horse, imitates the word, and James responds, "Yeah, it's a horse," and then makes neighing sounds. Dominique copies the neigh, and James laughs and imitates her, and they both laugh and look at each other, sharing smiles. He gives her a little hug and she turns the page to the next animal.

They have just carried out two joint activity routines, one with the blocks and one with the book. This is the kind of teaching interaction we work to create in the ESDM. There are eight important elements to note.

1. Child interest begins the activity.
2. The adult marks the important aspects with language and positive affect and follows the child's lead into the activity.
3. The adult makes it interesting and reciprocal through turn taking, imitating the child's actions, and adding interesting effects to sustain child attention and motivation for the objects and the actions.

4. The "topic" of the play develops as the partners co-construct this joint activity, each adding to the whole.
5. The adult elaborates the activity with theme and variation, which allows for extension of child attention and expansion into additional skills.
6. The adult weaves in target vocabulary, nouns, verbs, and prepositions, stimulates child imitation, develops symbolic aspects of the play, and maintains the activity as a dyadic and reciprocal social activity.
7. Positive affect dominates adult and child's experience.
8. Child communication, both verbal and nonverbal, occurs frequently, expressing multiple functions (request, comment, maintain interaction, protest, share emotion) in balanced exchanges with the adult.

How do we create this kind of rich learning activity with young children with autism? This is the focus of this chapter. We break the teaching procedures into two phases. The first is becoming a play partner. This involves first establishing your presence as helpful and reinforcing and then taking a more active role in the play. The second phase is developing the play into elaborated joint activity routines, both with and without objects. We end the chapter by describing therapists' preparatory activities for conducting an ESDM session.

BECOMING A PLAY PARTNER

Child Motivation

Child Interest Begins the Activity

When children are highly interested in something, they are motivated to attain the object, observe the spectacle, and repeat the exchange. The child is in "approach mode," and the energy for the object or activity and the positive emotions generated create the motivational window within which we can teach. Motivation is crucial for teaching and interacting with all children, but it needs to have particular emphasis when working with children with autism. They may show very different motivational patterns than typically developing children. The term *motivation* for our purpose here is demonstrated by interest and approach behavior: watching with positive affect or interest (as opposed to wariness), leaning or moving toward, or trying to attain something.

What Motivates Children with Autism?

Children with autism are typically less socially motivated than others. For them, social attention, social approval, and "being like" others through imitation does not seem to carry the same degree of reward, or motivational value, that exists for others (Dawson et al., 2005a). Their interest is typically focused on the physical environment around them. Their "spotlight of attention," through which all learning will occur, is quite attuned to the physical world. However, children with autism can be highly motivated to obtain objects, to handle favorite objects, to create interesting effects with objects, and to get help with objects they enjoy. Contrary to stereotypes about autism, many young children enjoy social activities involving physical contact: roughhouse, musical games, tickle games, running, bouncing, and swinging. To treat children in the ESDM, we need materials and activities that stimulate child interest, energy, positive affect (find the smile!), and approach—this produces the energy and the attention needed for learning.

To find out what motivates a child, put him or her in a situation where there are many age-appropriate objects, well organized and accessible; then watch what happens. The child's behavior will tell you what objects or activities are interesting and rewarding. A motivated child is a focused child, attentive and ready to learn. Strong motivation supports active learners rather than passive learners, and active learners show initiative and spontaneity—two characteristics that we want to nurture in children with autism.

Occasionally, there are very "low-drive" children who do not approach toys. Nevertheless, these children may respond to object spectacles. Object spectacles involve toys that create very interesting physical or sensory effects—bubbles, balloons, pompoms, wind-up toys that make little movements, water being poured in a basin, mardi gras beads, maracas, toy flutes or pianos, bells and shakers, and pinwheels. These objects may attract great attention and interest. In the ESDM, we call these "sensory social toys"—we say more on this later. If the child does not respond to any of these kinds of objects with interest, smiles, attention, or approach, then move to the child's body. Play gentle (or lively!) physical games—spin, "Creepy Fingers," bouncing on knees, hand and feet games, bouncing on a trampoline or small therapy ball, being rolled or wrapped up in a beanbag or dragged around the room in it—something that will help you "find the smile." If food is the only motivating object, then have a snack with the child, and add these little physical games to a drawn-out snack time. We have to begin by finding something that turns on the child's smile and interest and creates positive energy and approach behavior. To be able to teach a child, you need to find reliable ways to turn on that spotlight of attention and the motivation behind it.

There are a few, though very few, young children with autism who do not respond positively to any of these stimuli (Ingersoll & Schreibman, 2006; Sherer & Schreibman, 2005). These children may do better with a more adult-directed and didactic, discrete trial teaching approach to build up their interest and reward the value of interacting with objects and people. They can be managed in the ESDM by applying the decision tree, described later in this chapter.

Drawing the Child's Attention

It is not enough that children are focused on objects. In order to learn from people, children's attention has to be on people. We have to become part of the child's focus of attention—we have to step into that spotlight of attention. Thus, once we identify a child's object or activity interests, the next step is to draw the child's attention to our eyes and faces, our body actions, and our voices, sounds, and words. We need to be in that spotlight, too. How to do it? Here are some strategies.

Eliminate the Competition

The physical environment can be a powerful pull for children's attention. By observing children, we can often interpret what their attentional magnets are in a particular space. Video or computer images, toys, and moving objects can be powerful sources of competition for adults who are trying to capture their children's attention. If the child's attention is drawn away from you by something else, you will have to control and engineer the environment so that you have less competition for the his or her attention. Put the toys that you are not using away or out of sight, in closed cabinets or under blankets. Ideally, the room should be able to be arranged with nothing in it except a table and chairs and a closed or covered cabinet or shelves.

Other people can also be magnets for attention or for escape. If other people are present in the therapy session, they should be asked to be like furniture in the room. If children escape to a parent, ask the parent to be completely boring. He or she should respond to the child's communications but offer nothing extra. If the child wants his mother to give him his cup, have his mother give you the cup so that you can give it to the child. You need to be the source of everything interesting and desirable in the room.

Take Center Stage

Social communication occurs especially through eyes and faces. We need children to look at us, to make repeated eye contact, to have clear views of our face, expressions, gaze patterns, and mouth movements as we speak. That means we need to set up our interactions in such a way that children have a very clear view of our face, and we want to draw their attention to our face and eyes. As much as possible, we want to position ourselves so that we are face-to-face with children, at their eye level, and with the materials between us and the child, easily brought near the face. Both when playing together with toys and when playing socially, we want to face the child.

However, if children are averting their gaze, turning their head, or covering their eyes to avoid gaze, *move back*. The natural temptation is to move forward, to "get in their face" and increase the salience of the face. In our experience, this only increases gaze avoidance. Move your face farther away from the child as your first accommodation and evaluate the effect.

There are a number of ways to position yourself and the child so that this face-to-face position occurs easily. Sitting on the floor together facing each other brings you face-to-face. For small children, seating the child in a child-sized seat or on a little step stool while you sit on the floor facing the child is a wonderful position for sensory social routines. For book activities, and greeting and dressing routines, seating the child low in a beanbag or a toddler-sized chair with good back support, facing you, is a great position. While adults tend to do book activities with children seated in their laps, it is better to do them face-to-face. A small chair or soft beanbag chair is an ideal way to seat the child in front of you, with the book held in front of the child and your face and body right there ready to make animal sounds, give key words, point to pictures, prompt points, and provide sound effects. For lap games, children can sit on your lap facing you. Positions in which the adult is seated on the floor and the child is lying down on his or her back, either on the adult's legs or on the floor between the adult's legs, facilitate great eye contact and are wonderful for social games, finger plays, and little body movement songs and routines. These are great positions for "Creepy Fingers," "This Little Piggie Went to Market," "Peekaboo" and "Pattycake," "Round and Round the Garden," tummy tickles, and "Thumbkin."

A small table is a great asset. Children often like to sit or stand at a small table to do puzzles or pop-up toys, and the adult can position him- or herself on the floor or on a little chair across the table from the child, face-to-face. Seating a child helps with positioning because the chair supports him or her and keeps the child from easily moving away. When seating a child, make sure that the child's feet are flat on the ground and the back is supported (hips, knees, and ankles at 90 degrees); children are more comfortable when the chair fits them well and will stay put longer. Chairs with sides are often helpful in stabilizing a child in the chair. However, do not use a seatbelt to hold a child in a chair. We want children to sit voluntarily because they enjoy the activity. If they do not sit or stay seated willingly, then sitting for enjoyable activities becomes one of their learning objectives (it is an item on the ESDM Curriculum Checklist; see Appendix A).

Joining the child so that you become part of the activity in the child's mind requires a sensitive touch; we want to join but we need to do it in a way that the child's motivation is not lessened. Once a child knows us well, we have much freedom to add our own pieces to the play, but initially, children are often either wary of our presence, or they appear unaware of it. Adults have to adjust their level of participation sensitively by observing child cues in order to minimize signs of discomfort. We want to increase the child's comfort with our presence and add to his or her motivation for the activity by making the child's goal easier to attain or the activity more interesting. This builds the reinforcement value of our presence.

Watch and Comment

Position yourself in front and as close as is comfortable for the child. Then just watch the child with interest, nodding and smiling in a natural and approving fashion, while adding simple words and sound effects. Doing this conveys your presence and your attention. Narrate the child's actions with lively emotion using words or phrases that are appropriate for the child's language level. Add sound effects. Observe the child's goals and put words to them. Beginning in this way establishes that your close presence is not going to create any negative effects. This act of describing the child's play (without interrupting or changing the child's focus) can help to *maintain* the child's attention to the activity while providing opportunities for language learning.

Be Helpful

When the child is clearly comfortable with you close, in front, and admiring, start to assist the child in reaching his or her goals without requiring anything from the child. Offer one piece of the item that the child is reaching for or push it closer. Steady the object, move things closer, open containers, give materials, and help freely with any struggle the child is having. This establishes that your presence is actually helpful to the child in reaching his or her goals and that your handling of the materials will not impede the child. You are now developing a positive valence, a reinforcing value of your own. Continue being a helpful play partner, commenting, approving, and facilitating, until the child is readily accepting your help. Packaging toys in difficult-to-open containers gives you a great way to be very helpful. Use ziplock bags and clear-lidded containers with difficult lids, and open them for children before they become upset or frustrated.

The strategies just described provide a script of sorts for the first therapy session. Some children will be comfortable with your presence and ready for you to become more actively involved within a few minutes of interaction. Others, especially those who are avoidant or rejecting, may need you to be in this responsive and facilitating mode for a more extended period, 30 minutes or even longer, and they may need you to begin each of the next few sessions in this way before you become more active. The child's comfortable response to your presence and your interactions with materials tells you that it is time to take your own role in the play.

Taking a Role in the Play

Once children are comfortably accepting your presence and your handling of materials, once they will freely take things from you and do not show any avoidance or wariness, you can become a more active partner in the play. This phase allows you to demonstrate how interesting your activities are. In this phase, you will join actively and begin adding to the child's play theme, ending up in co-constructing the activity with the child. Several techniques help establish you as an active partner.

Imitate the Child

Pick up matching materials and do what the child is doing. By imitating, you create *parallel play*. Parallel play involves carrying out the same activity as the child with your own materials, right there in front of the child. Children with autism as a group demonstrate positive responses to being imitated (Dawson & Adams, 1984; Dawson & Galpert, 1990.) Some children are fine with this; others want to control all the materials themselves. If the child wants your materials, give them freely, take others, and start again. Don't get into a power struggle over the toys; just play.

Another way of imitating is through joining the child and creating shared goals, or imitating the child's use of the materials to accomplish the child's goal. If the child is stacking blocks, you add blocks to the child's tower, in between the child's turns. If the child is crashing cars, you gently crash a car into the child's. If the child is doing a puzzle, you put in a piece or two. This strategy of imitating the child's play and joining to share the child's goals helps to build awareness of the social partner and builds a framework for interactive, reciprocal play.

What if the child protests? Some children like being imitated and co-construction; others don't want you to touch their materials, in which case you can go back to parallel play. Do not get into any struggles around materials; avoid conflicts as much as you can in this early stage of treatment. You are trying to develop a relationship that will allow you to become more and more active. Try not to do things that will result in the child ignoring or avoiding you. Conflicts will happen; it is inevitable. If it happens, find a way to resolve the conflict fast, before there is any problem behavior. Becoming a cooperative partner and establishing a working relationship now will soon allow you to open up wonderful new opportunities for the child. As you play, continue to narrate, make lively sound effects and object effects, and observe in an interested way this fascinating little person in front of you.

Add Variations: Elaborate the Play

A final way to take a role is to make the activity more interesting by adding to it in some way. If you are building a train track together, you could add a bridge. If you are building a tower, you could crash down yours (don't destroy the child's!). If you are driving dump trucks, you could put pieces in. If you are pressing play dough, add a rolling pin. Elaborating the play keeps it interesting and novel and extends the length of time you and the child are engaged in the activity.

Becoming More Active

Once the child accepts you easily in this role of interesting partner, you can begin to be more active in the play. The timing of these transitions is very individual. Some children will move through these phases with you in a single hour. Others may need several sessions before they are comfortable enough with you for you to be more active. In this phase, you will need to add two more techniques that will give you the level of participation and control you need for embedding teaching into play: controlling the materials and taking turns.

Control the Materials

Once the child has selected materials and begun the activity, scoop up the rest of the materials. They may be puzzle pieces, balls, train tracks, blocks, markers, and so on. Having them in your possession and handing them over as the child needs them allows you control over powerful reinforcers and puts you squarely in the spotlight. This is a big step, so be sure to give freely until the child is completely at ease with your handling of materials in many situations.

Take Turns

This again involves handling the materials and completing steps yourself. But taking turns is a more intrusive action than any we have discussed; the child should be prepared by all the previous parallel play and object handling you have done. Turn taking begins when the child is engaged in a one-person activity, like banging a maze ball with a hammer, marking with a marker, shaking a maraca, and so on. After the child acts on the material for a minute or two, take a very brief turn by saying, "My turn," extending your hand, and taking the toy quickly to do what the child just did, and then handing it over very fast to the child again as you say, "Your turn" (of course, narrating your action as you did it).

This exchange of the object is necessary, but it may cause a struggle with the child for the object. Some level of struggle may be necessary at the beginning in order for the child to experience that the toy will be returned very quickly. If the child is not going to release the toy to you, hand him or her an alternative and make it a trade for a while, until the child realizes that objects that you take for a turn will quickly come back. The clinician has to gauge this; if the child leaves the toy or refuses to interact more, it is not the end of the world, and returning to less intrusive partnering will reestablish the foundation. However, if you have proceeded slowly through the preceding steps, the child is probably comfortable enough with you and with your use of materials that you can take a turn without upset. Take turns frequently in play; it is crucial for teaching new skills, as we discuss below. (*Note*: Do not use "taking a turn" to put something away or end an activity. This punishes the child for giving. If something needs to end, then it is "all done" or "finished." If you ask for a turn, always give the child another turn.)

JOINT ACTIVITY ROUTINES: FRAMES FOR TEACHING

A joint activity is an activity in which two partners are engaged with each other in the same cooperative activity, attending to the same objects, or playing or working together on a common activity (Bruner, 1975, 1977). The partners may be imitating each other, building something together, or taking turns at the same activity. They actively construct the activity together (co-construction). Joint activity routines are the frames for teaching in the ESDM and the social element of a joint activity is the richest teaching tool. In joint activities, partners look at each other, give each other materials, imitate each other, communicate with each other, and share smiles and fun. Silly games may begin, and sharing smiles and laughter may happen. Or the goal may be a serious one, of building a big tower together or crashing trains on a track.

Phases of Joint Activity Routines

Up until this point we have been mostly discussing single play acts: bouncing, building, puzzles, and so on. We use the term *joint activity routine* to discuss the entire envelope, or scenario, that surrounds the play acts with a social partner and provides for a whole teaching activity. In the ESDM, we consider a joint activity routine as made up of several phases.

- The *opening or set-up phase* involves the acts that precede the establishment of the first shared play activity—the theme of the play.
- The *theme* involves the period of the first play activity. The child and adult are engaged in a definable play activity, either object centered, like building blocks, pouring water, marking with crayons, or involving a social game like singing a song, dancing to music, or playing hide and seek.
- The *elaboration phase* involves variation on the theme to keep it interesting or to highlight different aspects of the activity. This keeps the play from becoming repetitious and allows more skill areas to be addressed. Variation and elaboration allow the adult to extend the child's attention, promote flexibility, develop creativity, and address a number of skill areas.
- The *closing* is the fourth and final phase when attention is waning or the teaching value of the activity is all used up. It is a time to put materials away and transition to something else. Closing allows for the development of nice transitions from one activity to another, with changes of location and tempo. Taking materials back to their places and choosing another activity marks the transition from one joint activity to another, from one closing to another opening.

An ESDM treatment session involves a series of joint activities, beginning with a greeting activity, then moving through a series of different activities, some more active, some at the table, some more object focused, and some more social, until the closing greeting routine ends the treatment session.

Teaching Inside Joint Activities

Teaching occurs at three points: (1) in the adult response to the child initiation, when the adult provides a model, a word, a gesture, or some other cue that serves as the stimulus for the child behavior that will follow; (2) in prompts, if they are needed, to ensure that the child responds with a target behavior to the antecedent stimulus; and (3) in the delivery of the positive consequence that follows the child response. These three acts are the instructional acts that will teach the targeted steps of each objective.

Teaching begins when you respond to a child's initiation. Children may initiate by walking to some material and reaching for it. A very common teaching activity at that point is to pick up that object and offer it to the child while naming it (language model) and waiting for or prompting a targeted communicative behavior from the child (e.g., point, word, phrase, sound, gaze as specified in the child's communication objectives) before handing the object over, which is the reinforcement for the child's communicative act. If there are multiple pieces of the material, you can repeat the communicative exchange and instruction with other pieces, accomplishing several repetitions.

Next, you and the child begin to develop a joint activity with the object that the child is holding. This phase of the play—setting the theme—will be a platform for a cognitive, imitative, play, or motor objective. You will follow the child's activity and then use one of the objects to model a target behavior from the child's objectives, waiting or prompting the child to follow your model, thus accomplishing the target skill. Once the child completes the modeled or instructed act, the child gains the material and a chance to play as he or she wishes (reinforcement for performing the target act). Next, you take another turn, repeating the same skill or targeting another, following the child's goal, and using the target acts to elaborate the play.

This pattern continues during the elaboration phase, as the two of you continue to act together on the objects, with the adult weaving additional target behaviors and/or materials into the play to develop the theme further, to practice additional targeted skills, and to return to favorite schemas, while continuing to teach and making interesting things happen until the child's interest starts to wane.

There are several different types of joint activities, including object-based routines used in the example above, sensory social routines, hello and goodbye routines, clean-up, and snack. We discuss these and other joint activities below.

Object-Based Joint Activities

In object-based joint activities, the materials provide the play theme. Both child and adult are attending to actions on objects, and the social element is woven into the actions on objects through all the techniques described above: imitation, turn taking, management of the materials, theme, and variation. The social aspects of object-based joint activities are extremely important, and social interactions with gaze and communication should occur throughout object-based joint activities. These activities set the stage for the development of joint attention, in which two partners share their own intentions, attention, and enjoyment of the objects with each other. Children demonstrate their awareness of joint attention through giving, sharing, showing, and pointing to materials, by alternating gaze between objects and partner, and by looking up from objects to share smiles with the partner (Mundy, Sigman, Ungever, & Sherman, 1986). Joint attention development is typically quite delayed in young children with ASD, and since it is an important foundation for language and social development (Mundy, 1987; Charman, 1998; Charman & Howlin, 2003), we emphasize the development of joint attention in the ESDM in joint activities with objects.

How to Do Joint Activities with Objects

Joint activities involve all the same techniques that we have discussed up until this point, with the addition of elaborations and transitions. In the set-up phase, narrate the activity as you follow the child's lead by naming objects, actions, and relations in simple language. As you and the child establish the theme of the activity, take turns with the child either by trading materials back and forth or by using double sets of materials, sometimes modeling a new action and having the child follow your lead, and sometimes imitating the child. These turns are marked by social communication acts and foster the shifting of attention from objects to people and back again—joint attention. These attention shifts should occur frequently in object-based joint activities, several times per minute. As one play theme or action becomes "played out," move to the elaboration phase and model new actions occasionally while encouraging the child to imitate you (Chapter 7 on imitation and play discusses in detail how to do this). The theme and variation quality of play allows you to elaborate the play to teach more objectives and hold the child's attention for a much longer time. As interest in the materials wanes, or as you have done all you can think of to do, move through the clean-up phase to a new set of materials and another joint activity routine.

Partner-Focused Joint Activities: Sensory Social Routines

We have coined the term *sensory social routines* to refer to joint activity routines in which each partner's attention is focused on the other person, rather than on objects, as in object-oriented joint activities and in which mutual pleasure and engagement dominate the play. A sensory social routine is a dyadic joint activity routine (partner and self), while an object-oriented joint activity is a triadic joint activity routine (object–partner–self). A sensory social routine is a dyadic activity in which two persons are engaged in the same activity in a reciprocal way: taking turns, imitating each other, communicating with words, gestures, or facial expressions, and building on each other's activity. In sensory social routines, objects are incidental; the theme of the joint activity is the social exchange. Typical sensory social routines involve lap games like "Peekaboo," "Here comes Mousey," "The Noble Duke of York," or "This Is the Way That Pony Trots"; song routines with motions, like "Eensy Weensy Spider" and "The Wheels on the Bus"; floor song games like "Motorboat" and "Ring around the Rosy"; finger plays like "Creepy Fingers" and "Round and Round the Garden"; and movement routines like "Airplane," "Swing," "Chase," and "Hide and Seek."

While a joint activity with objects focuses on parallel actions with objects, communication about objects, shared attention to objects, and taking turns with objects, sensory social routines draw the child's attention to the partner's face, voice, body movements, and gestures. While many of these activities resemble those found in RDI (Gutstein & Sheely, 2002) or DIR/Floortime (Greenspan et al., 1997), they were created independently and early in the development of the Denver Model (Rogers et al., 1986; Rogers & Lewis, 1989), long before our first exposure to either of these other models.

There are four main goals that sensory social routines accomplish:

- Drawing the child's attention to other people's social-communicative cues, especially eye contact and the face, but also physical gestures, postures, anticipatory movements, and facial expressions.
- Developing children's awareness of facial expressions and their ability to share emotional expressions face-to-face with another. Adults share smiles, make silly faces, add sound effects and expressions to all kinds of games, and draw children's attention to their face.
- Increasing children's communications to initiate, respond to, and continue social interactions through their eye contact, facial expressions, gestures, sounds, and words.
- Optimizing children's arousal, state, and attention. Sensory social routines can enliven a passive "tired" child and calm an overactive, overaroused child. Sensory social routines can alter children's moods, soothing an upset child or refocusing a giddy child.

Sensory Social Routines Foster Social Orienting and Communication

Sensory social routines teach children that other people's bodies and faces "talk" and are important sources of communication. Therefore, in sensory social routines, it is crucial that children be facing adults and be well positioned to focus on faces and gestures. Face-to-face contact is helped by having a child sit on your lap facing you, or in a little chair with you sitting in front of him or her, or in a beanbag facing you, or on a big ball that you sit or stand in front of to bounce him or her, as we discussed earlier.

Sensory social routines teach children to communicate intentionally to initiate, maintain, and end social interactions. Intentional communications involve both gestures, including gaze, postures, and facial expression, and vocalizations, including speech. In sensory social routines, adults set up interesting activities until the child is engaged, and then pause and wait for the child to signal them to continue. These signals may be quite subtle at first, involving looking, reaching, vocalizing, making eye contact, or making some other gesture. However, this signal marks the child's "turn," and the adult then responds by continuing the activity. Adults first draw out from the child simple, single nonverbal communications like gaze, hand gestures, or intentional vocalizations. They then shape these into integrated communications that involve directed gaze with gesture and vocalization, and then these are further shaped into word approximations and words. Many child communications occur in a single sensory social routine. With a skilled therapist, children are carrying out an intentional communication or other social act every 10 seconds on the average, somewhat more frequently than in object-oriented joint activities. It is crucial that the child is very active in initiating and continuing the activity in order to reap the potential gains that sensory social routines can offer as powerful teaching activities for communication and social objectives.

Sensory Social Routines Optimize Attention and Arousal for Learning

The type of touch, movement, and rhythm that the adult uses in the sensory social routine has fairly immediate effects on the child. In general, slow, quiet, calm, rhythmic movements and patterns are calming. Experiment with the child's reactions to a variety of types of touch—being held and squeezed in a bear hug, deep pressure, tickles, head and back rubs, being jumped, swung, spun, and bounced. Learn what types of actions are arousing, and what are quieting, for each individual child. Find routines that calm and routines that alert and arouse. The OT on the team will be of great help if these concepts are new or if the child is not very responsive to your efforts. Use these routines to help the child regulate and maintain an optimal state of attention and arousal during therapy. Use these activities as you see children losing an optimal state. The therapist's skill at helping the child to attain and maintain an ideal emotional state for learning is an important aspect of therapist behavior in the ESDM and is one of the fidelity items used to measure therapist skill.

Use of Objects in Sensory Social Routines

Sensory social routines often involve activities without any objects at all. However, sometimes objects are helpful as a prop for drawing attention to adults; this is especially the case for children who do not yet enjoy body games. Adult-operated objects like bubbles, balloons, pinwheels, or similar objects create exciting and interesting effects and draw attention to a person's face, supporting wonderful dyadic sensory social routines (and also joint attention and the development of joint attention behaviors).

For example, Lisa, the therapist, and Robbie, an 18-month-old with ASD, are looking through the sensory social toy box. Lisa pulls out a balloon. "Balloon," she says, and she blows it up and lets it fly through the air, to Robbie's delight, so she retrieves it and begins again. With each repetition, Lisa waits for Robbie to watch and anticipate. She holds the balloon to her mouth but doesn't blow, and Robbie watches with much anticipation and makes a little blow. Lisa immediately says, "Blow" and begins to blow, but gauges each blow to hold Robbie's eye contact and build his anticipation. After several repetitions of this game, the next time the balloon is blown up full, Lisa holds the balloon temptingly to Robbie but does not release it, and slowly says, "Ready, set, go!" and lets it fly. The third time she does this, she waits before saying, "Go!" and Robbie fills in "go!" before she lets it fly. Robbie now runs to fetch it and return it to Lisa's outstretched hand (Lisa makes sure that he does not put the balloon into his mouth). Lisa takes it, looks to Robbie, and waits. He smiles, makes eye contact, and blows again. She blows up the balloon and the activity begins again.

What makes this a sensory social routine rather than an object routine? The adult is manipulating the object to create exciting effects, and the child is communicating frequently and is attending intensely to the adult's face, voice, and body. There is excitement and strong positive affect that is shared between the two. The child does not operate the object; rather, the child's interaction with the object is limited to getting it and returning it to the adult. Most of the child's attention is on the adult. Sometimes the line between object-oriented activities and sensory social activities becomes very thin. What is important is the intensely social nature of the activity.

(*Caution:* When using objects, it is very important to keep the child's attention mostly on you rather than the object. That means that the adult must maintain control of the object. Even if the child requests it, keep hold of it and operate it for the child, so that you keep the child's attention on you. Treat the request as a request for you to activate the object rather than to hand it over.) In sensory social routines, we do not take turns with objects; instead, the child requests the adult to set interesting actions in motion or to continue them, and the child shares smiles and other communicative acts with the adult. Once the child's interest is captured, the adult pauses and waits for the child to communicate with the adult in order to continue the effect. If the child is so motivated to handle the object that the interaction becomes negative, change activities.

Beginning a New Sensory Social Routine

When first introducing a new sensory social routine, the adult may need to start and stop the activity several times without variation, so that the child learns what the routine is and what to expect. When introducing a new routine, children may not show immediate pleasure in it. They may seem dubious or uneasy. It is all right to persist in three quick repetitions of the game even if the child does not seem motivated, as a way to introduce the game. Over several days, the activity may become more and more interesting. However, if children are clearly uncomfortable or protesting vigorously, stop the routine or vary it to take away the negative element. We don't want the child to associate the routine with negative experiences. Be aware of subtle signs of negativity. Rapid eye blinking, a worried look, dampening of positive affect, startling, and stilling indicate that the child is uncomfortable just as clearly as withdrawal, physical avoidance, and seeking of the parent. *If you observe negative signs, decrease the intensity of the stimulus immediately.* If the negative signs do not decrease over each of three gentle demonstrations, stop the activity for that day. Try it again in the next couple of sessions, even more delicately than before. If the child continues to react negatively, then stop and find a different activity.

Turn Taking inside Sensory Social Routines

In a sensory social routine, the two partners should have many exchanges, or turns, but unlike object-focused joint activity routines, the turns involve only social or communicative behaviors. Children need to be active social partners, taking many turns to request, continue, imitate, or cue. The routine should look very reciprocal, with each partner acting in response to the other, and the child providing some social or communicative behavior every 10 seconds or so.

This is not a situation in which the adult is entertaining the child and the child is passively observing the adult. Rather, adult and child are in back-and-forth communication throughout, via movements, gestures, eye contact, sounds, words, or other actions. These reciprocal interactions are relatively balanced. Remember that the goal is for the child to focus on and communicate with the adult's face and body to initiate, respond to, or continue the sensory social routine. The adult will need to start, pause, and wait often, to give the child a chance for his or her communicative turn.

Building up the Child's Repertoire

We want to build up the child's repertoire of sensory social routines. As soon as the child has learned a communicative set of exchanges in one sensory social routine, we want to start another. Simple songs that involve simple hand movements are especially important to develop, because of their ritualized language, shared social content, and motor imitation. Begin songs as soon as the child will watch you while sitting or lying still for a minute or so. Introduce a song in a telegraphic format, emphasizing the gestures, and, if the child is interested, repeat it several times. Review it during each treatment session until it is a familiar source of pleasure and participation for the child. Then, add a new one. A goal in the first 12 weeks of the intervention is to build up a repertoire of 10 to 12 different sensory social routines that children enjoy and in which they communicate and actively participate.

Alternating between Object-Focused Joint Activities and Sensory Social Routines

In the ESDM therapy sessions, we alternate between object-focused joint activity routines and sensory social routines. The object-focused routines provide a platform for teaching cognitive skills, imitation, communication and language, fine motor skills, and toy play skills, while the sensory social routines focus on social skills, communication and language skills, and imitation skills. Sensory social routines draw children with autism into the social world and the pleasure of social exchanges; they regulate arousal and attention to the adult. They are a very important part of this intervention model and several age-appropriate sensory social activities should occur in every treatment hour, for all children, including older, high-functioning preschoolers (think birthday party games!).

Other Types of Joint Activity Routines

There are several other joints activities that we have not yet discussed: opening and closing routines, snack, clean-up, and transitions. These are not typical play activities, and so they do not lend themselves to the joint activity format straightforwardly. However, they are quite important activities for preschool and family life, and over time will become very important joint activities for your teaching.

Hello and Goodbye

Therapy needs to begin and end with greeting activities that also become joint activities. In the first one or two sessions, these may be no more than getting the child's attention, waving and saying "hi" or "Bye bye," and prompting the child to wave back. However, very soon this will be elaborated into a little sequence of activities involving sitting down, taking shoes and socks off and placing them in a little container, waving, saying, or singing "Hi" along with a hello song and imitated movements, and perhaps carrying out a sensory social routine. Hello–goodbye and book routines provide preparations for circle time activities in a group preschool setting. For a child who will soon attend a group preschool, adding a "circle time" to the schedule in which activities from the preschool are explicitly practiced provides excellent support for the preschool transition.

Receptive language objectives are also easy to work into greeting routines as you give instructions to sit down, stand up, give me five, take off shoes, get socks, and so on. Social objectives involving greetings and attending to another are also early objectives supported by hello and goodbye routines.

Snack

Snack is a wonderful communication activity with a high intrinsic reinforcement value for most children, and for children at the beginning of treatment, you can develop much intentional communication relatively quickly in snack. Following ESDM practices, we set up snack as a joint activity routine, which means that both therapist and child have a snack, and elaborate the activity through pouring, stirring, and using both finger foods, spoon/fork foods, and drinks. You can serve the child and have the child serve you. Narrate every step of the routine using the one-word-up rule. Review targeted receptive language objectives by asking for a napkin, fork, plate, and so on. Use utensils in ways that address fine motor skills. Use gestures that children can follow. Make "yummy" and "aah" noises when eating and drinking to encourage vocal imitation.

Once children have language or other symbolic means for requesting, snack becomes less necessary as a communication activity and it can address other goals. Bringing toy animals and dolls into snack helps it evolve into a symbolic play activity, involving mealtime for animals and tea parties for dolls. Snack may also become a complex and very interesting activity that can address multiple domains when you incorporate a multistep cooking or food preparation activity. Snack can address adaptive behavior skills like clean-up, table setting, pouring, scooping, and even spreading with a knife and cutting, for older preschoolers.

Clean-Up

Objects need to be cleaned up and put away at the end of each activity. The clean-up phase is important for several reasons. A primary purpose of clean-up is to keep the space relatively empty, so that you and the chosen activity can be the magnet for the child's attention. In the beginning of treatment, the therapist does the clean-up, and it may consist of no more than dumping the materials in a big container to be put away later. If children are moving from one material to another, you may need to do a fast clean-up so that you can move with the child to develop a new activity.

A second main purpose of clean-up is to add complexity to the activity and thus provide more teaching opportunities. Containers have to be opened, pieces inserted, containers closed, and then carried to their storage place. Pieces may need to be sorted or grouped by shape or color. Each one of these acts provides a place for language teaching, cognitive skills involving sorting, matching, and classifying, turn taking, and shared roles. Objects can be counted as they are put inside. Receptive language is easily woven into clean-up: "Hand me the block," "Put the hammers in the box and then put the box on the shelf," "Green goes here," and "Put it on the shelf under the markers." Clean-up activities are a natural activity for matching and sorting skills, and "creative packaging" on the part of the therapist can scaffold a variety of matching and sorting concepts, as well as preposition work, during clean-up. All kinds of cognitive matching activities can be carried out through clean-up: identity (dishes go here, spoons go there); color (matching colored lids on play dough containers or markers to close them); teaching that pictures represent objects (marking containers or shelves with pictures: pens in here, pencils in there; round blocks here, rectangular blocks there); and size and shape (big animals in the big box, little animals in the little box).

A third main purpose of clean-up is temporal sequencing and planning. Clean-up involves a temporal sequence—first this, then that. First we clean up, then we choose a new activity. First we put objects in the boxes, and then we put the boxes on the shelves. In a temporal sequence, we provide children with an introduction to the concept of future time. "What shall we do after we clean up the blocks?" "What next—art or tricycle?" "What will you make with the play dough?" "What book do you want to read today?" "What will we need to give the baby a bath?" This kind of verbal anticipation allows children to imagine the future and plan accordingly; clean-up gives opportunities all through the hour to plan one's next activity. Children with autism may be very present-focused, moving from one activity to another as their attention is caught by visual or auditory stimuli. Clean-up requires the child to inhibit the impulse to leap up and move to something else and instead to wait and work from a cognitive and temporal plan. If the child has expressed the desire to move to a new activity, he or she has to hold that new goal in mind, in working memory, and shift his or her thoughts back to finishing clean-up.

This act of holding a new goal in mind, and waiting while something else is completed, requires a very particular cognitive skill set—*executive function skills*—which are complex mental skills involving keeping a goal in mind and organizing oneself through a series of steps to reach that goal (Russell, 1997; Hughes, Russell, & Robbins, 1994; Pennington & Ozonoff, 1996). Executive function skills are mediated by the frontal lobe and are often affected by autism, particularly in older children (Ozonoff, Pennington, & Rogers, 1991; Griffith, Pennington, Wehner, & Rogers, 1999). The simple sequences involved in clean-up address key executive function capacities: inhibition, working memory, goal formation, and set shifting.

Clean-up also provides a wonderful opportunity to review the sequence of activities that just happened as materials are put away. "What did we do with the valentines?" "First we colored, then we cut the pieces out, then we smeared the glue, then we sprinkled the glitter." "Now they are drying." It prepares a narrative that the child can share with others.

A fourth purpose of clean-up is to stimulate language as a means of self-regulation. In clean-up, the adult is modeling the use of language to regulate oneself. By providing simple language to accompany the steps—first this, then this; after this, then that—the adult provides a script that the child can later learn as a means of self-regulation and planning—an important role of internalized language.

A final purpose of clean-up is to prepare children for the expectations of home, preschool, and kindergarten. In group education situations, clean-up is an important part of transitions between activities, and children are expected to carry out clean-up with some degree of independence. By teaching children appropriate clean-up routines during therapy sessions, we are teaching to the next environment.

Developing Clean-Up

Clean-up is a complex activity that develops slowly over repeated therapy sessions. With a child who is new to therapy, the adult carries out clean-up, either as the child watches or "on the run," to quickly remove materials and clear the space for a child who has already moved away. This marks the initial teaching phase of clean-up. The next phase involves a child who has been in enough therapy sessions to have a sense of the rhythm of therapy—moving together from one activity to the next. The therapist now expects the child to complete one or more steps of the clean-up activity. This might be putting a piece or two in a container, putting a lid on a box, or putting a container on a shelf. The therapist generally models the activity to be done and then hands the material to the child to complete, prompting if needed to imitate the adult's model (here is an object imitation task). The predominant language during this phase emphasizes the words *clean-up*. "Time to clean up" or "let's clean up" or "help clean up" labels the activity. The therapist will also narrate the steps in simple language close to the child's mean length of utterance (MLU)—"Put in," "Lid on," "Ball in," are typical narrative phrases, but we want to emphasize the more general term *clean-up* to mean putting away materials, whatever they are. So the child completes a few of the steps, often toward the end of the activity, and the therapist completes the rest of the steps, so the child sees the steps and joins the therapist for the final put away on a shelf or in a drawer.

Set-Up for Clean-Up

As much as feasible, have the materials "packaged" in bags or containers while they are on the shelf or at the choice point. Give them to the child packaged. In unpacking them, the child has a chance to preview the steps and the organization of the materials that will be involved in clean-up. Repacking makes more sense if you first have to unpack them. It makes clean-up less of an adult-directed and somewhat artificial request, and more of an intrinsic aspect of activities and materials.

Teach Clean-Up through Chaining, Like Any Other Multistep Activity

Clean-up is a multistep activity, like dressing, hand washing, or toileting and is taught in the same way. If the child has the attention span, we can use *partial participation* in each step of the sequence (Ferguson & Baumgart, 1991) for clean-up. Partial participation involves taking the child through each step, having him or her assist with an act in each step, and using a least-to-most prompting sequence to involve the child in each step. However, if there is much to clean up, if the child has a very short attention span or does not have object imitation skills to follow the model, or if the child is really wanting to change activities, we may ask the child to carry out only one step. For children who cannot stay with the clean-up long enough for partial participation and forward chaining, teach instead using a backward chaining approach or teach using most-to-least prompts to develop the sequence instead.

Consider the Reinforcers

The reinforcement for clean-up has to be considered carefully. Clean-up is generally a nonpreferred activity (though some children like placing the materials in containers, etc., and so some steps may contain intrinsic reinforcement). Nonpreferred activities require an external reinforcer. The external reinforcer for clean-up is the chance to choose a new activity. For children who have learned about clean-up, they know that the next choice of activities follows clean-up, and so it is the desire for a new pleasurable activity that motivates clean-up. However, for children who have not experienced this enough times, this association must be developed. The therapist has to motivate the child to the next activity via child choice. The therapist may provide the new activity and materials in one hand or just out of reach while having the child complete a step of clean-up, so that the presentation of the new desired object follows, and thus reinforces, the clean-up act that preceded it. This is an example of the Premack principle—when a more preferred activity follows a less preferred activity it serves as a reinforcer for the less preferred activity. The language used emphasizes this relationship: "First clean up, then ___________."

Transitions

Clean-up begins the process of transitioning from one activity to another. In the situations described above, the child is ready for something new, and the adult inserts the clean-up routine in between the old and the new activity. In general, we want children to move from one space to another for various activities. Some activities will occur at the table, some at the book corner, some at the hello–goodbye station, or some on the floor for physical activities. We want children to make these moves independently, without being led. Leading children from one place to another often means that the child does not know where he or she is going, or why. A child who moves through space independently and in a goal-directed fashion has a goal in mind already, knows where he or she is going and why, and is already mentally entering the activity, ready to participate and learn from you.

As the therapist sets up the rhythm for the therapy activities, children will begin to learn where activities occur. Art activities typically occur at the table. Ball activities occur in the motor area. Books happen in the beanbag. Hello and goodbye happen in the chair by the door. The child's transition through space should occur in relation to these activities. As the child chooses the art box, the therapist takes the box to the table and has the child help carry the box. This puts the child at the table. Or, the child chooses the box, the therapist says, "Let's go to the table," puts the box on the table, and the child follows the material and seats him- or herself at the table. In both these examples, the child moves him- or herself to the table and is being drawn to the activity—the material is a magnet for the transition. For a child who has been in therapy for a while, the child may choose the box, carry the material to the table, and seat him- or herself without any further cues, thus doing the whole transition independently. This is what we want to see.

Beware!

Signs that children are not independently engaged in a transition include adults leading children from one place to another, physically placing them on their seats rather than having them seat themselves, or physically lifting them to move them. Another sign that children are not mentally engaged in the transition occurs when an adult tells a child to sit at an empty table, and the child sits and waits without knowing what is coming next. Try not to seat a child at an empty table; the materials or choices for the activity should be obvious to the child so the child knows what to expect and is motivated by the activity that is about to unfold.

Transitioning Out of Repetitive Activities

There are times when the child does not want to change activities, and then transitions involve different challenges. Sometimes a child is getting much pleasure out of a very repetitive activity. When do you stop the activity and move on? You move on when you cannot think of anything else to make it a learning activity, or when you can't stand doing it anymore. Children may become upset by a forced transition, though we try to ease them through it. However, a possible upset is not a reason to avoid a transition. Our job is not to keep children happy; it is to teach them their objectives. Flexibility about changing activities is a very important objective for children whose long attention span allows them to continue a repetitive activity for a long time and who do not shift attention easily. Flexible shifting of attention is a cognitive skill that is often affected by autism, like other executive functions. Learning to shift attention when others ask you to is a very important skill for all of us.

Facilitating Transitions for Resistant Children

When children are quite resistant to changing activities or materials, the general sequence of teaching steps goes like this

- Stop participating in the activity so that social attention is no longer reinforcing the activity.
- Try to make the activity very boring. If the repetitive activity involves objects with multiple pieces (like building block towers or putting rings on a peg), start putting the rest of the objects away, so the child only has one or two pieces left, to make the activity less interesting.
- Bring another activity or two into the child's visual field. Call the child's attention and activate the material in an attractive way right in front of the child. As the child shifts attention to the new material, offer it to the child and try to elicit a reach.
- As the child reaches for the new material, surreptitiously slide the previous material out of the way and out of sight (this is not the right time to work on clean-up!)

As therapy progresses and a number of highly preferred object routines are built up, it generally becomes easier to help children move from one activity to another, and of course a clean-up routine helps mark this transition.

Other Object Interference Issues

Sometimes children enjoy one material so much that your best creative efforts cannot move the child to another activity. If a certain material begins to interfere with therapy, then before your next therapy session, remove it from the room. If it is interfering so much that you cannot teach during the present therapy session, and you have tried every way possible of transitioning, you may have to put the material out of reach or outside the door. This will very often result in a tantrum or period of child upset, but, managed well, the upset will pass and you can slowly move back into teaching. Better to lose 10 minutes to the upset than 40 minutes to the interfering material. Some children can be brought out of the upset by offering a new interesting material. However, often the upset child becomes more upset when you initiate another activity. In this case, managing the upset often goes better if you avoid offering anything else to the upset child, but rather move away from the child and do something interesting with an attractive toy by yourself. The child will eventually calm down and will often begin to watch you or your activity, either approaching or showing enough interest that you can now approach with the materials.

MANAGING UNWANTED BEHAVIORS

Unwanted behaviors lead to social consequences that are destructive to children's learning and development, and it is crucial that unwanted behaviors come to be replaced over time with behaviors that are more socially acceptable and understandable by others. However, it has been our experience that implementing the teaching principles and activities that we have discussed thus far, by themselves, is a powerful intervention that reduces many children's unwanted behaviors and replaces them with more conventional behaviors without specifically focusing on the goal of behavior reduction.

Thus, in this model, we begin by identifying unwanted behaviors and gathering frequency data on them. For dangerous or destructive behaviors, we immediately call in a behavior analyst or other person trained to assess the unwanted behaviors using a functional assessment/analysis and positive behavior supports approach. For behaviors that are not dangerous to self or others, our philosophy is to focus on implementing parent coaching and excellent treatment while keeping track of the frequency of unwanted behaviors intermittently. If problem behaviors do not decrease over the first month or so, then it is time to focus specifically on behavior reduction. At that point, the behavior analyst on the team would direct or oversee a functional assessment of problem behaviors (O'Neill et al., 1990) and the development of a positive behavior management plan.

Positive Behavior Supports

The general approach to unwanted behaviors that we use in the ESDM follows the principles of positive behavior supports (Carr et al., 2002; Duda et al., 2004). This is a way of applying the principles of ABA that focuses on the use of reinforcement strategies to teach children adaptive, conventional behaviors for meeting their needs and expressing their feelings, as well as promoting independent functioning. Twenty years ago, behavioral approaches to unwanted behaviors emphasized the use of negative consequences for these behaviors, either punishment (including verbal correction, overcorrection, time-out, response cost) or extinction alone (no consequences at all for the behavior, which leads to a large increase in the behavior—the extinction curve—before behavior reduction occurs). Today, positive approaches to unwanted behaviors are the approaches of choice.

These involve identifying the functions of the child's unwanted behavior, identifying a conventional behavior (usually a communicative behavior) that the child could use to achieve his or her goals (saying "no" instead of screaming, asking for a "break" instead of running away, signing "more" instead of grabbing, asking someone to "move, please" instead of pinching them). Once this new target behavior is identified, the child is actively taught to use the behavior through simulating the situation and prompting the behavior *before* the child has used the unwanted behavior. A combination of steady reinforcement for the new behavior and no reinforcement for the unwanted behavior results in a gradual increase in spontaneous use of the new behavior.

Two of the challenges in using positive behavior supports are (1) identifying the function of the unwanted behavior and the environmental cues that precede the unwanted behavior, and (2) choosing a replacement behavior that is already in the child's repertoire and can be as fast, easy, and efficient for the child to use to attain the goal as was the unwanted behavior. The child is using the unwanted behavior because it is the most efficient behavior the child has found to express his or her need or goal. The substitute behavior has to be even easier or more efficient in gaining the reinforcer than the unwanted behavior was, or it will be very difficult to teach the substitution.

The following outlines our ESDM stepwise approach for managing unwanted behaviors:

- Describe the unwanted behaviors according to parent reports and direct observation and gather frequency data.
- Is there a likelihood of injury or property destruction? If so, act now! If there is concern about injury to the child or others, and a history of such injury in the recent past, then call in your behavior analyst to conduct a functional assessment. (See O'Neill et al., 1997, for one well-described method for conducting a functional assessment of behavior.) The assessment will define the unwanted behaviors, their functions, their reinforcers, and their frequency.
- For children with severe self-injury, or a sudden onset of self-injury, seek the input of the child's primary care physician, and if needed, a developmental and behavioral pediatrician as part of the assessment phase. Self-injury, and sudden changes in any unwanted behaviors, can signal a biological condition that must be considered and ruled out or treated as part of the plan.
- Once a behavior plan is created, it can be implemented simultaneously with the implementation of the developmental and other learning objectives, but it should be implemented as a separate and specific behavior plan, with data collected and reviewed by the behavior analyst at appropriate frequencies to detect change. The behavior plan should be continued and modified as needed until it is successful at reducing the intensity and frequency of the behaviors. During this period, precautions for the safety of the child and others at risk of injury should be put in place and carefully monitored. All incidents should be recorded and modifications made as needed.
- If the behavior is considered very unlikely to result in injury or significant property destruction, then the therapist may proceed with the developmental teaching plan that has been developed without yet forming or implementing a behavior plan. Occurrences of the problem behavior should be noted on the Daily Data Sheet, in the behavior section that is part of each sheet. The therapist should be very aware of the functions of the unwanted behaviors that have been identified so that these behaviors are not reinforced in the treatment. Examine the data weekly in your sessions, both from the parents' data collected at home and that collected during your therapy session. If the

behavior is decreasing in both settings, and if the child is now using a more conventional behavior to attain his or her goals, proceed with the developmental treatment plan.

• Continue to track the behavior at least weekly. If, after 8–12 weeks, the behavior is still a problem, then it is time to add an additional plan that will target replacement of that behavior. The behavior may still be present because it serves multiple functions, not all of which have been addressed in the initial phase. Turn to the behavior expert on the team to plan and direct this intervention.

Autism can involve very specific abnormalities that are not primary to the core symptoms involving social-communicative and repetitive deficits, but rather appear to be secondary or related aspects of the disorder. Some of these include dyspraxia of speech, abnormal muscle tone, depression, seizures, severe self-injury, or intention tremor. Each of these conditions requires a disciplinary knowledge base in order to appropriately diagnose and treat the condition, and severe behavior problems are just as complex in their treatment as are seizures or dyspraxia. This is why we recommend that the behavioral expert on the team interact with the other disciplinary team members to carry out the evaluation, develop a functional understanding of the behavior, develop the behavioral treatment plan, and direct its implementation. Using expertise within the team supports the integrity and the priorities of the treatment plan. It is also much easier for families, who have already met these team members during the assessment phase, to see them again rather than to begin a whole new relationship with a therapist who does not yet know the child, the family, the history, the progress, or the plan.

Positive Attention and the Child with Severe Behavior Problems

Over time, children with severe behavior problems may receive less and less positive attention from family members, teachers, and others, because the strain of their problems is causing such stress to those around them. Part of an intervention plan needs to involve creating or reinstating high levels of positive, noncontingent interactions to ensure that children are getting positive social attention frequently throughout the day and from all the people around them. Help parents and all others around the child find times for fun interactions daily in situations that will not lead to conflict or problem behavior. Delivering high rates of unconditional positive attention and interaction is an extremely important part of the general approach for dealing with children with severe behavior problems, and should be implemented as part of any intervention plan.

Stereotypic Behavior

Stereotypies are another class of unwanted behavior that does not cause destruction or injury, but which interferes with learning and attending. Stereotypies are repetitive behaviors of the body or with objects. Stereotypies can occupy children's attention so that they are not watching and learning from others. They prevent practice of new skills with objects. They do not provide the child with any new information or ability, so they do not promote learning. They can be off-putting to other children and adults and can be a barrier to social interaction. And while it is believed by some that stereotypies provide children with ways of calming themselves or providing sensory input that they need, this view is not currently supported by empirical data.

In the ESDM, we seek to replace stereotypic patterns with more adaptive patterns. When stereotypy involves objects, we want to teach children to imitate more appropriate behaviors with the objects. We do this as follows: We take the object, model the desired behavior, prompt the child to imitate the model, and reinforce the child's imitation, in exactly the same way that we would if there was no stereotypy.

Hopefully, there are more powerful reinforcers for the child than engaging in the stereotypy. Since the stereotypic movement is the child's goal, there are probably no *intrinsic* reinforcers for that activity that are as powerful as stereotypy. So, here is a time that you will need an *extrinsic* reward, something that is even more powerful for the child than stereotypy. As you teach alternative actions with objects using powerful reinforcers, children will develop new schemas, and practicing these new schemas with the objects will weaken somewhat the connections with the stereotypy, since it is not being reinforced as often or as powerfully as the others.

Occasionally, there is really nothing as reinforcing to the child as producing his or her favorite stereotypy. In that case, eliminate the object from therapy. However, for children who shake or twiddle every single object, eliminating them is impossible. For them, being able to control the object as they want, and do their stereotypy, is reinforcing. So, you can require imitation of your act and reinforce with their control of the object and the freedom to "stim" for a brief period of time. (*Note:* This is a last resort response and will not be needed for most young children in the ESDM treatment.)

It is really difficult to completely eliminate stereotypy. Our goal is to increase children's spontaneous behavioral repertoire of adaptive and functional skills, not to eliminate all stereotypy. As this functional repertoire increases, stereotypy will represent a much smaller proportion of the child's activities with objects overall.

Behavior problems are often thought of as part and parcel of autism. However, focusing on building communication skills, following children's leads, and increasing the reinforcement value of social interaction may go a long way toward reducing children's behavior problems. This is because the interventions are teaching children adaptive ways of getting their needs met.

ORGANIZING AND PLANNING THE SESSION

Joint activity routines discussed above are the frames, or the stage, within which teaching occurs. In this section, we discuss how to organize the activities and teaching objectives within the therapy session.

Sequencing the Session Activities

An ESDM intervention session involves a series of joint activities, each 2 to 5 or so minutes in length at the start of treatment. Over time activities lengthen and may run as long as 10 minutes. In a 2-hour session, across the activities, all the child's objectives can be addressed, including a review of mastered skills—the maintenance skills—and multiple opportunities to practice the target skill—the current acquisition step for each objective.

There are several guidelines that we use to decide which activities to offer and in what order. Sessions begin and end with greeting routines that contain joint activity routines within them. Then therapists alternate between sensory social routines with object-oriented joint activities across the session to target the child's various learning objectives. As described above, therapists set up different activities in different locations in the room: hello chair with shoe box, table and chair for fine motor activities, beanbag for books, a floor area for gross motor activities, and a space for playing with objects on the floor (e.g., hello chair to floor to table, to beanbag, to floor). There is a frequent change of location with a change of activity, in order to keep children's energy levels and interest levels optimized. It is typical to change location with each change in activity, though it is not required. The pace also changes from activity to activity. A seated activity involving focus on an object is typically followed by a more active routine on the floor. A highly stimulating motor activity is followed by a less physically stimulating, seated activity. The amount of physical activity and excitement for each activity is determined by the adult, on the basis of the child's current level of arousal and what will be optimal for learning and attending.

Table 6.1 shows a typical sequence for a 1-hour therapy session for Landon, an 18-month-old, early on in the therapy process. On Landon's therapy schedule, you see many activities that fall under joint activities with objects and those that are sensory social routines. Joint activity routines are listed for working on gross and fine motor objectives, social, cognition, play, and communication objectives. For a child who has been in therapy longer and has developed a number of routines, those routines will typically lengthen, through experience and increasing elaboration. Remember that a key treatment technique is elaboration of child activities to work on more objectives from more domains. Thus, elaboration will turn routines into more complex sequences of activities.

For example, a drawing imitation activity may initially involve a 3- to 5-minute activity using markers and paper, perhaps with some stickers, glue, and glitter added for elaborations. However, a year later, the drawing objectives may use representational pictures, and the drawing activity may involve simple pictures of animals (circles for body, sticks for legs, and dots for eyes) that are tied to an animal book or song the child particularly likes (e.g., "Old McDonald Had a Farm"). This routine may involve first drawing a cat or dog, then singing "Old McDonald" with animal sounds, and then drawing an animal, choosing another animal to draw, singing, drawing, and so on, and then perhaps ending by drawing a fence and barn in the picture. Now, we have a 10- to 15-minute activity, with all kinds of objectives involved.

The hello, goodbye, and object routines, especially, will become longer because they will involve a lengthy sequence of steps and because clean-up and transition will also become a part of each of these. Thus, object routines will evolve into 5- to 10-minute activities, and sensory social routines will involve learned songs, dances, and circle games with increasing numbers of props, choices, verses, music, and other elaborations. The result will be fewer, more elaborated, multistep activities for older and advanced preschoolers that are very similar to those used in typical preschool classes and that support inclusion in typical preschools.

Planning Activities to Support Learning Objectives

Getting the most teaching into a session requires some planning and preparation. One of the most enjoyable and potentially difficult aspects of the ESDM is the lack of script-

TABLE 6.1. Typical Sequence of Activities for 1-Hour Therapy Session

Activity	Location	Activity	Objectives
Greeting Hello	Hello chair	Hello routine with song (and gestures) and shoes removal	Social communication, self-care, imitation objectives
Object Activity 1		Puzzle—object-activity routine	Fine motor, cognitive, play, communication objectives
Sensory Social 1	Moving on carpet	"Ring Around the Rosy"—sensory social routine	Social, imitation, communication objectives
Motor-Movement Activity 1	Standing on carpet	Throwing balls at Bobo doll—physical movement-gross motor activity	Imitation, gross motor, communication objectives
Object Activity 2	Seated at table	Block towers of matching colors—object-activity routine	Imitation, fine motor, cognitive, communication objectives
Sensory Social Activity 2	Standing on carpet	Popping and stamping bubbles—sensory social routine	Social, imitation, communication objectives
Snack	Seated at table	Snack—using fork for fruit pieces	Self-care, communication, social, fine motor, objectives
Motor-Movement Activity 2	Standing on carpet	Rolling therapy ball back and forth—object routine	Social, communication, imitation, motor objectives
Books	Seated on beanbag	Animal touch and sounds—book routine	Communication, joint attention, social objectives
Object Activity 3	Seated on carpet	Rhythm band with music	Communication, social, imitation, play objectives
Greeting Goodbye	Hello chair	Closing song and shoes routine	Self-care, social, communication, imitation objectives

ing of "teaching programs" for the therapist. While the objectives and developmental task analysis on the Daily Data Sheet dictate what *skills* should be taught in a session, the *activity* in which the skill will be taught is created by the therapist during a joint activity routine developed from a child choice. In other words, learning opportunities that target specific skills need to be created out of naturally evolving play routines. Doing this eventually becomes second nature for an experienced therapist. For therapists less experienced in the ESDM, 15 minutes of planning ahead of the session will help generate activities.

Keep in mind that there are several requirements that must be worked into every session:

- First, as stated earlier, you should try to target the acquisition and maintenance steps for every objective in each session (and of course keep data on them).
- Second, each activity should address objectives from multiple domains. This is an item on the ESDM Treatment Fidelity Rating System (Appendix B). As you plan your activities, look for multiple objectives from different domains to target within that activity.
- Every activity must target one or more communication objectives.

Planning the Flow of Joint Activities in a Session

When first using the ESDM, it helps to sketch out a rough plan for what activities you hope to create. We have developed a form for this, and a blank Intervention Session Plan has been included as Figure 6.1 that you can copy and use as a template.

1. Beginning with the child's Intervention Session Plan, teaching steps, and Daily Data Sheet in front of you, roughly sketch out one or two activities that would probably go well in each of the activity blocks on the Plan. For example, in Table 6.1, Landon's 1-hour session consists of 11 activity blocks. The session will begin and end with a greeting, with a snack somewhere in the middle, some book routines, alternating table and floor activities, and alternating object and sensory social joint activity routines. Each activity will last from 2 to 5 minutes for a younger child or a child newer to treatment, and 5 to 10 minutes for an older, experienced child, including time for clean-up and set-up, breaks, charting, and talking to the parent.

2. Examine each objective on the Daily Data Sheet for the session and use a colored highlighter to highlight the child's current acquisition step for each objective. (Note that the mastery step precedes the acquisition step for each objective. These are the two steps you will target for teaching and data collection.)

3. Start to fit the highlighted teaching steps for each objective into the various activities that you are considering in each activity block. Looking at each objective in turn, fit it into one or more activities and note it in the activity block of your Plan. Remember that you will work on objectives from multiple domains in each activity, so you can put two or three different objectives into each activity. One of these must always be a communication objective. For instance, dressing and undressing objectives may go into the greeting routines as well as water play activities. Hand washing and eating objectives are covered in snack. Picture-book activities go into the book routine activity. Fine motor activities like drawing can also involve communication (labeling the shapes you are drawing). A fine motor activity like block building can involve both a cognitive objective and a communication objective, as in building towers of different colors and having to match and sort by color and respond to receptive or expressive vocabulary targets regarding color names.

Continue working on the Intervention Plan until you have (1) two possible activities planned for each activity block on the Plan; (2) two or more objectives targeted for each

Child: ______________________________	Date: __________________
Materials needed:	
Greeting: Hello routine:	
Object activity 1:	
Sensory social routine 1:	
Object activity 2:	
Motor activity on floor: Ball activities:	

(*cont.*)

FIGURE 6.1. Intervention session plan.

Object activity 3:
Motor activity:
Books:
Snack:
Object activity 4:
Sensory social routines:
Greeting: Closing routine:

FIGURE 6.1 *(cont.)*

activity, allowing you to both review the maintenance step and teach the acquisition step; and (3) all objectives covered within the planned activities. You are almost finished planning. As the last step, list the materials you will need for each of the activities you have planned. This list will help you prepare the room before the child's session. List them at the top of the sheet, where it will be easy to refer to them as you gather or organize the items and furniture you need for this session.

Take this plan and your highlighted Daily Data Sheet into your session. The child may choose activities in a different order than you anticipated, but since you have already thought through what to do with each of the materials available, and how to work on all the objectives, it doesn't matter if the order shifts. Following the child's interests, varying the pace, location, and types of activities, and tracking your way through the Daily Data Sheet will ensure that you are working on the skills that are most important to teach.

Preparing the Room

Once your plan is ready, set up the therapy room. Gather all the materials you have listed and place them in the room, in containers, in drawers, on shelves, well organized, within reach of the child, and with all the pieces together that you need for a particular activity. Remove any materials that may derail your therapy hour: toys that the child wants to handle in a rigid way, toys that the child cannot easily part with or share, toys that do not contribute to any learning goal, or toys that are well below or above the child's developmental level. You want to have an environment in which anything the child chooses will allow you to create an activity that will target some of the child's objectives. Typically, we prepare the various locations in the room with one or two objects, so there are choices in each place. This generally facilitates child-initiated activities. Most of the materials should be out of the child's sight, but easily available to you.

Too Much Stuff?

For some children, the presence of the toys in the therapy room is a huge distraction, and the child darts from toy to toy without "landing" on any material long enough for you to create an activity. In this situation, shut away the toys and get them out two at a time, for each activity choice. Once you have finished with a material, shut it away again, or set it outside the room if you need to, so it isn't a distraction later.

Create Activity Zones

Organize the space and furniture into activity zones that correspond to the activity blocks on your Intervention Plan. Create a table activity space with a table and small chairs that fit the child well. You may want to put a small rolling cart near the table with the table activity materials in it so it is easy to have them near the table. Create a space for active play on the floor with a rug or mat and a therapy ball. Create a book area, with a beanbag chair, blanket, and books. You may want other sets of shelves or drawers by these zones. It helps tremendously to have the materials near the location you want to use them. Little ones often lose track of the goal they had when they first chose a material if they have to make a big transition across the room to a location. You want to quickly move from the choice to the beginning of the activity so that the child motivation is maintained, but you also want to vary locations for flexibility and energy.

WHEN CHILDREN AREN'T PROGRESSING: A DECISION TREE

No one teaching approach is right for each child. In this final section of the chapter, we discuss how to make decisions about changing the teaching approach in the face of poor progress. In the ESDM, we begin with naturalistic teaching because of its developmental appropriateness for young children to foster relationships, to foster social, communication, and play development, and also because of the collateral effects that naturalistic teaching has on initiation, motivation, positive affect, maintenance, and generalization. However, facilitating child learning and success is the core of the intervention, and if children are not demonstrating progress using the ESDM teaching techniques in a specified amount of time, we change teaching approaches to try to accelerate learning rates. We have typically defined progress as measurable progress on each acquisition step, as reflected on the Daily Data Sheets, in 3 to 5 days for children receiving 20 or more hours per week of individual teaching; in 1 to 2 weeks for children receiving 1 to 2 hours per day of individual teaching. Fostering learning is the bottom line. Do not let more than a couple of weeks pass without changing a teaching plan for an objective that is not showing any progress.

We have developed a decision tree to assist ESDM therapists who need to change their teaching procedures due to lack of progress on a specific teaching step of an objective. Figure 6.2 illustrates the decision tree. The section below takes you through the tree step-by-step. The initial decision to be made is whether the skill and the activities in which it can be taught contain an intrinsic reinforcer.

Is There an Intrinsic Reinforcer?

If yes, then it is appropriate for naturalistic teaching using intrinsic reinforcers. One uses the basic techniques laid out in the chapters on teaching. As long as children are showing measurable progress on a step at the rate defined above, continue to use naturalistic teaching.

No. There Is No Intrinsic Reinforcer for This Skill.

Many self-care skills have no intrinsic reinforcer (e.g., dressing, toileting, clean-up). A skill for which there is no intrinsic reinforcer will always need an extrinsic reinforcer. In this case, three separate variables can be manipulated to keep teaching as natural as possible. One adjusts teaching by adding reinforcement strength, adding structure and massing trials to the teaching episode, and adding visual or spatial supports. These are discussed in turn below.

Is There Measurable Progress?

Let us discuss this in more detail. What is the definition of *progress*? For once-weekly treatment, measurable progress may mean that the child has accomplished an acquisi-

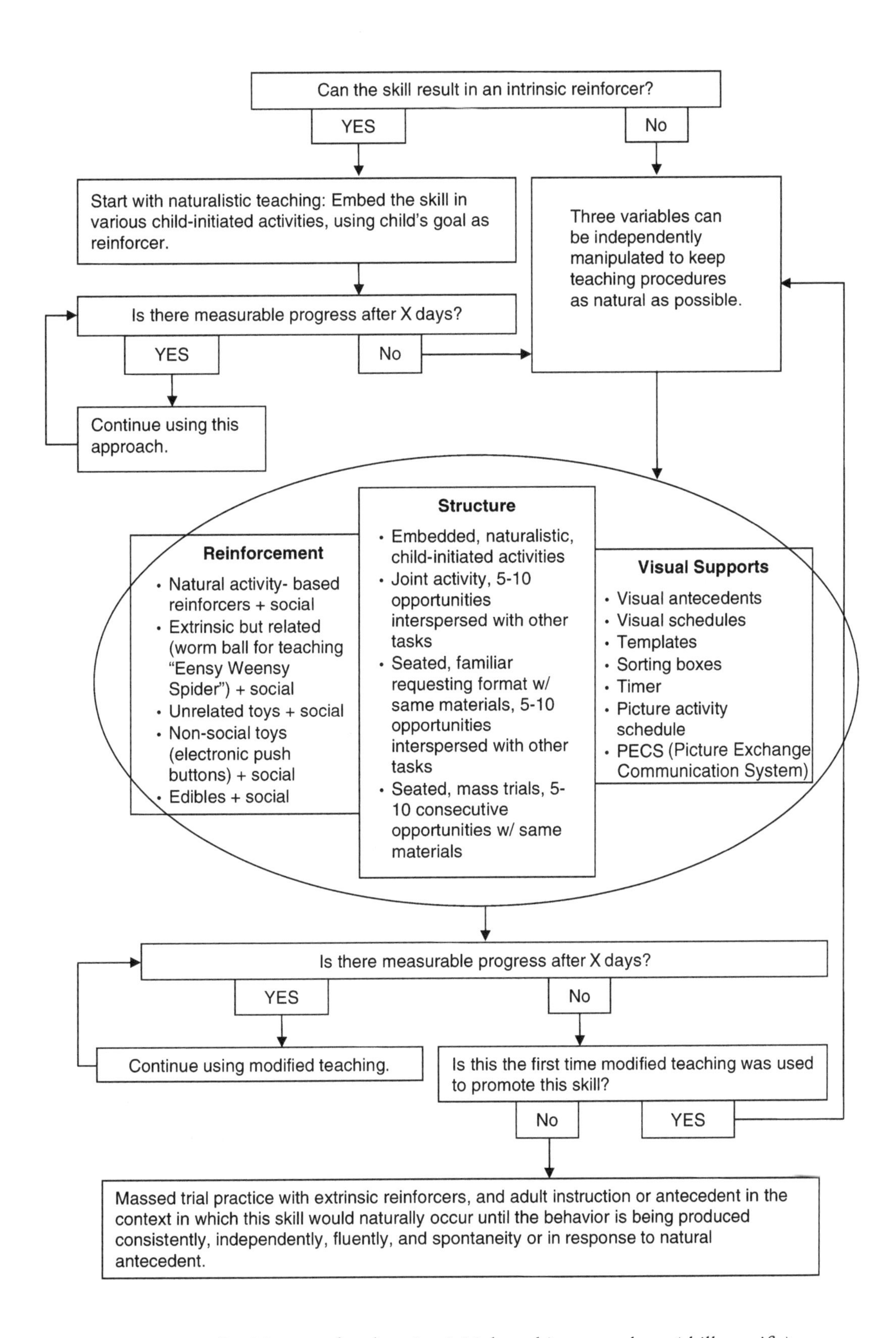

FIGURE 6.2. Decision tree for choosing initial teaching procedures (skill-specific).

tion step within two therapy sessions. If children pass each step of each objective within a 2-week period, assuming you have four to six steps for each objective, the child will completely master the objective during the 12-week period for which the objective was written—a quarter. For daily intensive treatment, one might expect a step to be mastered in two to three sessions, which may involve only 2 days. Each group using the ESDM should determine what definition of progress they are comfortable with and then establish that interval for the assessment of progress for each step of the objectives. (*Caution:* Do not let more than a couple of weeks pass without changing a teaching plan that is not showing any progress.) Continuing to work on steps for which no learning is occurring affects motivation for both children and adults.

What If There Is No Progress?

If children are not making measurable progress on a step, look at the circle in the middle of the diagram, where you will find the steps to adjust the teaching plan. There are three main ways to adjust teaching: by varying reinforcement strength, by adding structure and massing trials to the teaching episode, and by adding visual supports. Adjustments begin with a reinforcement strength hierarchy, by either finding more motivating natural reinforcers, or, if not possible, then working your way down the hierarchy to find strong reinforcers to motivate the child.

Reinforcer Strength

First consider the child's motivation for the reinforcers that are being used. Look at the hierarchy of reinforcers under the "Reinforcement" box in Figure 6.2. Is the child's motivation very strong for the materials or activity? If so, you are on the first level of reinforcement: natural activity-based reinforcers—the child's initial goal—and social attention. If the child's motivation is not very strong, the learning problem may be here.

When there is no highly motivating intrinsic reinforcer that can be developed for this teaching goal, the first set of adjustments begin with the second point under "Reinforcement," which is "extrinsic but related + social reinforcers." Our first option is to use activities as reinforcers, following the Premack principle. The Premack principle (Premack, 1959) states simply that higher-probability behaviors can be used to reinforce lower-probability behaviors. That is, a less preferred activity can be reinforced by following it with a more preferred activity. This is also known as Grandma's rule: Do your homework before you go out to play. Eat your vegetables before your dessert. In other words, for a skill such as undressing, we would follow it with a favorite activity, like water play. Similarly, we would have redressing precede a favored activity like snack. Other examples include having hand washing occur right before snack, or having toileting precede playground activities. Provided that the more preferred activity immediately follows the less preferred activity, this option generally works well for children who have been in treatment for a while and who thus anticipate activities in the schedule and enjoy these activities.

However, at the beginning of therapy, before the child has begun to anticipate or enjoy the activities, the child may progress farther and faster if you hand over preferred objects; those steps involving "unrelated toys + social reinforcement" or "electronic toys + social reinforcement," using reinforcer strength as the criterion for choosing. For children who are not very motivated by objects but are very motivated by food, then tiny bites of nutritious foods can be used along with social reinforcers. In all these examples, pair extrinsic reinforcers with social reinforcers, and use the Premack principle (Premack, 1959) to order activities. This will allow you to shift reinforcers and reinforcement schedules over the course of the child's acquisition of all the steps of a certain skill. Make plans for increasing reinforcement strength in your next session using the hierarchy above. Note these plans on your Daily Data Sheet. If the child is showing excellent motivation for the reinforcer and is consistently performing the maintenance level step for the reinforcer, then the teaching problem probably lies elsewhere.

Teaching Structure

Teaching structure refers to the level of structure in the teaching routines. We increase the structure of the teaching by adding more trials, by decreasing the variation in materials and antecedents being used, and by decreasing the number of different actions and events that are occurring in a joint activity. By decreasing the variation and increasing the consistency of the child's experience, we hope to increase the rate of child learning. Each step on this hierarchy adds adult structure to the teaching. When making these adjustments, first implement the top item in the hierarchy for the particular objective that is not progressing well. Do not change the structure for other objectives that are progressing well. Make a note on your Session Plan for changes in teaching this skill in next week's session. Implement the new step for three to four sessions and examine learning rates. If progress hasn't occurred, make the next adjustment. Continue to follow the steps involving increased structure until you determine the level of structure at which progress picks up. If you have moved through all the steps and there is still no progress, move to the next box: "Visual Supports."

Visual Supports

This is the final level of teaching adjustment. You would not reach this step until you have completed the hierarchy of steps under Teaching Structure. In this adjustment, you will consider how to change the teaching stimuli. How can you make the discrimination that is being called for in the teaching step more salient to the child? Will adding information from another sensory modality help? For auditory discrimination tasks, add visual or tactile information. For visual tasks, add tactile or kinesthetic information. For learning symbolic play scripts, add video modeling. Can you add visual clarity to the task? For receptive language tasks, can you add visual symbols? For sequencing, can you add a TEACCH-type workbasket or picture schedule approach (Schopler et al., 1995; Hodgdon, 1995)? For sorting, matching, and counting tasks, can you add visual templates? This is where the use of picture, word, or symbol schedules, picture systems, Picture Exchange Communication System (PECS) (Bondy & Frost, 1994), Treatment and Education of Autistic and Related Communication-Handicapped Children (TEACCH) adaptations, and other supports for self-regulatory or independent performance can be brought into the plan (Koegel et al., 1992; Stahmer & Schreibman, 1992; Kern, Marder, Boyajian, & Elliot, 1997).

It may seem counterintuitive to wait so long to add visual supports, massed trial teaching, or external reinforcers. However, our preference is to teach children skills that will be useful to them in everyday life and in multiple settings with multiple people. Our goal is not to develop skills so that children can perform well in the therapy session. Our goal is to develop skills that will transfer easily to home, Sunday school, and typical preschool settings. Thus, we begin by teaching children with the materials, reinforcers, and antecedents that occur in typical life settings—natural environments. We feel that this maximizes participation across environments (and thus ongoing practice of skills), maintenance of skills via the natural reinforcers available in the environment, and generalization of skills.

One reason for not using pictures to accompany language from the beginning is because we want children to develop auditory discrimination for speech. If the picture is there, then it becomes the stimulus for the behavior, and the accompanying language is neither a stimulus nor a prompt—it does not need to be attended to. By using language, gesture, or some other typical social communication as the stimulus, and carefully fading prompts, we know that children are learning to discriminate speech. While there is certainly evidence that some children with autism learn verbal language as they use picture-based systems, there is no evidence that they learn verbal language faster using PECS than using a verbal system (Yoder & Layton, 1988; Yoder & Stone, 2006)

It also takes a lot of time to implement a visual system well. Using PECS (Bondy & Frost, 1994) or using the TEACCH approach requires considerable teaching over many months. There is no evidence demonstrating that these approaches are *better* than others for developing language and other skills. Possible downsides to these approaches involve the artificiality of the materials, which limits the environments in which children will use them. A second cost is that time spent learning a visual system is time not spent learning to speak and understand speech and gesture. We feel that it is more beneficial to children to put the teaching time directly into language learning, as long as there is progress. Our data for speech development using the ESDM approach are convincing. Eighty percent or more of children treated according to the ESDM and the Denver Model principles became verbal. In our most recent study of children ages 2 or younger at the start of intensive ESDM treatment, 90% or more of children receiving the ESDM acquired verbal communication before age 5 (Dawson et al., 2010). For those few children who will not quickly progress, the decision tree will take us to the use of visual systems if they are needed to stimulate progress. Thus, we see visual and other supports and alternative communication systems as necessary for some young children with autism, but only for a few, not all.

CONCLUSION

Joint activity routines, both those with objects and those without objects, provide the platform for teaching in the ESDM. A certain type of relationship is being developed during these first steps, in which you are becoming a fun partner in the child's play, and play is becoming more fun and more interesting because of your presence. Your positioning, activity, and narration pull the child's attention toward you, and your contributions to the play are turning a solo into a duet. Have fun with these. Joint activity routines depend on positive relationships. Be creative. If an activity is becoming boring, change it. Alternate between object and sensory social routines. Vary the location of each activity. Move from the floor to the table and to the beanbag. Vary the activity level as well, from seated to moving, from more attentive to lively. Change the pace, objects, and locations with changes in sensory social routines. It helps children to stay alert, attentive, and engaged. You'll know when you are successful—the child will be watching you, extending objects to you for help, and waiting as you take a turn. Play activities are evolving into joint activity routines, marked by reciprocity, enjoyment, and shared control. The activity structure of the hour is emerging. Once we have the quality of relationship and attention and the patterns of interaction, we need to focus more specifically on instruction within these routines; we can shift to greater focus on teaching the objectives.

Developing a plan for a treatment session ensures that materials are available to support the objectives and the development of the joint activity routines that will be the frame in which you teach the objectives. The plan allows the therapist to think through activities that will target all the objectives on the Daily Data Sheet; both the current maintenance and acquisition tasks. Smooth, independent transitions between joint activities involve children in making choices, as well as in finishing and cleaning up after themselves and in planning what will come next, fostering concept learning, temporal sequences, self-regulation, and personal independence.

The structure underlying this "naturalistic" therapy is now clear. To an observer, it may look like the therapy just evolves naturally from the interaction of the child and adult. However, the playfulness of the moment belies the degree of planning and preparation that have gone into the session and the active teaching embedded in the play.

However, the bottom line is child learning. If children are not progressing steadily, the teaching strategy for that objective needs to be adapted to attain maximal progress. We have provided a decision tree that supports a systematic method for varying the instructional frame in order to attain the most rapid progress possible.

Chapter 7

Developing Imitation and Play

While all developmental objectives receive focused teaching during therapy sessions, five domains are weighted very heavily in the Denver Model: imitation, nonverbal communication (including joint attention), verbal communication, social development, and play. These receive strong emphasis first because of their role as primary, autism-specific impairments during early childhood (Rogers, 1998) and, second, because these are the fundamental tools for social learning in young children (Bruner, 1972) (and, with perhaps the exception of play, probably fundamental for social learning in humans of all ages). This chapter describes teaching approaches for imitation and play using joint activity routines.

TEACHING IMITATION

Imitation is a powerful learning tool across the age span. Once we have observed someone else act in a certain way, that behavior becomes a part of our own skill set via a process that learning theorists call observational learning (Bandura, Ross, & Ross, 1963). Imitation does not require conscious intention; we imitate automatically, outside of consciousness (the chameleon effect) (Chartrand & Bargh, 1999; Niedenthal, Barsalou, Winkielman, Krauth-Gruber, & Ric, 2005), a process sometimes called mimicry (Whiten & Ham, 1992; Tomasello, 1998). Our imitative abilities allow for easy transmission of skills, feelings, and even thoughts from one person to a social partner, and across generations. Imitation is a foundation of cultural learning, as is language (Carpenter & Tomasello, 2000). Our brains are wired for imitation in a special way, with brain cells—the mirror neurons—that link actions that we see others make to our own action patterns, just by watching (Iacoboni, 2005, 2006).

Imitation Occurs in Many Domains

Though we most often think of imitation as involving actions with objects, it actually involves a number of different types of behaviors. Through facial imitation, the child reproduces others' expressions, which appears to facilitate emotional attunement (McIntosh, 1996). Through vocal imitation, the child explores and acquires new sounds and words that will serve as a base for spoken language (Bates, Bretherton, & Snyder, 2001). Through gestural imitation, the child learns the power of communicative gestures both to express him- or herself and understand others' communicative acts. Through imitation of actions on objects, the child expands his or her thinking abilities and understanding of how humans use objects to act on the world or to express the self. Through imitation with tools, children prepare to take on adult roles involving tasks for occupation, recreation, and daily living imitation.

Imitation also involves a turn-taking exchange, in which the model and the learner alternate or reciprocate. In playful interactions, young children and their parents use imitation as a way to share topics, and they elaborate their imitations to keep the play interesting. This turn taking and theme and variation that occur in imitative exchanges between young children resemble the structure of conversation among adults. Thus, imitation in play may be important in laying down the structure of a conversation and some of the pragmatic rules (topic maintenance, taking turns) long before children have enough language to converse (Nadel, Guerini, Peze, & Rivet, 1999).

Imitation in Autism

Young children with autism, on the other hand, are not very imitative (Rogers & Williams, 2006). They are much less inclined to imitate words, gestures, and actions of others than their agemates (Rogers et al., 2003). This lack of imitation may drastically reduce their learning opportunities, and if it continues, it can be a huge impediment for learning from teachers, parents, therapists, and other children. We don't know yet why there is such a problem with imitation in autism, but we do know that young children with autism are capable of learning to imitate a wide range of behaviors in a variety of domains. Because of its important role in social and language learning, building imitation skills in youngsters with autism is a critical component of the ESDM intervention. We target (1) imitation of actions on objects; (2) imitation of body movements without objects, which we refer to as gestural imitation; (3) oral–facial imitation; and (4) vocal imitation of sounds and words. We recommend this sequence for teaching imitation.

How Do We Teach Imitation?

The basic teaching approach involves capturing children's attention with a motivating activity, modeling an action, then prompting the child to imitate before continuing the rewarding activity. We follow a series of teaching steps that come from developmental science and represent the stages that typically developing toddlers and preschoolers follow as they develop imitation skills (Piaget, 1963; McCune-Nicholich, 1977).

Actions on objects occur throughout an ESDM session, so there are many opportunities to target imitation in play. Similarly, language and vocal sounds occur throughout the session, providing many opportunities to model and imitate speech. Gestures, body postures, and facial movements require a little more planning. Facial expressions can be worked into snack and pretend play involving food: big smiles for "yummy," disgust face for "yucky." Facial expressions also work well in stories, when the adult is exaggerating the emotions involved and displaying them on both face and in voice. Using pictures in books where a character is making a clear facial expression gives the therapist the opportunity to name the emotion and model it, encouraging the child to model it.

Making silly faces can become a social game. Imitating body postures and movements can occur in games of pretense: imitating different animals (walking on all fours like a lion, hopping like a kangaroo). Pretend play also allows for pantomime, which involves imitating gestures.

Using double sets of toys can be *very* helpful for teaching novel imitations and for building automatic and rapid responding to models. Having two sets of the materials and sitting directly in front of the child provides a powerful stimulus for the child to watch your imitations of the child, as well as attending to your actions and copying them (Nadel & Peze, 1993). For some children, using the double toy scenario is the most powerful way to teach imitation. However, if the child is too focused on his or her own toys to attend to your actions on your toys, then either trade materials back and forth using a turn-taking frame, or hold back the second set until you have modeled with the first—then give the child the second set to use for imitation.

There is no particular verbal instruction for imitation. We want the adult model to be the stimulus for the imitation, not a particular verbal instruction. We may say "Look," "You do it," "Your turn," or we may not give any instruction, instead relying on the nonverbal request implicit in the demonstration to convey that the child is to copy the adult.

When teaching imitation, adults should mark the act they are modeling with language or some type of vocal sound effect. Adults typically narrate their actions in imitation tasks the same way they narrate their actions in other object play activities (discussed in more detail in the following chapters). Imitation is often about actions, though in some types of tasks (e.g., matching, for instance), it is about nouns. Mark the most salient aspects of the act with a word or short phrase that fits your language to the complexity level of the child's. Typical words are *in* or *put in, take out, bang, bounce, shake, throw, roll, stack* or *build,* and *on top*. But also, *fast, slow, big, little, clap, squeeze,* and others. Sound-effect words like *zip* work well when there is no conventional word to mark an action. For example, when modeling how to shake a pom-pom, the adult may say, "Luke, shake shake shake," in rhythm to the actions. Then, in giving the pom-poms to Luke, "Your turn," or "You do it." And then, as he shakes, "Yes, shake shake shake." Verbal children may imitate both the action and the word, *shake, shake,* and the adult would then respond with an expansion, "Yes, shake pom-pom." In the following sections, we discuss teaching approaches in more detail.

Object Imitation

For a nonimitative child, learning imitation generally progresses most rapidly in object imitation, because it has the most meaning for the child (he or she can experience the effects of the action), and it is easy to prompt. By contrast, vocal imitation is very hard to prompt. When beginning to work on object imitation, use actions that are already in the child's repertoire. You can determine these by simply observing the child in play to see how he or she handles and manipulates the objects or materials.

For example, if the child is hammering, you take a turn, hammer, and give the hammer back to the child. You might say something like, "My turn," and then "Bang bang bang" as you hit the hammer. Then, give the hammer back to the child. If the child hammers again, respond positively and say something like, "Yes! Bang bang." Let the child continue to have the hammer for a bit—don't take it back for a turn right away. That would not be a positive consequence for having imitated! If the child does not hammer, then quickly prompt the action with a full physical prompt, adding the sound effects, and then letting the child have the hammer after you have prompted—to reinforce. Is the child truly imitating you? Not necessarily. He or she may be continuing a behavior of his or her own, but is experiencing the synchrony of two persons doing the same thing; this is where imitation begins.

You would stay at this level of skill until the child is consistently imitating you after you have first imitated him or her, for many different actions. A good rule of thumb is to use 8 to 10 different actions as a criterion for when to move to the next level of difficulty.

After the child is consistently imitating 8 to 10 or more different actions that you have modeled after the child has first made the action, it is time to move to the next level of difficulty. This involves the child imitating an action that is in the child's repertoire but in response to *your* initiation of that action (e.g., in the previous step, the child first initiated the action). Now, you would model banging when you first present the hammer, before the child has had a chance to use the hammer (but of course after the child has made a choice for it, so that you know he or she wants it). Then, you would give the child the hammer, saying "You bang it," or some such phrase. If the child imitates banging, he or she gets to play with the hammer for a while. If he or she doesn't, take it back, demonstrate again, prompt to be sure imitation occurs, and then let the child have the hammer. Continue at this level until the child is imitating 8 to 10 actions in his or her repertoire when you initiate them. This represents complete mastery of the ESDM Curriculum Checklist, Level 1, Imitation item 1 (Appendix A). (See Ingersoll and Schreibman, 2006, for additional description and evidence of the effectiveness of naturalistic teaching for action imitation.)

The next level of object imitation is imitating novel actions on objects. This involves modeling an unusual (but simple) action on objects: sticking a tinkertoy stick into a play dough ball, tapping a shaker with a stick, putting a ball in the bottom hole of the maze instead of the top—simple, unusual, but interesting actions. You teach this in exactly the same way as described above. Materials that work very well for working on imitation at the level of novel actions include play dough, art activities, and complex arrays of things like train tracks and cars, blocks and cars, tinkertoys, and pretend play props. This is also a great time to bring out brand new toys for which the child has no set schemas, and everything you model will be novel. Materials that don't work well for teaching object imitation are those that the child has a very set and repetitive way of handling. Once the child is imitating well, you can then incorporate toys that are handled repetitively and use imitation to introduce more varied and flexible ways of playing with them. However, when first teaching imitation, learning will occur more quickly if you choose actions and objects that the child is more likely to handle flexibly.

Imitate and Elaborate

Once a child can imitate simple acts, imitating will be more interesting if there is some variety. Adding a new element to the imitation is often a strong attention attractor. This involves initially imitating the child's behavior and then introducing a new component to extend the play interaction and encouraging that imitation. This also supports imitating and playing with objects using multiple, flexible schemas.

For example, as the therapist and child are imitating rolling their cars back and forth, the therapist begins to drive his or her car a little closer toward the child's car and introduces some car noises (e.g., "vroom, beep beep"). Or the adult may vary the rolling action, driving his or her car in fast movements with quick stops, or crashing into the child's car or another obstacle. Another example is a pom-pom game: the adult models shaking a pom-pom and the child imitates. After this repeats a couple of times, the adult puts the pom-pom on his or her head and labels the body part (receptive language objective) while prompting imitation. The therapist then puts the pom-pom on his or her belly, labeling and prompting, and then models the pom-pom on his or her toe. The child imitates, and then the therapist puts the pom-pom in front of his or her face and pulls it away saying, "Peekaboo," which the child imitates, and the two play "Peekaboo" back and forth. The child has imitated a series of actions, each different than the last, demonstrating rapid and flexible mirroring of the adult; this level of performance represents the Curriculum Checklist Level 2, Imitation item 6. In addition, this theme and variation imitation game has become a very reinforcing sensory social routine!

To summarize, the teaching steps for object imitation will be dictated by the developmental task analysis that you write for an individual child, and each step laid out above will likely be broken down further for a child who does not imitate actions on objects yet. However, the general teaching steps involve the following:

1. *Continues an action after the model imitates it.* The adult takes a turn inside the child's actions with an object, imitates the child's action, returns the material to the child, and the child imitates the same act. Goal: Child imitates 8 to 10 different actions.
2. *Imitates a familiar action first modeled by the adult.* The adult models an action that is in the child's repertoire with this toy, not one that the child has just been using, and hands the material to the child. Goal: Child imitates 8 to 10 different familiar actions.
3. *Imitates simple novel actions.* The adult models a simple action within the child's ability but one that the child has not used on this particular object before, and hands the material to the child. Goal: Child imitates 8 to 10 different novel acts on objects.
4. *Imitates a series of different but related acts.* The adult provides a series of three or four different one-step actions, pausing between each one for the child to imitate (using double toys may facilitate this). Goal: Child quickly imitates each act in turn, and can do so for a number of sets of materials. (*Note:* The actions should fit the functional or conventional use of the materials.)
5. *Imitates a series of counterconventional acts.* This is the most mature level of object imitation that we teach preschoolers. It involves imitating actions that are at odds with the real function or conventional use of the object. Preschoolers do not prefer to do this, and it works best in a "silly format"; for example, in a pretend eating scenario with dishes, spoons, cups, and dolls, and at some point, put the bowl on your own head and call it a "hat."

Gestural Imitation

We teach gestural imitation, or imitating body movements, during meaningful activities. The two situations in which gestures are most often taught are sensory social routines, especially song routines, and conventional communicative gestures like head nods and shakes, pointing, "mine," and so on. As the child's repertoire develops, using and understanding descriptive gestures can be taught in object play to tell others to act on objects in certain ways. Typical descriptive gestures communicate put in and take out, place, turn, wait, put it here, tall, short, long, big, and little.

Imitation of Gestures in Songs and Finger Plays

Build up the child's enjoyment of your ritualized gestures in "lap games" like "Peekaboo," "So Big," "Pattycake," "Open, Shut Them," and simple songs. As soon as the child recognizes and enjoys the song or routine, begin to prompt the child to make the movements along with you, using the routine of the song itself as the "reward" for imitating the movement. Be careful about moving children through all the steps of the song by operating their hands. This can quickly develop into a passive routine, or it can lead to avoidance if the child is wary or doesn't like to be handled so much. Focus on just one movement at a time, and move from full physical prompts to partial physical prompts very quickly—after just a couple of trials or so. Prompting from the wrists, elbows, or upper arms rather than the hands can also help avoid prompt dependence.

Beware!

If children are offering their hands to you (instead of trying to make the correct gesture) during a song at a point at which you always provide a hand-over-hand prompt, you know what has happened! Lack of prompt fading! One way to fade is to move your hands up the child's arms, away from his or her hands. Do this quickly, as soon as you have moved his or her hands a few times.

Don't keep prompting to get the child's imitations more accurate. It is better that the child is making the imitation sloppily independently than making it perfectly but need prompting for a long time to do so. You can always shape a sloppy imitation later. Getting children to independently imitate gestures as quickly as possible is the most important part of the teaching in the beginning phases.

When teaching children to put an action into a song, stop the song after the modeled gesture and wait for the child to imitate it (prompting as needed) before continuing the song, so that the continuation of the song is the reinforcer for attempting the imitation. (Pick songs the child really likes!) Children who can produce some sounds will often begin to hum along and imitate some words of the song. As they begin to pick up the words, we can prompt them to imitate a word or fill in a pause in the song, waiting for them to speak before continuing, and thus develop a language routine as well as an imitative gesture routine in the song.

Beware of dragging out the song while waiting for the child to respond. Slowing the song and waiting may make it boring and so may lose the child's interest. Prompt fast while you are singing, or put your model slightly earlier in the song so the child's imitation happens on the right beat. Then, you don't have to stop and wait.

Oral–Facial Imitation

Oral–facial imitations are quite difficult for many young children with autism to learn. However, we have found them to be quite important for developing vocal imitation for children who do not do this spontaneously. In such children oral–facial imitation needs to be carefully developed.

Begin after the Child Imitates Many Manual Actions

We have found it most successful to begin to emphasize facial imitation after the child fluidly, independently, and consistently imitates 8 to 10 or more body actions. We provide stimuli for facial imitation from the beginning: in exaggerated blows for bubbles, in song routines, in making funny faces and animal noises during book routines, mirror play, and so on. If children begin to imitate these, they are always reinforced.

Use Activities Involving Body Parts

An easy frame for beginning to teach oral–facial movements is to use games and activities involving body parts. Teach children to touch their nose, touch their tongue, pat their cheeks, pat their mouth, pat their ears, pat their head, touch their teeth, or blow a kiss as part of songs and body part games. These can be developed as joint activities supported by a variety of activities in which body parts are a theme: books, bath activities with dolls and animals, and songs ("If you're happy and you know it, touch your nose!"). Some therapists find a mirror a useful additional tool for teaching oral–facial imitations, but others find using mirrors more difficult than teaching face-to-face, because the child now has two stimuli to attend to—the therapist's face in the mirror and the child's face in the mirror. However, if progress is not coming quickly, by all means try a mirror! Also, if the child already makes facial movements in a mirror, then use the mirror as a scaffold for developing imitation with you.

Use specific oral–facial gestures with the sensory social toys and begin to expect the child to imitate them as a request. Model actions like puffing cheeks and blowing before you blow a balloon, bubbles, pinwheel, or a feather. Over time, children will generally begin to imitate these facial gestures as a way of requesting the blowing action. Many children with autism will enjoy your silly displays of raspberries, tongue wiggles, lip smacks (during eating routines), and snorting with your nose when making pig noises, and these can become antecedents for facial imitation as well. Blowing kisses and giving hugs at the end of the goodbye routine can be a good activity for imitating kisses and other affectionate behavior.

Teach Gestural Imitation for Conventional Gestures

After children can imitate novel gestures of face, head, and body, they have the prerequisites for learning conventional gestures through imitation. To teach them, pair the gesture to be taught with the communicative behavior the child already has to express that pragmatic function (if the child has not developed a natural gesture to express basic communications for protest, request, interest, and social interaction, those should be developed first—see Chapter 8 on nonverbal communication). Set up an activity that will allow you to elicit the child's existing communicative gesture that expresses that function (like pushing away an unwanted food). Once the child produces the communication, hold back the reinforcer, model the desired gesture (exaggerate it), and prompt the child to imitate you. Reinforce immediately. Now you have paired the child's existing gesture with the new, conventional gesture, and the reinforcer has followed the conventional gesture. After repeated trials, once the child imitates the gesture easily, begin to fade your model (the prompt), but be sure to use the gesture in your own communications frequently. The communicative intent is the actual antecedent for the gesture. Don't require gesturing at every opportunity; that would be unnatural.

For example, Nicky has learned to say "No" when offered an unwanted food. The objective is to teach the conventional "no" head shake. During snack, Kayla offers Nicky a carrot (which he dislikes!) while asking, "Do you want a carrot?" and he says, "No." She models, "No carrot" with an exaggerated head shake, while continuing to offer the carrot. He then says "No" again and shakes his head a little, so she immediately withdraws the carrot, while shaking her head and saying, "Nicky said no-o-o carrot." (Note that withdrawing the disliked carrot is a negative reinforcement paradigm.)

If Nicky had not imitated the head shake, Kayla would have prompted once again. If he again had said, "No" without the head shake, she would immediately give an imitation instruction involving the head shake. She would say, "Nicky, do this," while shaking her head vigorously. As soon as he imitates the head shake, she will withdraw the carrot while repeating, "No carrot," with head shake, and then she would offer the choice of a preferred food.

Vocal Imitation

Vocal/verbal imitation is probably the single most important skill we can teach to a nonspeaking child, but for a child who does not imitate sounds, it is one of the hardest skills to teach. Vocal imitation is necessary for learning to speak. For the relatively silent child, vocal imitation is built up over a long series of steps.

Increase Vocalizations

Highly arousing sensory social activities are often the best ways of stimulating any type of vocalization. "Creepy Fingers" games and others involving high suspense often stimulate children to vocalize. When the child vocalizes, imitate the child immediately and provide the reinforcing action. If you can elicit a vocalization in a sensory social routine, incorporate your imitation of the child's sound into the game. For relatively silent children, be sure to reinforce any vocalization other than crying, screaming, and fussing, and reward the vocalization more strongly than any other child behavior (differential reinforcement of vocalizations). Make sure that the vocalization gets the strongest, fastest reward, and the rewards are the desired object or activity. This is true even if the sound the child made seemed unintentional. For children who seldom vocalize, teaching vocal imitation will require that you first increase the rate of vocalizations and develop intentional vocalization.

Imitate Child's Actions and Vocalizations

Imitate children when they are acting on objects and vocalizing. When we imitate them, we capture the child's attention and create the opportunity for an imitation game in which child and adult imitate each other back and forth. They seem to become more aware of the other person and more inclined to imitate the other person when the other person is also imitating them (Dawson & Galpert, 1990). Once this game becomes familiar, the adult can begin the schema that has been the basis for the imitation game and the child will join in. Through these repeated exchanges, the child will learn to imitate more and more behaviors and sounds.

Develop Imitative Vocal Rounds

As the child's vocalizations increase and you are consistently imitating them, you will begin to recognize vocal rounds occurring, in which the child vocalizes, you vocalize in response, and the child then vocalizes again. This is a very positive step and of course you will differentially reinforce these with the desired object or activity. However, your vocal response itself may well be the reinforcement. If the child is looking at you, waiting expectantly for you to imitate, and then repeating it, you know that your vocalization is the reward. Note that this step parallels the initial step of teaching action imitation, in which the therapist imitates an action that the child has just made. Once vocal rounds occur consistently, you are ready to take the child to the next step: imitation of sounds in the child's vocal repertoire.

Initiate Well-Established Vocalizations

Up until now, the child has been beginning the vocal rounds. The next step involves the therapist beginning the vocal rounds, using sounds from the rounds that you and the child have been doing previously, to see whether the child will imitate the sound. To initiate the vocal round, use the same type of physical game or physical positioning that supported these sounds before. Position the child for the activity, get the child's gaze, produce the vocalization, and look expectantly. If the child doesn't produce it, try it again, with a little of the accompanying action. If still no luck, then proceed with the game as usual and continue your work on the previous step with imitative vocal rounds. Eventually, the child will begin to imitate you when you begin the vocal rounds.

Increase Differentiated Vocalizations

In order for children to begin to imitate speech, we need both frequent vocalizations and a range of vocalizations, both vowels and consonants, which should be spelled out in the child's objectives and on the Daily Data Sheet (see Chapter 5, Figure 5.2). Listen and record the vowel sounds and the consonant sounds you hear in each session. For new sounds just coming into a child's repertoire, differentially reinforce them with the preferred object or activity. In addition to imitating children's sounds as the child produces them, try to work the child's new sounds into the narrative of your play. That is, try to fit the child's sounds with a conventional word used in a favored activity. If you are playing cars and the child babbles "za za," imitate it right back and then work the sound into "zoom zoom" combined with a fast zip of the car toward the child. Make the vocalization a part of the object game, paired with the action. If the child makes a "bababa" vocalization, interpret it as "ball," "balloon," or "bubble," imitate it back, and immediately get the favorite material to begin the activity. If you are modeling "more" and you get "aah," switch to "yeah!" and try to get another imitation, which you then reinforce.

Don't expect the child to imitate novel sounds. Vocal imitation should always build from sounds already in the child's repertoire. Picking your targets for vocal imitation from the child's already existing vocal repertoire allows the child to focus on producing a familiar sound in a specific context.

When the Child Does Not Produce Phonemes

If the child does not spontaneously produce phonemes (i.e., speech-like syllables that contain both a consonant and a vowel), you will have to build them up. It is possible to help children develop new phonemes using their own ability to imitate some sounds and combining this with oral–facial imitation. In all these cases, work with a speech pathologist to choose the best sounds with which to begin. (*Note:* If the child needs intensive help to produce phonemes, he or she may well benefit from a speech therapy approach like PROMPT [Hayden, 2004], which targets speech dyspraxia.) Refer the child to a speech pathologist who is skilled in treating children with severe difficulty producing speech sounds. Then, incorporate the recommendations from the speech pathologist for developing phonemes in your treatment.

Use Meaningful Contexts and Sounds

The purpose of building vocal imitation is to develop meaningful speech related to activities. Vocal imitation should fit meaningfully into a joint activity. The vocal imitation should highlight a word or a sound effect related to the routine. If the context is a joint activity with objects, the sound needs to resemble a word or sound effect that is congruent with the routine. Of course, vocal imitative play is an enjoyable social routine for many toddlers developing speech, and it can be a sensory social routine in its own right. Remember to reinforce all sounds with a desired object or activity.

Don't Emphasize Articulation

There is a very wide range of imitative accuracy in vocalizations among beginning speakers. Don't expect children to have mature articulation; reward vocal approximations strongly. Remember how long it takes typically developing children to speak clearly. The speech pathologist on the child's team should see the child at regular intervals. Direct concerns about articulation to the speech pathologist, who has the expertise to evaluate the child's articulation and to treat or guide the treatment of articulation if needed. Articulation improves over time, through experience with speech. Learning to produce more sounds and words is the primary way that articulation increases in beginning talkers.

Don't Emphasize Imitating Multiword Utterances for Beginning Speakers

For children with excellent verbal imitation skills, it is very tempting to use their imitation to chain together multiword sentences. *Don't do this!* For children who primarily imitate speech rather than initiate it, the most important thing you can do is to foster single-word initiations. Follow the one-up rule that states that the therapist's mean length of utterance (MLU) should equal the child's MLU + 1. This refers to the child's spontaneous, generative verbal productions—not echoed phrases. We feel that using imitation to build sentence length in primarily echolalic speakers actually reinforces echoing and impedes the child's ability to learn the communicative power of speech.

Repeat but Don't Drill

Motor actions require repetition in order to establish and strengthen the neural connections underlying them (Vidoni & Boyd, 2008; Remy, Wenderoth, Lipkins, & Swinnen, 2008). In both gestural and vocal imitation, try to get several repetitions quickly. However, if the task has been difficult for the child, don't ask for it to be repeated immediately. Shift to an easy action (remember to alternate acquisition and mastery). Do not worry if the child needs some prompts after he or she has done a difficult imitation once independently—reward these fully. Be sure to keep motivation very high with strongly preferred objects and activities. If motivation is flagging, don't try to get an imitation. Shift your focus to building up the child's motivation. Try to prevent failures from occurring; add a prompt or target an easier imitation quickly. Imitation is such an important skill that we have to make sure it does not become an unpleasant or overly difficult activity for children.

TEACHING PLAY SKILLS

Teaching play skills is actually a subset of teaching imitation on objects. We use imitation as the primary tool for teaching play skills, inside the same child-initiated format described above. Sensorimotor play is part and parcel of the routines used for teaching object imitations, and sensorimotor play and object imitation fit together nicely in joint activities with objects.

Teaching Spontaneous Sensorimotor Play Acts

Teaching sensorimotor play follows exactly the procedures described above for teaching imitation of actions on objects. The only difference is that the goal of sensorimotor play is child initiation of the action pattern. In object imitation, the goal is imitation only. To teach specific sensorimotor play schemas:

1. First, use the object imitation format described above to teach the child how to do the target action on the object.

2. Once children can imitate the target action, present the materials without modeling the target act, in order to give the child the opportunity to initiate the action spontaneously. If the child does so, reinforce with continued play by giving an additional object, helping or imitating the child, and providing social attention.

3. If the child does not initiate the target act, model the action briefly, or pantomime it, or begin it without finishing, so that you are using the least amount of prompting the child needs: a least-to-most prompt hierarchy. Continued play with the toy is the reward for demonstrating the target act.

Teaching Functional Play Acts

A functional play act involves using an object in a socially conventional manner. This is an important step in play development, because it means that the child has learned certain actions from watching other people and/or from self-experiences with others (like having one's hair brushed by the parent). Thus, in functional play, the child carries out these social uses of a toy or other object, rather than more perceptually based actions (like stroking the brush bristles with the fingers). The object now has a culturally defined meaning for the child as opposed to a perceptually based meaning.

For example, consider a tissue. The most interesting perceptual attribute about a tissue for a young child is either the fact that it shreds so easily or the fact that when one is pulled out of the box, another pops up and can be pulled out. Thus, when a toddler pulls a tissue out and puts it to his or her nose, instead of doing one of these more perceptually based actions, we see him or her acting out a social convention with the tissue, which illustrates our definition of functional play (Ungerer & Sigman, 1981).

To teach a child to use a functional play act, introduce the functional play schema as a *variation or elaboration* of sensorimotor play. Offer the child a container holding functional play objects like a car, toy animal, comb, brush, cup, fork, tissue, hat, beads, mirror, sunglasses, toothbrush, toy food, and so on. It's helpful to have doubles of these objects in the box, so that you have an identical object to use for modeling—the "double toy" or parallel play approach. If the child shows interest, allow him or her to choose an object and explore it, just as in any other object play routine. If the child uses it conventionally, the adult admires and imitates the child. If the child does not, for the adult's turn, the adult models a conventional action with the object, using relevant words or sound effects (e.g., "brush hair"; "zoom zoom" while rolling the car fast; drinking noises with cup, "yum, good juice"), and then hands the object back to the child to imitate, prompting, shaping, and fading prompts just as in teaching any object imitation, until the child imitates the functional action easily and independently.

Once this happens easily through imitation, begin to work on spontaneous production of the functional play act, in the same way we just discussed involving spontaneous sensorimotor play. Present the object to the child and wait, or make the sound effect. If the child produces the functional act, show enthusiasm and imitate or elaborate it into a dyadic game (using double sets of materials will be quite helpful for this). If the child does not produce the functional act spontaneously, then take a turn, model the functional act very briefly, and give the object back to the child. Use least-to-most prompt hierarchies involving modeling to foster spontaneous use of functional schemas in children's initial exploration of the task. If the child produces them, mark them enthusiastically with sound effects and praise, and elaborate it, using your own response, or acting it out on dolls or animals, as a way of elaborating the play.

Role Reversal in Functional Play

As you model functional play acts, model on both yourself and the child. As the child takes the object, prompt him or her to act on you with the object, as well as on him- or herself. Encourage role reversal games where you put the hat on the child, and the child puts the hat on you. Hats, beads, brushes, cups, and spoons work very well for role reversal. Experiment with double toy sets and see whether they are helpful. As you practice the role reversal of these, use proper names or pronouns, depending on the child's objectives in this area. After the child is successfully imitating these actions and also initiating these functional actions on objects on the self and with you, bring a large doll or a teddy bear or other animal into this play. Model functional acts with these toys, always with simple narrative language, and encourage and prompt the child to "feed Poo," "brush teddy," "hat for baby, hat for me," and so on. Now, you have the fundamentals that you need for teaching symbolic play, as well as for simple interactive play. You also have a great frame for teaching pronoun use and agent–action–object relations!

Parallel Play Skills

Parallel play is one type of peer play that occurs frequently in toddlers. It essentially involves two children, each with similar materials doing similar actions in parallel (Parten, 1933). It appears in the curriculum as a Level 3 skill. In your imitation teaching using a double toy scenario you have already taught the child to carry out parallel play with you. The work that you did on imitation of familiar actions, novel actions, and actions in a series has already taught the child how to carry out parallel play with an adult. Once the child has developed that foundation, you can transfer, or generalize these skills, to focus on another child as the play partner.

Using a double set of toys is *very* powerful for focusing the attention of the child with autism on the peer; this is the natural format for parallel play in typically developing children. Position the child with ASD across from their typical peer at a small table so that each child is at eye level with the other and near enough to touch each other's toys. This reduces the visual attention shifts required of the child with ASD to observe the peer and seems to enhance the salience of the peer's actions for the child with ASD. Let the children choose materials and give them each the same materials. Adults should then reduce their activity so that there is no source of interference for the children's attention to each other. Wait a little and see how the play begins. Provide additional props or play ideas for the typical peer if the play starts to seem repetitive or boring, and if needed, help focus the child with autism's attention on the peer. If the peer has highly interesting materials and is combining them in interesting ways, the child with ASD is likely to imitate spontaneously, since this will have been very well mastered with adults during Levels 1 and 2. If not, then the same teaching approach will be used as has been used previously, with adults prompting peer imitation, rewarding it by giving the child freedom with the materials, and differentially rewarding spontaneous imitation of the peer. Be sure that the child with autism also has interesting props so that the typical peer will imitate him or her. In parallel play, the leader and follower roles shift fluidly.

Teaching Symbolic Play Acts

Symbolic play involves building more abstract representational aspects of conventional play (McCune-Nicholich, 1977), and you will teach symbolic play in a similar fashion as we have just discussed for functional play. There are three classes of symbolic play schemes on which we focus: (1) using dolls and animals as agents, (2) making symbolic substitutions in which an object is used as if it were something else, and (3) symbolic combinations in which the play contains several different symbolic actions sequenced together in a meaningful way (McCune-Nicolich, 1977). When teaching these, use an interesting set of realistic props and a large doll and stuffed animal so that there are enough materials that you can create an interesting scene. Use multiple nonidentical objects to promote generalization. Embed the target skill you are teaching into a little play scene with the props; create a richer format than the child can currently produce. As in other naturalistic teaching, you will embed the teaching into a joint activity that you and the child will co-create with the materials.

Using Dolls as Agents

To teach acting on dolls or stuffed animals, the adult first models a functional action that is already in the child's repertoire. The action will involve a functional act directed first to the adult and then to a particular "other," and the adult will name both action and the other ("feed kitty," "give baby drink," "comb Poo's hair"). Next, hand the object to the child, and verbally prompt the child to follow through: "Joshua feed kitty," Joshua give baby a drink." If the child does not respond to the verbal request, follow through with prompts, and then fade prompts until the child acts independently.

To go from imitation to spontaneous acts, begin when the child has mastered these acts as imitations. Provide the materials and other related realistic props to the child without modeling, and wait, looking interested. Provide a verbal script (e.g., "It's dinner time." "Baby is hungry!" "Baby wants to eat!"). If the child produces a spontaneous act, comment on it and join in with a related act. If the child does not spontaneously produce a functional action on the other, then prompt, using a least-to-most hierarchy involving verbal instructions, then a brief model, and so on. Such acts constitute the beginning of symbolic play.

Once the child easily produces multiple spontaneous acts in which the child is acting on a doll or animal, begin to model how the "other" can be the actor. Now, the doll or the animal does the feeding, combing, playing, coloring, to you and to the child with an appropriate narrative. Take the child through the same steps as above, first developing the child's ability to imitate this, and then fostering the child's spontaneous acts involving the other as an animate being.

Teaching Object Substitution

To teach use of substitute objects, choose a theme and props that are very well understood by the child. Spoons, cups, and baby bottles are the type of extremely common objects that work well when beginning this teaching. Set the stage for the play by first setting up a play theme with appropriate objects and agents (e.g., dolls, animals, self, mother, child) and have the child spontaneously or imitatively produce the target act with real objects to set the theme. Then, repeat with miniature but highly realistic materials.

If the child easily uses the miniature as a realistic substitute, immediately repeat the target action but now with a neutral, or placeholder, object—an object that has no specific function of its own and is roughly the same size and shape as the object it represents. A cylinder-shaped block is a neutral object. A cylinder-shaped cup is not; it has a functional definition as a drinking utensil. As you repeat the target action with the neutral object, continue to narrate the acts. For example, if the goal is for the child to use a small cylinder block to pretend it is a baby bottle, have the block, bottle, and baby present. First, model feeding the baby with the real bottle, and have the child imitate. Then, immediately follow with the miniature bottle. If the child plays appropriately with the miniature, follow with the placeholder, modeling feeding the baby with the block, calling it a bottle, and have the child imitate. Using a mix of real, miniature, and neutral objects in pretend play activities facilitates symbolic play.

After children use neutral objects easily to substitute for real ones, you can use the same process to go from neutral objects to pantomime—the use of objects represented only by gesture (imagine a 2-year-old feeding you an "invisible" cookie from a plate; that is pantomime). Practice with the realistic object first, with the child imitating, and then model the pantomimed action on the child with your hand, and have the child imitate the pantomime to you. Using one's hand as a hammer, toothbrush, baby, comb or brush, spoon, or keys are common early pantomimes for preschoolers. Since the child has already learned to imitate gestures in the imitation program, and since you have brought these concepts carefully along, this is not a huge leap, and children with ASD should move smoothly through this sequence, taught in Levels 3 and 4 of the ESDM Curriculum.

To move from imitated to spontaneous acts, provide the child with a set of toys in which most are realistic but a key object is missing, although an ambiguous object that could be substituted is present (e.g., in an eating scenario, a spoon might be missing but a tongue depressor is present). Give the child the props and begin to construct a relevant play scene. As the play evolves, see whether the child uses the ambiguous object symbolically. If not, hand the ambiguous object to the child and ask the child to feed the baby, comb the baby's hair, and so on. Children generally prefer to use realistic props rather than ambiguous ones, so you may have to set the stage a little in order to encourage the child to use the prop as a substitute. You can also feign ignorance, as in, "I need a spoon to feed the baby. There are no spoons. What can I use?" Hopefully, the child will produce the prop. If not, hold it up and ask, "Can this be a spoon?" and see whether the child will then use it.

Teaching Symbolic Combinations

The last category of symbolic play is symbolic combinations, or sequences of related play acts that together play out a theme from life. Begin to teach this once children have mastered imitating and are spontaneously producing several different single symbolic acts to a specific object—the prerequisite skill for combinations. In your turn, model two linked acts—acts that occur together in the scenario you are acting out (e.g., pour from pitcher to cup, then drink from the cup), while narrating, "Pour the juice, drink juice, yum, good juice," and then give the child the props and cue the child, "Get some juice," using prompts as needed to ensure success. Double toys can work well here to prompt the child through imitation. Since you have been using thematic play as the joint activity for all these symbolic acts, you will have been demonstrating combinations to the child for quite a while. It is not a big leap for children to move from single acts to sequenced acts, especially when they have been observing and participating in elaborated play routines for a while.

Through all these activities, consciously elaborate and vary them, so the child is learning many appropriate pretend play schemas that can be used flexibly in elaborated pretend play. Elaborate by adding more props and characters to the scene, like when eating and drinking, involve pouring and stirring the drinks and serving the food to be eaten. You can also elaborate by adding related schemas—setting the table before the food, or cleaning up and washing dishes after (use real water and soap in a plastic dishpan and see how much fun that is for the child!).

Choosing Themes for Symbolic and Functional Play

The child must have already lived through the scenarios and know the actions and objects in real life in order for them to have meaning in play. Choose materials to fit a real-life theme, and choose as themes life events that the child has lived through many times. Meals, baths, cooking, bedtime, hairbrushing, toothbrushing, singing songs and doing finger plays, and playing with toys are themes that young children with autism know well. Doll routines have special meaning for children with infant siblings at home. Knowing what activities the child has experienced in real life helps build skills. Play out a zoo theme after the child has gone to the zoo. Play out a doctor visit after the child's annual physical and birthdays after a birthday party. Favorite books contain stories that children will know. Routines learned at preschool or therapy can be scripts: circle time, snack time, and various songs.

Once the child has learned to use substitute objects, link schemas together, and carry out acts on dolls, we want to give children many scenarios or scripts for symbolic play activities, so that they can participate with other preschoolers. (See Goldstein, Wickstrom, Hoyson, Jamieson, and Odom, 1988, for a detailed description. Scripts can also come from books, and books can also be an excellent intermediary between real-life experiences and symbolic play as another way of helping children learn the scripts.)

Teaching Role Play

For some adults, creating the scripts for symbolic play comes very easily, and they have no problem thinking about what props to use, what to say, and what actions to model. For others, this is a difficult task. However, there are several steps therapists can take to prepare themselves. Over time and with experience of many different scenarios, this becomes much easier. Here are some suggestions for preparing for symbolic play activities.

Develop the Story Line

How do you build a story line or play script? A script lays out a life event from the child's perspective: the actions, objects, words, people, and interactions that define this activity and make it different from all others. Think it through from the child's perspective. Going to McDonald's involves at least three people: child, parent, and counter person. The main actions are (1) walking in through the door, (2) standing in line behind other people, (3) asking for your food or giving your order to the counter person, (4) giving the money to the counter person, (5) getting the food from the counter person, (6) walking to a table with your food and sitting down, (7) opening the food and eating, (8) standing up and throwing away your litter, and (9) leaving. Each of these involves a few words, a few objects, and another person. Write them down for yourself, along with the essential props and words that mark each action. Once children can do all the above routines, they are ready to learn more elaborated thematic play including roles. Here are some steps for teaching it.

Build a Storyboard

Together with the child draw a storybook or make a felt-board story. We use the McDonald's scenario above as an example. This is a good way to prepare a child for the experience. Draw nine pictures or take nine photos of the child, the other person, and the relevant object, each with a phrase or sentence to describe the action. The length and complexity of the phrases or sentences should be based on the child's current language level. You have now produced the script for this pretend play scenario.

Preparing simple storyboards with children is excellent preparation for complex symbolic play scenes, and you have also produced a "social story" for the child (Gray & Garand, 1993). Assemble the pictures in a book and "read" it through with the child several times to familiarize him or her with the sequence. Once the child knows the book, take the pictures out and mix them up. Then, have the child help you order them, using "first," "next," and "last" terms: "What do we do first? First, we walk into McDonald's. Then, we stand in line," and so on. Ordering the pictures emphasizes the temporal sequence.

Next, Act It Out with Characters

You can act out this story with characters and props in treatment. The first time, act it out for the child, using small dolls to represent the people, and dollhouse furniture and blocks for props. After you have read through a storybook with the child a few times (allowing the child to fill in words and narrate as he or she learns the story), act out the book with the characters and props. Go fast enough to hold the child's interest. The child may say some of the script as you go along. Use the same ritual phrases that you used in the book. Adhere tightly to the book when you first act it out. After the child has seen it a couple of times, begin to shift some of the script and props to the child. Have the child start to fill in some of the child's role, and you take the counter person's role or parent's role. After the child knows the rudiments of the child's role, have the child be the counter person, taking on both script and actions. You can use the first, next, and last language that you used with the pictures to narrate.

Finally, Act It Out Yourselves

Set up the therapy room so there are the essential props: a counter with cash register, tray, bag with some props inside, table, chairs, and trash can. Walk the child through it, switching between the adult roles of parent and counter person while the child takes the child role. Prompt the verbal script and the sequence of events. Make sure the child eventually learns all three roles. The child can learn the parent role and eventually use a doll for the child.

Use This Approach to Prepare for New Experiences

Once children understand symbolic play, have some language, and can generate acts independently, you can use this kind of symbolic play to prepare children for unfamiliar real-life events. Practice birthday party, practice dentist and doctor visits, and practice greetings between dolls so children can learn the social scripts that go with these routines. Practice empathy responses when a doll gets "hurt." Pretend play routines can also be used to practice fearful situations and provide some desensitization for phobias: a first airplane ride, a trip to the hospital, first day of a new group program, going to church, a new baby in the family, or adjusting to a new pet. Symbolic play can also be used to help children practice group games and activities. Learning the rules for "Duck, Duck Goose," "Hello Circle," or "Musical Chairs" can be fun and extremely helpful when written up as a storyboard, played out with dolls, and roles played with familiar people. Children can use imitation to learn both the action scripts and the verbal scripts. (This is how we all learn social scripts, but most children learn the scripts from natural life examples. Children with autism need more practice than most children). Preschoolers tend to enjoy dollhouse dolls and furniture, and these materials can be used to play out all kinds of events and scripts that occur in daily life for typically developing children.

Symbolic play, once developed, can thus have the same functions for children with autism that it does for children without autism—assimilating real-life situations.

CONCLUSION

We have laid out the main methods for teaching object, gestural, oral–facial, and verbal imitation, and we have described how to use imitation skills to build sensory motor, functional, and symbolic play. This approach uses meaningful and preferred activities, with appropriate language and careful use of ABC teaching in which the reinforcing consequences involve access to preferred activities and objects. We have not been explicit about the need to keep the affect lively and positive, and the need to maintain children's levels of arousal and attention at optimum levels for learning, but this is only because we trust that the readers understand that to be a part of all treatment inside the ESDM.

Chapter 8

Developing Nonverbal Communication

While most people think of communication as synonymous with verbal language, there is much more than speech involved. Infants and toddlers develop a variety of ways to communicate before they begin to speak. They use eye contact, facial expressions, gestures, body postures, and vocal sounds to get their message across, and they become very skilled communicators in this nonverbal communication system before formal speech develops. Speech becomes an additional communication system. It is built on top of an already very functional nonverbal communication system involving "talking bodies." Gestures—nonverbal communication behaviors—provide an expressive system for children to convey their meanings to others. Gestures involve motor acts of fingers, hands, whole body, and face, displayed with the intent to communicate to a partner (Crais, Douglas, & Campbell, 2004). Toddlers also learn to comprehend others' nonverbal communication signals, reading their "talking bodies," and interpreting a partner's meanings and intentions. Reading bodies means reading minds!

Intentional communication sends a message about what is in the speaker's mind, and the thoughts, feelings, and goals of the speaker in communicating. The speaker's goals in communicating are the pragmatic functions of the speaker's communications. Some common pragmatic functions that we express to young children include gaining their attention, sharing interest and other emotions with them, interacting socially just for the pleasure of interacting, providing help to them, and placing demands on them to change their behavior in some way. Teaching communication to young children with ASD involves teaching not only the forms of communication—the sounds, words, gestures, and their combinations—but also the range of messages, or pragmatic functions, that can be communicated. Young children's early communication goals also include sharing interest, attention, and emotions about events (these serve the pragmatic function of joint attention); interacting socially (the pragmatic function of social interaction); and demanding certain behaviors from us (the pragmatic function of behavior regulation) (Bruner, 1981b).

This chapter describes the main teaching procedures used in the ESDM to develop intentional nonverbal communication and coordinated attention skills to express these three main pragmatic functions in young children with ASD. Chapter 9 addresses verbal communication.

COORDINATING ATTENTION UNDERLIES COMMUNICATION

The large body of research on the early development of communication indicates that coordinated attention between infant and caregiver is foundational to communication development. Typically developing infants as young as 3–6 months of age sustain short episodes of coordinated attention with their caregivers (Legerstee, Markova, & Fisher, 2007). They exchange social signals through gaze, voice, and facial and body movements in coordinated and reciprocal exchanges that convey emotional information to their partners, even though infants have not yet developed intentional communicative acts. Infants also pick up emotional messages that their partners send to them. The very act of attending to a social partner via eye contact and shared attention is considered to be the beginning of enveloping a child in the "common culture" of social interaction. This forms the basis of communication and the basis for passing on a culture from one generation to the next (Vygotsky, 1978). This dyadic capacity to attend to a partner and interact reciprocally has typically not developed well in young children with autism (Maestro et al., 2002), and it marks the initial communication and social skill that will be taught in the ESDM curriculum.

Coordinated attention is a precursor to joint attention. The latter may be described as an opportunity for a child and a communication partner to share a focus of interest to include a common object or event. Bruner best explained that "joint attention is not just joint attention, but joint participation in a common culture" (1995, p. 12)

Joint attention involves an intentional communicative act. The child has something in mind that he or she wants to share with another person, and intentionally behaves in some way to capture the other's attention and convey the message the child wants to share. Thus, joint attention involves sharing of mental states with another and demonstrates the toddler's awareness of the mind of the partner (Bruner, 1995). Joint attention is a main vehicle for learning language from others, because the nonverbal meaning that is being shared in the exchange maps onto the words that are being used. When a child directs an adult's attention to something of interest to the child, the adult responds with the relevant spoken language, and the child can map the new words onto the meaning already present in the child's mind. Conversely, when an adult directs a child's attention, the child's attention to the adult and understanding of the event the adult is sharing provides the meanings that the child needs to map onto the words that are being heard. Joint attention is an area of weakness for children with autism. Thus, not only do children with autism demonstrate ineffective communication with others, but they are isolated from the common culture of social interaction (Mundy & Neal, 2001). Joint attention is specifically developed inside the curriculum, as soon as children have learned to coordinate and sustain attention with an adult.

The ESDM develops joint attention and builds nonverbal communication skills in two stages. In the first stage, the focus is on developing natural gestures that the child can use for all three main communicative functions—behavior regulation (requests and protests), social interaction (beginning and maintaining dyadic social activities), and joint attention (sharing attention with a partner about an object or event). In the second stage, children will learn conventional gestures—those that anyone in our culture recognizes—head shakes and nods for no and yes, respectively, pointing, and shoulder shrugs, among others.

DEVELOPING USE AND UNDERSTANDING OF NATURAL GESTURES

The first stage involves eliciting natural gestures from children by consciously beginning activities that involve a motor component and then, once the activity is set up, "extracting" natural gestures from children. For example, one might offer an item to a child part way, but then hold back until the child extends a hand to grasp it, or hold up a choice of two items just out of reach so the child has to gesture toward one or the other, or offer things the child does not want so the child will actually push them away. We want to develop a repertoire of natural actions that allow the child's desires and intents to be much more obvious. Of course, all of these actions will be accompanied by simple language—single words for preverbal children.

Here is an example of a sensory social activity that elicits several natural gestures from 18-month-old Landon, whom we met earlier. He is a very passive toddler who does not yet communicate intentionally in any way.

Landon, barefoot and clad in shorts and a T-shirt, is lying on his back on the floor, playing with his feet. The therapist moves over to him and sits at his feet, facing him. She takes a bare foot in each hand and starts to pat them together rhythmically while singing a version of "Pattycake," called "pattyfeet" for this song. She sings, smiling and looking at his face, while she pats his feet together. He looks at her and smiles (both the eye contact and the smile communicate his desire—these are natural communicative gestures), so she claps his feet together, sole to sole, firmly. At the end of the song, at the line in the song "throw it in the pan," she tosses both his feet up toward his head and then lets them fall to the ground. He smiles brightly and maintains eye contact throughout. She picks up his feet again and takes him through the song a second time, and he continues to respond with lively smiles and consistent eye contact. The third time, she holds her hands toward his feet (her gesture), but does not take them; instead, she looks at him and says, "Pattyfeet? More pattyfeet?" He raises his feet to her hands (natural gesture) and she begins again. At the end, she waits and he claps his hands together (natural gesture). She interprets this as an imitation of sorts of what the feet were doing and responds, "More pattyfeet?" She holds her hands to his feet (her gesture), he offers (natural gesture), and she repeats. Again, he claps (gesture) and she goes through the song.

In this little sensory social routine, the therapist quickly develops a game from the child's own repetitive actions and then elicits a number of communicative gestures, including smiles and eye contact, and hand and foot movements that act to continue the game. Landon takes several turns, communicating through body movements his desire for the game to continue. The therapist acts contingently upon each gesture, and over the course of the game, Landon uses many gestures to request and continue the game.

Underlying Intervention Techniques for Natural Gestures

There are several teaching techniques that we lean on heavily to develop these natural gestures from the child.

Do Less So They Do More

The lack of directed communication from a child easily leads adults to guessing the child wants or needs and providing it in the absence of communicative cues. This eliminates any need for the child to act on his or her needs in an intentional manner. We need to hold back from giving things to the child and doing things *to* the child and *for* the child, and instead, expect and make sure that the child is initiating as often as we are in play routines and daily living routines. When we wait, children use their bodies to communicate and in so doing learn what communication is all about.

By doing less, we help children develop "talking bodies" and give them a chance to do more. Doing less often means acting as if we don't know what they want, offering things rather than giving them, offering more than one choice, offering things children don't want. It means we need to *wait* for a gesture, for eye contact, or for a vocalization. In the beginning of therapy, these child behaviors may be extremely subtle, and they may not be intentional. It is the adult's interpretation of these behaviors as potential communicative acts, and the reinforcement of them as communicative acts, that allows these to evolve into communicative gestures inside the play routines.

Shape Subtle Gestures into Clearer Gestures

Initially, we look for toddlers with autism to use eye contact, a gesture, or a vocalization to express their intentions and meanings. We find ways to elicit child actions that indicate his or her goals or intentions, and then use reinforcement and shaping techniques to establish these as stronger, clearer, more meaningful gestures. For example, we want children to indicate their desire for objects out of reach. To shape this, we begin by eliciting children's reach to proximal objects we offer them and then wait for the child to reach before releasing the object. Once children are reaching as a request gesture, we frequently offer a choice of two or more objects, still proximal. When children can communicate choice, we begin to offer objects that are out of the child's reach, so that the reach gesture does not make contact with the object, we pause for a second, and then give the object. Next, we offer choices out of reach, so the child's reach to the preferred object does not result in contact, and we deliver the chosen object after a clear reach. Finally, we select the attractive object, position the object prominently on a table or small shelf in front of the child, but out of reach, and wait for the child to reach toward the object before we deliver it. Now, we have used shaping to teach the child to make clear reaches to request distal objects.

Choosing Which Gestures to Target

In typical infants, gestures appear in a somewhat consistent order and this sequence can be a guide for choosing which gesture to target. Table 8.1 shows a rough order for typical non-

TABLE 8.1. Average Age of Emergence of Intentional, Communicative Gestures in Typical Development

Age	Behavior regulation	Social interaction	Initiates joint attention
5–6 months	Looks and vocalizes.		
6 months	Pushes away, reaches for pickup.	Shows interest.	
7–8 months	Reaches with whole hand.	Anticipatory behavior.	Looks to adult and vocalizes.
8 months	Pushes away both hands.	Waves in context.	
9 months	Reaches with open/closed hand.	Participatory behavior, claps.	Gives objects.
10 months	Touches adult.	Waves to prompt, initiates social games, dances to music.	Shows objects.
11 months	Points.	Shows function of object.	Points to comment.
12 months	Gives objects, alternates gaze from object to person to object.		
13 months	Shakes head "no."	Hugs objects, claps with excitement.	Points for request ("Where's the light?").
14 months	Takes adult by hand.	Points to request information.	
15 months		Smacks lips, blows kisses.	
16 months		Nods head "yes."	
17 months		Shrugs shoulders, "shhh."	

Note. Data from Crais, Douglas, and Campbell (2004).

verbal gesture development for infants from 6 to 8 months until around 18 months for the three main functions of early communication, based on research by Crais et al. (2004).

Elicit Coordinated Gaze and Gesture

Gestures are often, but not consistently, accompanied by eye contact during the first 2 years of life. For gestures other than commenting and requesting, typically developing toddlers from 12 to 24 months accompany gestures with eye contact less than 50% of the time (Blake, McConnell, Horton, & Benson, 1992). While we teach children to use natural gestures at first without requiring eye contact, once they have learned to use each of these behaviors separately, we then want them to combine gaze with gesture in their requests. How do we add eye contact to these gestures? Here is an example.

Luke has learned to give an object to an adult for help. Nancy, the therapist, sits in front of him and hands him a small jar with the lid screwed on tightly. Inside the jar are five matchbox cars (a favorite object). He takes the jar, tries to unscrew it, cannot, and extends it toward her hand for help. Usually she takes it, saying, "Help. You need help!" But now she doesn't take it, and waits instead. Luke looks up at her to see what is going on, and the minute he looks at her she says, "Sure. I'll help you," while taking the jar, opening it, and removing one car. When she opens it, he reaches for the car. But she does not release it, instead holding onto it. He again looks up at her to see what is happening, and she immediately releases it while saying, "Here's the car," and also hands him the jar. They repeat this sequence several more times, until he has all the cars out of the jar. The last time he offers Nancy the jar to open, Luke hands it over and glances up at her, combining gesture and gaze for the first time.

In this segment, we see the adult waiting for eye contact as well as the gesture before she helps or gives objects to the child. She uses prompting techniques she knows will elicit eye contact in this child—waiting, blocking, not responding at times when he is very accustomed to her responding. If she needed to, she could call his name during the wait in order to get eye contact. In these situations, Nancy needs to be sure that she provides the reinforcer following eye contact, rather than the communicative gesture alone. Once Luke is consistently following her prompts with gaze, she needs to fade the prompts, using partial prompts, verbal prompts, or waiting, to get spontaneous gaze coordinated with the gesture. In following these procedures, she is using prompting, fading, and chaining techniques—chaining the gesture and gaze together, and reinforcing at the moment both behaviors have been expressed. A note of caution involving coordination of gesture and gaze: Objectives regarding conventional gestures should not require coordination of gesture and gaze more than 50% of the time for mastery, based on research in typical children (Blake et al., 1992; except for commenting and requesting).

Helping Children Read Other People's Gestures

Young children with autism are often remarkably unaware of the meaning of other people's nonverbal communication. It is not unusual to see a child who does not understand the "give me" gesture of an open hand, or the meaning of a point when you want a child to place an object in a certain location or look at an interesting object. He or she may not understand the significance of an angry facial expression on another person. We need to teach young children with autism what body movements mean in a focused way. How? Here are some ideas.

1. *Highlight and exaggerate the targeted gestures* in joint activities with objects. Accompany gestures with simple language, but emphasize the gesture and require the child to follow through by making the gesture before he or she attains his or her goal. Prompt the child to make the gesture and then reinforce him or her vigorously both socially and with immediate access to the preferred object or activity. In the case of teaching the "give me" gesture, be sure to give the object back immediately so that the child doesn't lose the object, and thus be inadvertently punished for handing it over. Use gestures with high frequency. Insert them into actions the child is about to make

anyway, like pointing to the object that the child is about to pick up, as you say, "This one"; pointing to the top block on a block tower while saying, "Here" or "Put it here" as the child is about to stack the block; or pointing to the hole into which the child is about to insert a puzzle piece and saying, "It goes here." Highlight gestures in routines to ask children to give or pick up pieces, to set up or clean up an activity, or to take the next turn.

2. *Add lively gestures and facial and vocal expressions to steps and sequences in joint activity routines with objects.* For example, build a tower and then use a gesture to signal time to knock it down. Make these a part of the game—the social script that goes with the activity. As the child's imitation skills come along, teach the child to imitate the gestures and words in these little scripts. This is an important way to make object routines social and increase the fun.

3. *In sensory social routines, highlight facial expressions and body movements to cue the games.* Exaggerating affect and gestures or body postures mark sensory social routines, and these become "labels" for the child when you offer a game. Playing these games in a rather ritualized way helps children learn to associate the gestures and expressions with the games and to begin to focus more and more on adult faces, gestures, and bodies.

4. *Provide interesting visual discrimination toys and tasks* that are too hard for the child to complete independently (such as a puzzle or shape sorter), and then *use your point to indicate to the child where to put the piece* while saying "Here" or "Horse goes here." Having the piece go in immediately meets the child's goal and is the reinforcer. Be sure that the piece goes in easily and fast; help it in if you need to—if the child has to struggle, you have lost the reinforcement for following your point. Over time, this will teach the child the salience of your point.

TEACHING CONVENTIONAL GESTURE USE

As shown in Table 8.1, conventional gestures follow natural gestures in typical development. We follow this sequence with toddlers with ASD. We begin to teach conventional gestures once a child has a variety of natural gestures that he or she uses to regulate others' behavior, to initiate and continue dyadic social interactions, and to coordinate attention to an object or event with a partner. When choosing conventional gestures to teach a child, one needs to be sure that the underlying communicative function of the gesture is one the child expresses, so that the gesture you teach has meaning for the child. A useful way to teach the meaning is to introduce the gesture in your own actions first by highlighting it and the accompanying language in context. Incorporate it into routines that you and the child already carry out. The gesture might be part of a social script that you have developed surrounding a favorite joint activity with objects (like calling an animal in a barnyard game by wiggling your finger in the "come" gesture, saying, "Lion, come here, come here," and having the lion walk to you). Or it might be part of a natural household routine, as in snack, when you have some yummy food out that you eat with exaggerated pleasure, head nods, and smiles, as well as a contrasting "yucky" food that you taste with exaggerated displeasure and then push away with strong head shakes saying, "No, no sauerkraut. No sauerkraut!" You can add gestures to a favorite song, as in the goodbye song, adding an exaggerated sad face when you sing, "Bye, bye, Nathan, bye, bye, Nathan, bye, bye, Nathan, I'm sad to see you go." Such gestures develop meaning for the child through the routine. Table 8.1 provides ideas for basic gestures to teach; observing typical toddlers in interaction will provide more ideas for gestures to model and teach to toddlers with ASD.

To teach conventional gestures, we rely on gestural imitation skills covered in Chapter 7 under "Teaching Gestural Imitation." In general, we set up an opportunity for the child to express a conventional gesture in a natural context, and then we prompt the child by modeling the conventional gesture, prompting the child to imitate the gesture, and then providing the reinforcing object or activity after the gesture has been expressed. The adult needs to set up many times to practice this and use appropriate prompt fading techniques to establish these as independent spontaneous gestures. While it is often the case that we will teach a gesture in one particular situation, the adult needs to be attuned to other times during the treatment session that the child is expressing that same communicative function. Then, the adult needs to elicit the gesture in multiple situations. This allows the child to learn the generalized meaning of the gesture over time.

Teaching the appropriate words to accompany the gestures occurs in the same way, through pairing verbal language with the gesture. Be careful not to overteach this or require both gesture and the accompanying words in every single possible opportunity. We do not want children appearing scripted in their gestural use.

Teaching Conventional Hand/Body Gestures

After enough time spent working with children with autism, we often forget how frequently gestures are used in typical communication. These include "gimme," shoulder shrug, head nods and head shakes for yes and no, respectively, and hand gesture to reject. Take the opportunity to observe typically developing children with the same level of verbal language as the child with autism you are treating. Watch how that child communicates; note the gestures and the postures that accompany that child's speech in the grocery store, the restaurant, and the park. Here is your source for the repertoire of gestures, postures, and facial expressions to target in the child you are treating and also your guide for what to model yourself.

To teach these, use the same teaching approaches that we have discussed thus far. Set up a situation involving choices for preferred and nonpreferred objects or activities in which you can induce in the child the underlying meaning of the gesture ("more," "no," "I want," "I don't care"). For the requesting gestures, offer a highly desired object. For the rejecting or protesting gestures, offer a choice between a highly preferred and a nonpreferred object. For the "I don't care," offer two low-interest objects. Once you make the offer and get the "meaning" expressed in the child's behavior, prompt the target gesture through imitation or physical prompts. Once the child makes an approximation of the gesture, follow through with the motivator that will serve as the reinforcer. For requesting behaviors, that will be the desired object. For protest or refusal and I don't care gestures, it will be the removal of the nonpreferred object and the immediate choice of a highly preferred object. (See Ingersoll and Schreibman, 2006, for a description of the effectiveness of a very similar procedure.)

Teaching Expressive Facial Expressions

Teaching children to make facial expressions begins in the work on facial imitations discussed in Chapter 7. Teaching children to copy "funny faces" as imitation games should include aspects of facial expressions as well—laughing, pouting, frowning, and scrunching up the face. Because you cannot prompt facial expressions, you have to rely on shaping to improve them over time. Mirror games can be developed as fun ways to practice facial imitations; the immediate feedback of the mirror allows you to prompt the child and reinforce child approximations.

After children are good imitators of individual facial movements, add facial expressions to the "game," labeling them as you do them: happy, laughing, sad, and so on. As you begin to do this inside a facial imitation game, it is time to begin highlighting emotional expressions and emotional experiences in many aspects of the treatment. Use books with big emotional expressions like *Where the Wild Things Are* (Sendak, 1963) so that you can imitate the pictures in the books.

Highlight emotional experiences that happen in the treatment session and use exaggerated emotion to pair the expressions with the affective experiences that the child is having at the moment during therapy. Things happen that make you and the child feel happy, sad, mad, and scared during therapy. Use these natural events to link affect words and expressions together in yourself and model these for the child's experiences of affect. You can also draw these out with exaggerated affect elements in simple faces as you recount the experience. Make a little picture of the event and narrate it as we described under "Symbolic Play Acts" in Chapter 7. Then, as you review the event, add the affect voice and face. Encourage the child to imitate these, and then later to "read" them to you, adding facial expressions to the script. Play out emotionally intense scenes with dolls, animals, and puppets, so there are appropriate "scripts" in play for acting out emotional expressions. Add emotional expressions to your greeting songs—happy expressions for "Hello, I'm glad to see you" and sad expressions for "Goodbye, I'll miss you."

Developing Joint Attention Behaviors

As previewed earlier in this chapter, joint attention behaviors are very special communicative skills that begin to emerge in the 6- to 12-month period and increase in frequency and range of behaviors used in the second year of life in children without developmental difficulties (Legerstee et al., 2007). Joint attention involves a communication shared between two persons about an object or event. Before joint attention develops, children focus their attention on either an object or a person during a play interaction, but they don't seem to be able to focus on both at once. Joint attention marks children's ability to focus on both—the partner and the object, at once, through gaze shifts between the person and the object. It's a triangle of communication: child, partner, and object. The child is communicating *with* the partner *about* the object.

Many communicative meanings can be shared through gaze and affect. The child may be expressing interest, intention, pleasure, desire, or wariness. The product and goal of joint attention behaviors is the sharing of one's mental state with a partner about an object or event.

Joint attention generally involves several specific behaviors. Gaze shifts from the interesting object or event to the partner and back again are the first and earliest expressions of joint attention. During gaze shifts, the child may also direct a particular facial emotion to the partner, conveying his or her feelings about the target of interest. When using joint attention to share emotions, the child looks at the object and then looks at the adult with a smile or frown, and thus communicates his or her feelings *about* the object or event.

While joint attention displays involve expressing one's own thoughts or feelings—sharing something about one's state of mind—they also involve reading a partner's cues and understanding the partner's desires or feelings about the object; that is, reading the partner's mind. Children respond to others' joint attention communications by reading their gestures, facial expressions, and their focus of gaze. Thus, children both initiate joint attention behaviors and they understand them when their partner expresses them.

How do we teach joint attention? We've already discussed increasing children's eye contact and positioning ourselves in front of children to assist with eye contact. We have also discussed highlighting gestures and eliciting early gestures in general. Once we have increased eye contact to us, we need to target several of the gestures that specifically mark joint attention: giving, showing, and pointing.

Giving to Get Help

We teach children to comprehend the meaning of an outstretched hand as a cue to give an object. Our earlier focus on turn taking has provided a good foundation for this. There are two pragmatic functions that are often communicated through giving. One is giving to get help—a way to influence others to help you reach your goal (behavior regulation, in the language of Bruner, 1977). This is an easy gesture to teach because the reinforcer is built in. We get the child to give for help by setting up activities that require our assistance: bubble jars, juice boxes, and toy containers to open, kazoos to blow, and markers or jars with lids that are too tight for the child to open. We give the child the desired object and when the child struggles, we elicit the give for help with an open hand.

Our goal is that the child will initiate giving for help, so the open hand is a prompt that we want to fade quickly. Each time you repeat this, wait longer before you extend your hand (a time delay procedure) and minimize your hand gesture. Increase the distance from the child's hand to yours. Each time, do less and wait a little longer. Your goal is that the child will hand the object to you without you making any movement at all. We discuss getting gaze later. Right now, it's only about giving to get help. When the child places the object in your hand, say, "Oh, you need *help*," "Help me," or "Open," "Open box," or "I'll open." Then open, hand it back saying something like, "Here's the cracker," or "Marker is open."

Giving to Share, or Show

Teaching children to give to share (show) means giving the object right back with a big attractive emotional display, or activating the toy once to create interest and handing it back to the child.

1. Prompt the give with an open hand, take the object and show it to the child, respond with something reinforcing like a big smile and eye contact, say "Wow, cool car!" run it along the child's tummy, and then hand it right back—"Here's car."
2. As you repeat these behaviors, watch for the child to begin to pick up the object and look expectantly to you for the reaction. Respond by gesturing for "give" and providing the full display.
3. As this occurs over repetitions, wait for the give before you gesture and respond. Now you have a give to share. *Be sure to always give it back after your display.*
4. The final shaping step here is to take it from "give" to "show." When the child offers you the toy, don't take it, and instead provide the full display to the child's give gesture. (If needed, stabilize the child's hand so the "offer" continues until the end of the display, but don't take the toy.) You have now prompted and reinforced a "show."
5. In addition to teaching the child how to show, we need to teach the child to show in response to the verbal instruction, "Show me." To do this, pair the words, "Show me" with a "give me" gesture directed to an object the child is holding or facing. Hold your hand out to prompt the child to give the object. *But once the child offers, don't take the object; just admire it enthusiastically, providing the same reinforcers you used for the spontaneous shows.*

Don't change your expectations involving coordination of gaze and gesture. To do so would violate the rule about mixing maintenance and acquisition tasks, and you would run the risk of extinguishing giving. Instead, start to require gaze intermittently; perhaps one out of every four times. Once the child is coordinating give with gaze more frequently, then begin to elicit it every second to third give. After the child is consistent at that level, move to expecting it most times and not reinforcing gives that are not accompanied by looks. Be careful to monitor the frequency of gives during this teaching: Do not ignore the child's gives or you run the risk of extinguishing gives. Be sure to reinforce strongly.

Pay attention to how typically developing children use gaze with gives to share or get help: That is our model!

One final step in this sequence is persistence. Occasionally, do not respond to the child's first full request, even with gaze. Pretend to be looking elsewhere. Wait for the child to repeat the request. Reinforce on the second bid instead of the first. Shape the child to position that toy right in front of your face and persist. Continue to shape until you have built a strong and persistent request.

Frequently direct your own joint attention behaviors to the child. As the child is learning these routines, be sure to also give objects to the child to help you, and to share, so you can model these behaviors and help the child learn how to respond to these as well as how to produce them. Use the typical ways of teaching we have discussed, providing the bid (the antecedent), prompting the child to respond (the behavior), and then reinforcing by giving the object to the child to use as he or she wants. This develops the child's receptive as well as expressive understanding of joint attention, and it fosters the role reversal and coordination that occurs between social partners.

Pointing

We must teach children both to comprehend pointing and to produce it. To teach its meaning, we use our own finger to point and draw children's attention to something: to the place for a puzzle piece to go, to the tower for block stacking, to the button on a button-activated toy, to pictures in a book, to the Goldfish cracker that we want them to pick up next. We need to see children learn to follow our point with their eyes and demonstrate that they understand the meaning of the point through their actions. When they intentionally act at the location that we are pointing to, in a variety of situations and with a variety of materials, then we know they are learning the meaning of point.

Pointing to Indicate a Request

To teach pointing, we first need children to be able to reliably reach toward distant objects to request—to indicate choices and desires. If the child does not yet use a distal reach to signal a choice, develop that first, as described in the earlier section of this chapter.

When teaching pointing, we actually elicit a proximal reach to a desired object and then very quickly mold the hand into a point. We have the child touch the desired object with the point and then give the object to the child. Use the instruction "Point." Putting little round dots or stickers on objects for children to point to can help them learn. As soon as the child spontaneously and consistently points to these dots to request, peel the dots off while continuing to prompt pointing through a physical prompt or word if needed. The child will point to these objects. We can get lots of opportunities for practice by controlling multipiece materials like puzzle pieces, pieces for a shape sorter, pegs for a pegboard, and having children request with their point.

A very powerful way to get a point is to use a cup during snack time, with a dot or sticker on it and a little food in it. The child should see you put a treat in the cup. Show the child the food in the cup, or use a transparent cup. Hold the cup to the child with the dot facing the child and as the child reaches for the cup, mold his or her hand fast so that the index finger touches the dot. Immediately turn the cup to the child and let him or her reach in and take the treat. Once the child spontaneously touches the dot, use the dot on other things the child is requesting as well.

Once the child is consistently and spontaneously pointing to proximal objects to request, make it a distal point by holding the objects out of the child's reach, so the child is pointing toward the object but cannot touch it. Systematically increase the distance until the child is pointing from several feet to make a choice consistently and spontaneously, in response to the question, "Which one do you want?" or just to a visual offer of two choices without any verbal language.

Adding Eye Contact to Points to Request

As with the give and show gestures, we teach the point gesture first without requiring eye contact. Once the gesture is mastered and used spontaneously, we start to require eye contact after the gesture by waiting to give over the object and thus violating the child's expectations or, if needed, perhaps by calling his or her name. Then we begin to expect pairing of gaze plus point to request, first intermittently, and then with greater frequency. Thus, after the child points reliably to request, we begin to work for coordination of eye contact with point as well.

Pointing to Comment

Children use pointing to express several meanings (pragmatic functions). It may mean "I want this" (requesting), "Do this" (directing), "Look at this" (the showing, or commenting function). The commenting function is especially important for language and vocabulary development because parents typically label objects and events of interest. We have already talked about teaching pointing and giving as ways to request. How do we develop commenting at the nonverbal level for young children with autism?

One of the best ways involves developing commenting routines around books with several clear pictures on a page, picture albums, and puzzle pictures. In these routines, the adult (facing the child) points to each picture in turn, and when the child looks at the picture, the adult names the picture. The adult may also produce sound effects to add interest. Adults must make sure the child is attending to the item being labeled. When the child's interest wanes, the activity is finished. Doing the same books in the same way each time builds up the child's learning about the routine and the child's interest and attention expands.

Once the child demonstrates that he or she enjoys this activity, the adult begins the activity as usual, makes the point to get the child's attention on the object, but then waits to name it. The child will likely look up to see why the adult isn't naming the object; when the child looks, the adult names the object. With this variation, we have reinforced the child for using eye contact to get someone to produce a label—that's commenting. If the child doesn't look up or signal, but instead begins to turn the page, block him or her from turning and wait for the look that follows the block or, if needed, prompt the look more directly with a name call or a gestural prompt. Then, continue the game.

Now teach the child to use a point to get the comment. To do so, add this variation to the routine. Rather than the adult pointing, take the child's hand and have the child do the pointing to each picture, while the adult provides the verbal label as before. As this becomes the routine, the adult provides less and less help until the child is leading the activity by pointing, and the adult is responding to the point with the word. The final elaboration of this step occurs when the adult is sitting in front of the child (of course), so that when the child points, the adult waits for eye contact and thus violates an expectation. This will often elicit the look, and the adult will then provide the word after the child makes eye contact. The child is now combining pointing and gaze to request the label—just as it occurs in typical development.

CONCLUSION

In the descriptions above, we have provided directions on how to teach children to both use and understand gestural communication for all three pragmatic functions. Giving for help involves behavior regulation. Responding to sensory social routines by maintaining and continuing a game involves dyadic social interactions. Teaching children to point, show, and give to express interest involves joint attention. You now have strategies to develop a wide range of nonverbal communicative gestures that mark typical communication development in the toddler period.

The above techniques, combined with the techniques for teaching imitation of gestures described in Chapter 7, can be used to develop all kinds of communicative gestures. The procedures are always the same. Identify the gesture to be taught, model it in a contextually appropriate way within a relevant, preferred activity or social routine, require the child to imitate it back before the routine continues, and prompt the child as needed. As you teach these, be sure to use them extensively during therapy, along with the typical language that accompanies the gestures. As children begin to produce them spontaneously, differentially reinforce these. However, continue to reinforce productions that do not involve all of these gestures. We do not want to create abnormal and rigid use of gestures inside communication routines.

In developing the nonverbal communicative repertoire described above and working your way through the ESDM Curriculum Checklist (Appendix A), you will also be increasing children's intentional, communicative vocalizations through their integration of eye contact, gesture, and vocalization. This prepares them well for moving into verbal language, the topic of the following chapter. However, as you progress into verbal language, be sure to continue to work on nonverbal communication. Nonverbal communication *always* accompanies verbal communication in typical development and lack of appropriate nonverbal communication is a well-known symptom of autism, even in highly verbal persons with ASD. Continue to work on gesture through pantomime, games like "Guesstures," and many other activities throughout the treatment of ASD.

Chapter 9

Developing Verbal Communication

Verbal communication is comprised of expressive language and receptive language. Understanding language is part and parcel of using it, and thus we expect receptive and expressive language to develop concurrently. In this chapter, we focus on how to foster development of the foundations of expressive language, limiting ourselves to the techniques involved in promoting development of spontaneous, generative verbal communication up to the two-word stage.

Useful, communicative speech results from several foundational skills: understanding the pragmatic utility, or social effects, of verbal communication; having appropriate maturity and intentional control of the speech production system; the ability to imitate other people's speech in order to acquire the forms; and the ability to learn word meanings. Verbal language is not an isolated communication system; rather, it is combined with nonverbal communicative behaviors like gaze, gesture, and intonation patterns that add meaning. Building these "packages" of verbal and nonverbal communication is the focus of this chapter.

As with nonverbal communication, a main goal is to teach children to use speech to convey a wide range of pragmatic functions: commenting, joint attention, affirmation, protest and negation, greeting and attention getting, as well as behavior regulation (Bruner, 1981a). In the ESDM, verbal language teaching occurs inside joint activities that also target the nonverbal pragmatic communications described earlier. Within these joint activities, treatment first targets the development of intentional vocalizations, followed by consonant–vowel combinations (e.g., syllables that imitate word production), then single-word approximations, and finally, multiword combinations. All are taught within shared activities to provide the content and functions of child communication.

To already developed nonverbal communication "packages," we now focus on adding intentional vocalizations. Building speech occurs in exactly the same way as nonverbal communication. The following sections describe how to build up a repertoire of intentional sounds, stimulating the child's development of verbal communication and his or her intentional control of voice. This work will be done within the context of joint activity routines by highlighting sensory social routines as a starting point. As children become easily able to produce sounds intentionally and to imitate some sounds, the adult will use prompting to add these sounds to the nonverbal communications the child already expresses. This same process will be used to turn sounds into words, and single words into multiword productions. The work will occur within joint activity routines, building on the pragmatic functions the child already uses and new functions as they come up in the interactions between child and adult. "Early words develop to fulfill the social functions originally conveyed by gestures" (Owens, 1996).

Thus, the pragmatics of communication continue to ground communication developed and expanded through ongoing experiences, adult models, and naturalistic teaching techniques. Adults will *follow* children's interests and motivations in joint activity routines with relevant language and supports for child communications. For both typically developing children and children with ASD, adult language teaching techniques that follow children's leads and focus of attention have been found to be more successful than directive means for enhancing language development (Hart & Risley, 1975; Siller & Sigman, 2002). This is one of the strengths of the ESDM: the solid grounding of communication teaching in the pragmatics of communication.

STIMULATING DEVELOPMENT OF SPEECH PRODUCTION

Speech develops from a child's intentional vocalizations. Essential building blocks of this development are the ability to produce an increasing number of phonemes (speech sounds) and to imitate others' speech productions.

Typical Speech Development

Infants first develop new sounds unintentionally, through exposure to their native language, vocal play, and neurological maturation of the speech mechanisms. Infant speech productions follow a characteristic order in typical development, starting with the production of primarily middle and back vowel sounds, followed by babbling (vocalizing strings of consonants and vowels [CV] or vowels and consonants [VC], often in response to the speech of others).

With greater maturity comes increased variation in intonation and vowel productions, as well as the addition of new consonant productions. As typical development continues, infants demonstrate CV or VC syllable repetitions, or reduplicative babbling (e.g., *ba-ba, di-di*) and then begin to imitate those around them, including the intonation patterns of adult speech production. Next, variegated babbling emerges, which refers to babbling in which the CV–CV or VC–VC sequences are not identical (*ba-da, da-di*), and the sequences may also include CVC or VCV combinations (*pop, aba*). A final stage in early speech production occurs when infants start to produce long strings of sounds with adult-like intonation patterns known as jargon.

In typical development, nasal phonemes (*m, n*), plosives (*p, b, t, d*), and approximants (*w, y*) constitute the majority of consonants in infant vocalizations (Leonard, Newhoff, & Mesalam, 1980); however, productions at this stage are neither fully formed nor necessarily accurate. Therefore, one must also consider the typical age of *mastery* when determining intervention targets.

Mastering all the sounds of our language normally takes many years and typical preschoolers may still demonstrate developmental errors on the most mature sounds (e.g., *th, r, j*). Often, some of the earliest mastered phonemes include *p, b, m, n, h,* and *w*. These sounds are often followed by mastery of *k, g, f, d, y,* and *t* (Sander, 1972). As such, when working with a child with autism who is just starting to develop spoken language, keep these developmental speech patterns in mind when choosing intervention activities and materials, and pick targets that use the sounds in the first position of the word that is appropriate to the child's level of speech production development. Young children with ASD appear to demonstrate the same repertoire of phonemes, or speech sounds, as do typically developing children (McCleery et al., 2006).

Developing a Repertoire of Sounds

Some toddlers with autism produce very few sounds, especially consonants. Clinically, we observe that their vocalizations are few in number, the number of different sounds, or phonemes, they use is small, and their intonation patterns may be quite unusual. The typical pitch and melody of infant vocal play are often missing. Their voices may be unusually quiet or loud, unusually high or low in pitch, and their intonation patterns may be rather flat and monotonic, or they may be unusual in their stress patterns and unlike typical speech (McCann & Peppe, 2003).

For children who produce reduced rates and variety of sounds, our initial goals are to increase the frequency and variety of sounds the child produces. We do this by finding activities in which children tend to vocalize and by reinforcing vocalizations whenever they occur. Sensory social activities involving movement activities are often especially helpful in stimulating unintentional vocalization in children.

Imitating children's vocalizations often has a reinforcing function (although it can also stop vocalizations—be very aware of the impact of your imitations on child vocalization). For children who do not produce many sounds, differential reinforcement of vocalization is important and will be helpful in increasing their frequency. That is, regardless of what target behavior you were seeking to elicit in the interaction, if the child vocalizes, he or she should receive immediate reinforcement for vocalizing. One natural, contingent reinforcement of speech is for one's communication partner to respond. The adult might immediately stop what he or she is doing and vocalize in response or imitate the child (again, while being aware of the child's response to the adult's imitations) and follow through by providing the child with whatever his or her pragmatic goal was being expressed via the vocalization.

In the chapter on imitation, we discussed ways to stimulate increased frequency and diversity of vocalizations. Adults build up a child's repertoire of speech sounds through little sound-making games, through adding ritualized sound effects to our play routines with toys and books, and through sensory social routines. Imitating children's sounds back to them and developing vocal games involving rounds of imitation are extremely helpful kinds of activities. Refer to Chapter 7 for ways to build a repertoire of intentional vocalizations through imitation games. Those are prerequisite skills for developing speech. Their goal is to build from the child's spontaneous productions, using imitation of the child's sounds to help those sounds become intentional, and then using adult-initiated imitation to get the sounds fully under the child's control. Once children are reliably vocalizing in response to adult sounds, the adult starts shaping those sounds into words.

Moving from Sounds to Words

The adult will use two processes to mold sounds into words. First, the adult will match the child's sounds with related words in relevant activities. Here is an example:

Molly produces the syllable "ba"—and consistently imitates when her therapist, Jill, models it. Jill now begins to choose activities for which the production "ba" is relevant—bubbles, ball, balloon, bottle, baby, and bath. Jill offers a large ball to Molly for her favorite bouncing game. "Want ball?" Molly reaches and looks to request. Jill repeats, "Ball? Ba?" And Molly imitates "ba." "Yes, ball" says Jill, picks her up, and immediately begins the bouncing game. She bounces her briefly, stops, and holds the ball still. Molly wiggles her body to continue the bounce. "Ball?" asks Jill. "Ball?" Molly replies "ba," and Jill nods, smiles, says "Yea, bounce!" and begins to bounce her again. This stop and go routine occurs for six rounds On the sixth round, Jill waits for the word before modeling it, does not get "ba" spontaneously, so whispers "ba," and Molly responds, "ba, ba." "Ball," says Jill, as she bounces her for a long time.

In this episode, the adult has set up the activity so that the adult model results in the child's imitation of the word to request and she provides the reinforcement immediately after the child has spoken. In this situation, "ba" is being associated with a particular event and is in transition to becoming a word.

A second strategy is to shape sounds in the child's repertoire to be more word-like. Once the child produces the well-mastered sound for the activity, the adult begins to model a somewhat modified sound that is closer to the real word but still within the child's repertoire. To return to Jill and Molly, the sound "ba" is also used in their bubbles game and balloon game. During a bubbles activity, after the "ba" has been well established, Jill will begin to hold back reinforcement for the single syllable while modeling "baba" for bubbles, and differentially reinforcing a two-syllable production from Molly to shape "ba" into bubbles; this is referred to as successive approximation. The child's production is shaped successively closer to the adult-like production of the word.

Similarly, within the balloon game, Molly is also capable of imitating "ooo." Thus, after "ba" is well established as a request for balloon, Jill will then model "balloon," and when Molly responds with "ba," Jill will then model and elicit "oo." She will continue to elicit "ba" and "oo" in the balloon game, and as Molly consistently imitates each, Jill will start to expect to hear both syllables after her model "Ball-oon." She will differentially reinforce this combination and over time Molly will become more consistent at imitating "balloon" by saying "ba oo." Prompting, shaping, and fading procedures are being used to move from sounds to words.

Imbuing Spontaneous Productions with Meaning

As children learn to vocalize intentionally to accompany their gestural communications, adults need to start to treat those vocalizations as attempts at words and begin to model simple words in return. One technique involves responding to a child's spontaneous verbal productions with real words, appropriate to context, that match the phonemic patterns of the child's production during the interaction.

For example, Jason produces multiple-syllable utterances containing consonants and vowels with a speech-like intonation. He babbles "zaza" in vocal play during a joint activity routine with cars, which Laurie, his therapist, immediately incorporates into "zoom zoom" and reinforces with a lively and interesting car action. Laurie then stops the car and looks expectantly at Jason. She asks him, "Zoom zoom?" and waits for him to produce the "zaza" with the car routine as the consequence. If he does not produce it, she will model it by saying, "zaza," waiting for him to say it again, and then proceeding with the game, whether or not he produces it again. In this way, she has imbued his spontaneous vocalization with meaning by pairing it with "zoom zoom" and the car game, a preferred activity.

Imbuing Imitated Productions with Meaning

The same exact process will occur using productions the child imitates. Vocal imitations occur as part of meaningful joint activity routines in the ESDM. To add semantic meaning to the imitations, the adult chooses models for imitation that fit a key word in the activity and consequates the child's imitation with the preferred activity. This is quite similar to the example above with Jill and Molly, but the goal here is to add meaning to the child's sound rather than to shape the child's sound. Here is an example:

The therapist, Diane, has taught Kerry to imitate "ba" to request balls and bubbles. In a floor activity, Diane offers Kerry bubbles or a drum, while labeling each. The child reaches for the bubbles and the adult says, Bubbles, bubbles," emphasizing the first syllable and looking expectantly at her while holding onto the bubbles. Kerry does not produce "ba," so Diane models "ba." Kerry produces "ba" and Diane expands immediately to "ba-bubbles" while handing the closed bubble jar to Kerry. Kerry hands the jar back to Diane to open, and Diane models "help," seeking an imitation (approximation). Kerry produces "ha" and Diane responds, "Help, sure, I'll help," and she opens the bottle and dips the wand in the liquid and gets ready to blow. "Blow?" she asks, and Kerry says "ba," to which Diane replies "Blow" and blows a long stream of bubbles. Kerry jumps up to bat at them and Diane shares in the bubble play, popping bubbles and saying "Pop, pop," as she pops the bubbles with her finger. The child produces "ba" and pokes and Diane says "Bubbles, pop bubbles."

In this example, we see child imitations always consequated by the child's goal and we see the adult responding repeatedly with target words that fit the phonetic pattern the child produces. The child's imitated sounds are imbued with meaning by the adult's actions with the objects as well as the responsive language being produced.

Because communication happens inside joint activity routines in the ESDM, there is always a function and meaning to the child's communication. We are assured that the child's sounds and word approximations have semantic meaning when the child produces them spontaneously in the presence of the target object or action, when the child requests those objects or actions in their absence, and when we offer the activity or object verbally and the child immediately acts in such a way that it is clear he or she understands. Thus, when the child demonstrates that he or she understands the meaning of the words, we move away from the imitation format and move to spontaneous speech and receptive language acquisition. This is the next topic.

Getting to Spontaneous Words from Imitated Words

Facilitating development of spontaneity involves establishing a routine of modeling words and then fading the model over trials. For this goal, the words need to be unvarying and repeated in a chain. Here is an example:

Therapist Greg is stacking blocks with Lee to make towers that they then crash into with a car, which Lee loves. Greg is controlling the materials and eliciting the approximation "ba" as a request for a block via modeling, "Block?" as he offers a block to Lee. They are sitting on the floor facing each other and Greg has the block container in his lap. He provides a block or two to Lee and begins to stack two blocks on the floor between them. Lee stacks his block on this base. Then, Greg stacks a block and offers another block, "Block?" Lee responds with "ba," Greg releases the block while repeating, "Block," and Lee stacks. Greg repeats this sequence two or three more times (full prompts), and then the next time he offers Lee a block, he does not model the word. If Lee says "ba," Greg gives the block and says, "Block." If Lee does not say "ba" but instead tries to take it, Greg whispers, "Block," gets Lee's "ba," and hands Lee the block. Greg has provided a partial prompt instead of a full prompt. He will continue to fade the prompt until Lee produces the "ba" in response to the offered object, without any adult language preceding it.

This is the general procedure for moving from verbal imitation to spontaneous production of words. Set up the communication routine with numerous one-word repetitions and begin to fade the verbal models. This involves a fair amount of repetition, and while in other sections of this manual we have discussed elaborating joint activities through turn taking, changes in language, elaboration, and so on to prevent too much repetition, in this particular situation, we need the repetition to create "behavioral momentum," to lead the child into spontaneous speech production. Thus, we will use the same word four to five times in a row, "Ba blow," having the child imitate the "ba" each time before we blow. Then on the sixth trial, we will hold back from saying "ba," instead looking expectantly at the child for the "ba," and perhaps forming our mouths into the "b" shape, waiting for the child to say "ba" before we blow the bubbles. We proceed in this more repetitive way to support the child's spontaneous verbal initiation. We can elaborate, or vary, the joint activity routine after we have several spontaneous productions, or after the child's attention and motivation are starting to wane.

Don't be discouraged by overgeneralization. Children typically overgeneralize their first words to multiple objects or requests (Rescorla, 1980). It's as if they have learned the power of the spoken word, but don't understand the limits of the first word's meaning. When a child uses the wrong word to request something, simply provide a model of the correct word in order to elicit an imitated approximation that is different from the word the child used, and hand over the requested object. As the child's expressive and receptive language skills continue to develop, this issue will eventually work itself out. The important thing to remember is to reinforce the child's expressive initiation.

However, keep the number of words you are working on very small but work on them a lot. Continue to target just a few words using powerfully attractive objects and much repetition; things will progress. Asking parents to keep a list of words that the child uses spontaneously at home will help you track vocabulary and know what words to target in your session. Also, keep in mind that as a child's vocabulary grows, his or her productions do not have to be adult-like in accuracy to be considered valid gains in language and vocabulary growth. Consistent use of a speech approximation for a particular object, person, or action indicates that the child has a representation (a word) for that, even if it may not yet sound exactly like an adult production. These productions should be included in that inventory of words as well. Finally, use nouns and verbs for these first words; avoid overuse of words like "more" or "yeah" that are very general themselves.

Using Spontaneous Speech to Make Choices

Once the child clearly has the word–object link down, demonstrated by using spontaneous word approximations to request some objects, we want to provide opportunities for discrimination. For Lee, who has learned to spontaneously request blocks in the tower activity, the adult now needs to offer a choice of two objects for which the child knows the labels, while stating their labels, "Block or spoon?" If Lee echoes "Spoon," he will get a spoon; not what he needs to make a block tower. Getting the spoon should frustrate him a little. Make another offer, this time saying, "Spoon or block?" He should ask for "block." (Children tend to echo the last word they have heard. You are going to use this tendency to teach.)

Vary the order of the choices you model so that you allow the natural consequences of echoing (i.e., getting the wrong object if he says "Spoon") assist in teaching the child how to think instead of echo. As this episode plays out, Lee will likely make the mistake several times. When Lee says "Spoon," offer the spoon, and when he looks unhappy but before he takes it, pull it back, say "Block. You want block." and give the block as he says "Block." Be careful with this: Don't allow the child to make too many mistakes or you will lose motivation. However, this discrimination step is important to facilitate development from imitation to spontaneous verbal language. Children's nonverbal communications may also be helpful in interpreting their meaning. If their gestures indicate that they want one object and they are saying the name of the other, be sure to label what they are reaching for and hand it to them. We want to honor their nonverbal communication rather than ignoring it.

Deciding What Spontaneous Words to Target in the Teaching

There are a few rules to follow in deciding what words to target for spontaneous speech:

- Target words that are associated with things children like a lot.
- Target words that the child already has the sounds to approximate.
- Target developmentally appropriate words (e.g., words that do not combine multiple consonants together in blends).
- Target words that are common across multiple environments.
- Target the words for the requests the child routinely makes nonverbally.
- Don't forget to include action words sometimes!

Build up a simple vocabulary of words that refer to important things for the child and use those words frequently until the child learns them. Typically developing toddler's first words are generally animals, food, and toys (Nelson, 1973). Provide simple labels for all main interests of the child—favorite social games, foods, toys, people, and animals. Actions are important to highlight, as well as names of things, though actions come into toddler vocabularies a little later than labels and are much less frequent than nouns (Nelson, 1973). Words for colors, numbers, shapes, and other concepts come later. There is no need to highlight those nouns in this early language learning phase. In the beginning, target labels and actions using simple, but specific words: cup, ball, hop, and eat.

Finally, try not to target general words that can be used for a large number of requests. For instance, try to avoid the word *more,* or if you need it for a particular reason, try not to let it become too universal. Otherwise, it will take the place of a lot of different words that could be taught. Instead, try to elicit approximations of the specific nouns or actions themselves—juice, cookie, book, and bubble. Early words come into typical toddlers' repertoires slowly initially, but as they approach 50 words, their rate of word learning picks up significantly—"the language explosion"—as it's often called. It is that period in typical development when children seem to add vocabulary daily and effortlessly.

Developing Action Words: Verbs

As children's vocabularies grow toward the 100-word mark, verbs become a larger part of their repertoire (though still small) (Bates et al., 1994). We foster verb development just like noun development—through imitation, choices for action routines, discrimination, and prompt fading during requests for interesting activities. But now we have to emphasize action choices instead of noun–object choices in the joint activities. Some activities lend themselves very well to working on verbs:

- Physical games with children can involve "hop," "push," "swing," "run," and "hide."
- Play dough routines can involve "poke," "roll," "pinch," "cut," and "wiggle."
- All kinds of activities can involve "stop" and "go."
- Ball routines can involve "throw," "kick," "spin," "bounce," or "roll."
- Physical touch can involve "pat," "squeeze," or "tickle."
- A child's play toolkit or workbench has great objects for emphasizing actions.

Choose target verbs that the child has the sounds to approximate. Then, develop with the child a fun routine built around the target verb action. Model the action with the word as you develop the activity. Give the child a choice of actions and within that choice get the verbal imitation to the verb model, and consequate—reinforce—with the desired action. Thus, you are using the same procedures to teach verbs that you used earlier to teach nouns. You will also use the procedures described above for spontaneous production of nouns to help the child progress to spontaneous production of verbs.

Building Multiword Utterances

When is it time to expect two-word combinations from a child who consistently produces one-word productions in spontaneous speech? Communication science does not provide us with a universally agreed-upon guideline for this (Tomasello, 2006). However, it is clear that there is a positive relationship between expressive vocabulary size and sentence length. In both English and other languages, toddlers begin to demonstrate growth in word combinations and other evidence of syntactic development as their vocabularies approach 100 words (Caselli, Casadio, & Bates, 1999). In the ESDM, we begin to target two-word utterances when the child has at least 60 to 80 spontaneous words in his or her repertoire and is using words spontaneously at a high frequency (i.e., speaks multiple times per minute in a social interaction). Many young children with autism who have developed single-word speech to this level will spontaneously begin to imitate two-word phrases that adults are using and will move into multiword speech as a result of the enriched language environment that is provided in the ESDM. However, if the child with autism has that number of words and is initiating verbal communication with high frequency, but not yet combining words by imitating your two-word utterances during joint activity routines, then we need to adopt additional strategies.

Adults should use the child's already developed verbal imitation skills to use imitation to elicit these two-word utterances. However, do not require children to produce longer sentences by teaching them to imitate each word in turn: "I I," "want want," "juice juice." Our experience indicates that this fosters echolalia and interferes with spontaneity and syntactic development. Instead, use the child's already developed imitation skills within joint activities.

There are several ways to do this. First is through a change in expectations. Up until this point, the child has been speaking in one-word utterances and you have been modeling two-word utterances because you were following the "one-up" rule, discussed earlier. Many young children with ASD at this point in therapy will have already begun to imitate your two-word utterances. If this is the case, you can now begin to differentially reinforce two-word utterances. If the child has not done this spontaneously, you can use the child's existing imitation ability and require that he or she imitate your model before achieving his or her goal. If you typically ask, "Blow bubbles?" and the child responds "Bubbles," say, "Blow?" If the child imitates "Blow," then ask, "Blow bubbles?" and see whether the child attempts to imitate both words. By changing your expectations and emphasizing both words, the child will likely begin to imitate the two-word utterance. If not, do not shift to this kind of model: "Blow? Blow." "Bubbles? Bubbles." Instead, stay with the two-word model.

Another technique is to set up choices in which two words are necessary for the child to express his or her meaning. Here is an example:

Within a building activity in which you are building towers, offer two blocks, one of which is the same size as the other blocks in the tower, and one that is the wrong size—too small. Then, when the child asks for "block," offer both sizes and ask, "Big block or little block?" As the child says "Block" and reaches for the big block, hold it back and say, "Big block," and use imitation to elicit the two-word utterance, delivering the correct block as soon as the child approximates the two-word utterance.

In this example, the two words are necessary to capture the child's meaning. Setting up the activity in this way emphasizes the utility of two-word utterances for expressing one's thoughts. You can think of countless ways to offer these useful two-word discrimination models: Big cookie or little cookie? Drink juice or stir juice? Feed baby or feed Pooh? Drive car or crash car? Poke dough or roll dough? Red marker or blue marker?

Going Beyond Two-Word Utterances

Going beyond the two-word sentence involves teaching syntax. It is necessary to have an S-LP direct the language interventions for children who are ready to move into three-word utterances. Consult with the S-LP on your team regarding the semantic and syntactic objectives to address within the ESDM intervention, as well as the child's broader, overarching social communication needs; continue using the joint activity frame for teaching.

Adult Language Affects Child Learning

How adults talk to children has tremendous influence on child language learning throughout the infant and preschool periods (Huttenlocher, Vasilyeva, Cymerman, & Levine, 2002; Hart & Risley, 1995). We have not yet discussed in any depth the adult's use of language with children, though we have given many examples. There are several practices that we follow, based on empirical findings of child language learning. One involves the way we have suggested that adults choose the target word to model in order to elicit the child's expressive language. We have said that adults should choose target words that contain an initial sound that is already in the child's spontaneous and imitative repertoire. We have also said that adults should use target sounds that are the early ones that new talkers produce. In this way, we are using the child's own phonological development and following the principles of phonological development from developmental science.

A second main practice in the ESDM is the "one-up" rule described earlier. Use the same number of words as in the child's spontaneous productions plus one. For a child who doesn't speak any words (i.e., the child has an MLU of 0), adults need to highlight and model one-word utterances in their communications to the child. For a child who produces single words consistently and spontaneously (MLU of 1), the adult needs to emphasize two-word utterances. The adult will use one word "up" to model, to expand, and to comment. The child is hearing the next step that the child will produce, and is hearing it in syntactically appropriate ways. Very often, children who are well on their way to mastering verbal language at their current level will begin to imitate spontaneously the adult's expanded (by one) language production. From immediate imitation, the child will begin to display occasional, and then more frequent, spontaneous use of the new combination.

The main exception to the one-up rule is for children with a primary expressive language impairment as well as ASD. These are children who demonstrate significant speech production deficits compared to their superior receptive language abilities. It is clear that specific language disorders also occur in some children with ASD (Kjelgaard & Tager-Flusberg, 2001). For such children, consult with the team S-LP. These children's needs are quite special and go beyond the general plan outlined here.

A third adult language practice involves adults' responses that "recast," or restate, the child's speech while correcting errors. Typically developing children respond to recasts by imitating the correct form more often than other types of adult responses to their errors (Farrar, 1992). Recasts allow the adult to model the phonology, or articulation, of the word; the semantics, or meaning of the word; or the syntax, or grammar, of the multiword construction. Recasts are not corrections, in that they do not require the child to change his or her utterance and copy the adult before he or she achieves the goal of his or her communication. Rather, it's a restatement that the adult makes while providing the child's goal. Recasts are what the adults say as they deliver the child's goal, rather than the response "Good talking," or "Good saying ____________," or "Good asking." We restate the child's production in a way that models appropriate articulation, syntax, or semantics (if the child has used the wrong word). Recasts emphasize again the relationship between the word or word combination and its meaning; they let the child know that his or her communication has been successful, and *powerful*; and they let children know we have understood them and are following through.

For an example of a phonology: Two-year-old Sylvie comments "bu bu" while viewing the bubble jar that her mother, Nancy, shows her. Nancy recasts the immature articulation by saying, "Bubbles! Here are bubbles," and then blows some. Three-year-old Max reaches for markers extended to him for a drawing skill, requesting, "Want bwue marker" as he reaches for the red marker. His therapist Paul provides a semantic recast by saying, "*Red* marker, you want *red* marker" as he hands over the red marker. As an example: Two-year-old Sasha, playing with stuffed toy kittens, brings their faces together and comments, "K'y kiss." Her older sister, Becca, responds with a syntactic, or grammatical recast: "Yes, the kitties are kissing" and makes a kissing noise. In each example, the adult stays within the one-up rule and recasts the child's language by restating the child's production in a slightly more mature form as the adult responds to the child's communicative goal. These are not corrections. The adult is not saying "I want red marker," before delivering the marker.

Adult Language with Echolalic Children

Children who primarily echo rather than speak spontaneously have a great strength—the ability to imitate speech easily. They may also use their echoing for intentional communication, conveying pragmatic functions like requesting, social interaction, or protest (Prizant & Duchan, 1981; Rydell & Mirenda, 1994). However, it seems that they have not yet figured out that speech is about combining words that represent one's own meaning for others to decode. They seem to think that speech is about imitating. There are four main interventions to use to support the use of spontaneous rather than echoed speech:

- Reduce the complexity of your speech. *Do not apply the one-up rule to echoed speech phrases.* Apply it only to spontaneous speech. That means, if the child never produces spontaneous speech (i.e., MLU = 0 for spontaneous speech), your MLU should be at a one-word level, even if the child can echo three- or four-word utterances.
- Try to have other primary adults in the child's life apply this MLU level.
- Don't require imitation to make requests. The child will imitate spontaneously, but don't push it or expect it. Use one-word utterances communicatively in your joint activities, and respond to the child's one-word utterances as if they were spontaneous and fully meaningful.
- Apply the teaching strategies laid out above for getting to spontaneous words from imitated words, fading your single-word model each time until you get a spontaneous production.

In summary, then, when working with a child who primarily uses echolalic speech, proceed according to the principles laid out above, as if the child did not have speech: Differentially reinforce spontaneous speech, work within a limited vocabulary of preferred activities, and slowly build up a solid, simple foundation of spontaneous, meaningful nouns and action words. Also, wait—wait for children to produce their own utterance, and then imitate only or imitate and expand. Follow the one-up rule for the child's meaningful, spontaneous speech. The child's spontaneous language should right itself under these conditions.

Children Who Do Not Progress in Speech Development

Occasionally, there are children who are rapid learners in object and manual imitation, simple instructions, and play skills, but who appear unable to produce speech. These children are rare, in our experience, but they appear in clinical practice. Dealing with this level of speech production deficit is beyond the scope of this text and beyond the scope of those not professionally trained in S-LP. These children's speech development programs need to be directed by an S-LP. In conjunction with the speech pathologist, you would follow the decision tree shown in Figure 9.1 to alter the teaching approach, and if the child continues to have difficulties, you would end up with the need for a visually based alternative system. At this point, you would shift to a nonverbal approach for developing word associations, using manual signs, pictures, or written words. The child's own proclivities will help the speech pathologist and you figure out which of these means is best. Figure 9.1 is a decision tree to be used in decision making about what alternative or augmentative systems to use.

Once you have chosen the alternative language learning route, you essentially follow all the steps outlined in the ESDM curriculum and the objectives, but use the alternate language system. The adult essentially uses total communication, pairing speech with the alternative system for all activities. In our experience, children can progress through all the same steps as verbal children would, including multiword utterances, both expressed and understood, using pictures assembled onto word strips connected with Velcro. We have tested the decision tree in Figure 9.1 in our University of Washington project on children 18 to 30 months old at the start of 2 years of intensive ESDM (25 hours per week). Twenty-two of 24 children, or 92%, developed spontaneous, communicative speech during the treatment period. Thus, this approach has been tested and found to be successful (see Rogers et al., 2006, and Vismara et al., 2009, or additional short-term outcome studies that demonstrate the success of this approach for developing speech).

RECEPTIVE LANGUAGE

The majority of young children with autism have big difficulties in learning to understand speech, and their receptive language development tends to be as delayed as their expressive language development (Lord, Risi, et al., 2005; Stone et al., 1999; Rogers & DiLalla, 1991). Their lack of understanding may be expressed in several ways:

1. *Children may be responding to nonverbal cues.* They may appear to understand more than they actually do, because they learn to read the whole situation and make good guesses about what will happen next based on their past experiences. This is a common stage for all young children developmentally, when they employ receptive language strategies, such as looking for contextual cues or following routines, to determine what to do when given a verbal instruction. Children with autism may continue to use these strategies long after this developmental stage has passed because they continue to demonstrate difficulty understanding the verbal instruction without the cues. For example, a mother may say, "It's time to get in the car," and the child may head to the garage, and Mother assumes the child understands what she has said. But, the mother

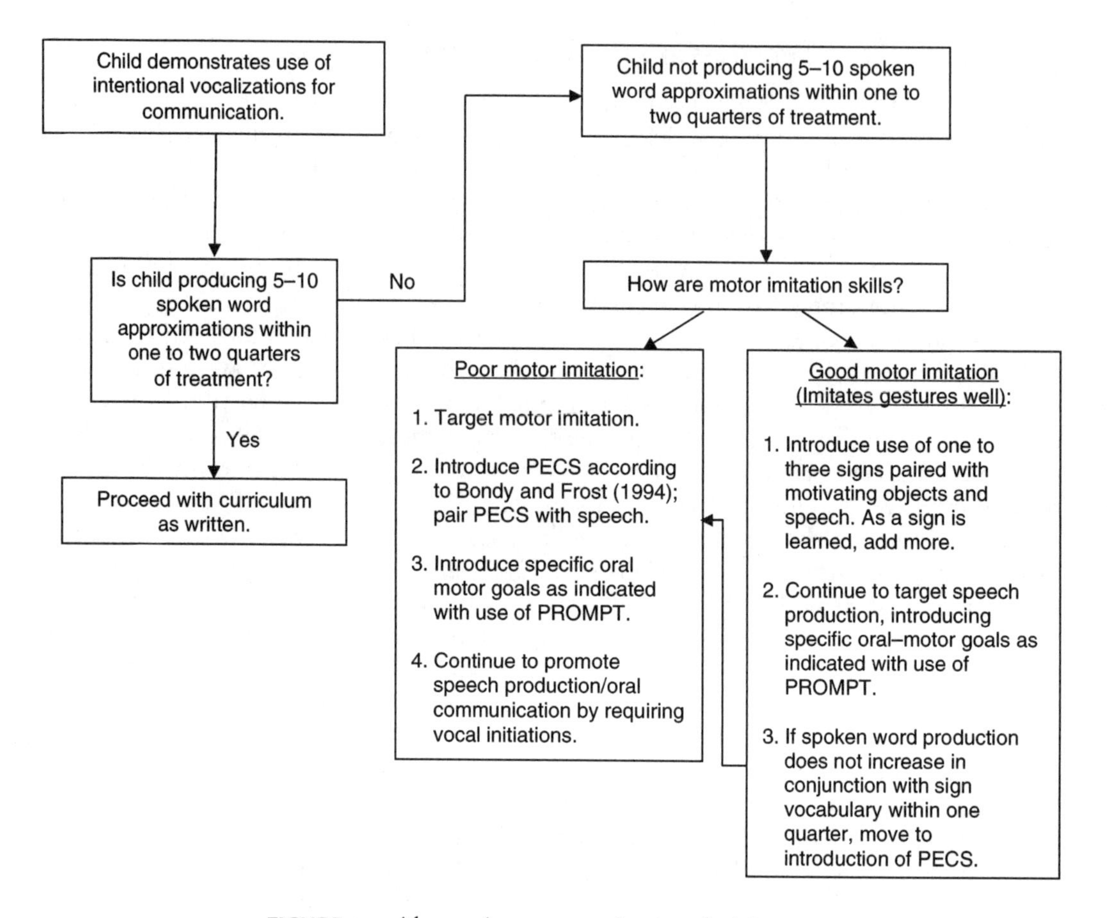

FIGURE 9.1. Alternative communication decision tree.

has also picked up her keys, her purse, and her jacket, and so these may be the cues the child is interpreting.

2. *Children may ignore verbal language.* Sometimes, young children with autism appear to ignore the speech that is being directed to them. Adults may do a terrific job of narrating play, using the one-up rule, and providing excellent language input, but the words may not "penetrate" the child's attention. It is not unusual to see an adult ask a child for something and have the child completely ignore the request.

We must teach children that verbal language is important, that they must respond when instructed, and that they need to listen and attend to what is being said. To a very large extent, all of the techniques that we just discussed about developing expressive verbal language will simultaneously be teaching children the meaning of our verbal communication. Teaching expressive communication using naturalistic strategies is also teaching receptive communication. However, in the ESDM there are a few specific practices that we adopt to highlight receptive language development.

Expect and Require Responding

Give the Instruction within the Appropriate Sentence Length for the Child

Then wait briefly for a child response. If there is none, quickly physically cue the child to the correct response. This teaches the child what the instruction means and that he or she needs to respond to speech.

Don't Take Too Long!

We run the risk of losing the child's attention and interest when we hold back the object and deliver some type of instruction. Therefore, we need to move fast and prompt with something very important to the child. Then we want to be sure that as soon as the child responds to the instruction, even if we prompted him or her to do so, that the child then gets what he or she wanted in the first place.

The turn-taking routines that we discussed earlier are great examples of this concept. When the adult needs to take a turn, the adult can extend his or her hand, say, "Give me," or "My turn," wait briefly for the child to give, and prompt the child to place the object in the adult's hand. Then, the adult takes a very fast turn and gives the object right back, so that the child ends up with the object he or she wanted in the first place. Making easy frequent requests or instructions *within the context of the activity* and requiring follow-through is a crucial teaching technique for developing children's understanding of words and developing their attention and responsiveness to adult language.

Following Verbal Instructions

The main receptive language learning situation that we have not yet addressed involves following verbal instructions. There are several points to consider:

1. *Make sure that the instruction is short* (don't forget the one-up rule!) and use typical, child-directed language. Use the same instructions that others would use in other settings.

2. *Make sure that the verbal instruction precedes the gesture, prompt, or object.* In order to learn the meaning of words, the child needs to hear the word and immediately experience its meaning.

> Consider this scenario. You want to teach a child the instruction "Sit down." If you prompt him or her to sit, and then say, "Sit down," the words don't add anything to the sequence. The child has sat because of the physical prompt. The words are neither an antecedent or a prompt; they have little meaning.
>
> Now, consider the opposite. The child hears "Sit down" and then experiences a hand that gets him or her down into the chair and a desired object or activity that follows. This sequence happens every time the child sits. "Sit down" is the antecedent, and the physical maneuver is the prompt. Then you fade the prompt, so that the antecedent is associated with the behavior through the power of the reinforcing consequence.

3. *Follow through.* If you say it, you need to follow through. It is amazing how often people give instructions to children with autism without expecting or requiring a response. The child has to learn that speech is meaningful, that there is reason to attend to the sounds coming out of the people around them. This does *not* mean that we will become engaged in battles around compliance, or that we will physically bring a child who has made a spontaneous transition to another useful activity back to a past activity to clean it up. We want to be reasonable and maximize the opportunities for teaching. Rather, it means that adults should gauge their timing around instructions so that there is time to prompt and follow through within the "teachable moment"—while children are still attending and interested.

4. *Reinforce*! Have a toy or object ready to follow a "Sit down." Sitting down to have shoes removed or the start of a goodbye routine is generally not a strong enough reward until those routines become very reinforcing. Be ready to deliver a fast and powerful reinforcer.

CONCLUSION

Throughout this manual we have emphasized the use of adult language within meaningful contexts, at simple syntactic levels and with limited targeted vocabulary and accompanying gestures. Verbal language accompanies every activity, and in all activities children are hearing appropriate speech production models. The procedures we have laid out for teaching nonverbal communication and expressive language will also result in receptive language learning.

In the same way that expressive communication is woven into every activity, receptive language is also woven into every activity. Every choice that is given is a receptive language activity. Every instruction, every comment, every model, and every expansion is a receptive language learning opportunity. The careful pairing of context and experience with language provides as powerful an opportunity for receptive language as for expressive language. For the majority of young children with autism, their receptive language and their expressive language will develop in parallel.

Young children with autism present severe difficulties in expressing and understanding verbal communication, as well as intentional nonverbal communication. Yet these children are capable of making enormous gains in these areas. Crucial adult techniques involve adults creating many opportunities for the child to intentionally communicate throughout the day; facilitating the child's expressive language development from vocalization through multiword utterances by means of vocal play, imitation, modeling, and shaping within a variety of joint activities; and facilitating the child's receptive language development by simplifying and directing his or her language to the child using both nonverbal and verbal communication, and expecting the child to respond. As we help children develop nonverbal and verbal communication inside meaningful communicative exchanges, they are learning functional language skills, based on their own thoughts and feelings. This is how most children learn to use and understand spoken language (Tager-Flusberg, 1993; McCune, 1995; Tomasello, 1995; Prizant & Wetherby, 1998; Yoder & Warren, 2001; Charman et al., 2001; Csibra & Gergely, 2005).

We began this book by stating that autism is at its heart a social disorder. It may appear as if we have not addressed social objectives in the chapters on imitation, play, nonverbal communication, and verbal communication. However, if you examine the items on the ESDM Curriculum Checklist (Appendix A) under the Social domain for Levels 1 and 2, you will see that we have discussed teaching every single behavior listed. Social behavior does not stand alone; it occurs in interactions involving play, requesting, sharing emotion and attention, greetings and goodbyes, and sharing materials. The key social behaviors are part and parcel of these other activities and will be embedded in your work on the four areas that we have covered in such depth.

Two content areas that we have not yet discussed in detail include peer relationships and self-care skills. We discuss these areas in the next and final chapter, in the context of designing and implementing the ESDM in a group classroom setting.

Chapter 10

Using the Early Start Denver Model in Group Settings

Thus far, descriptions of the ESDM have highlighted 1:1 interactions of adults and children using the ESDM. However, as stated in Chapter 1, the ESDM involves a curriculum and a set of teaching procedures that can be used in a variety of settings, including group preschool classroom programs, and that is the focus of this chapter. The model began as a group model in a specialized preschool, and the data for the first four Denver Model efficacy papers came from children in group settings (Rogers, 1977; Rogers et al., 1986, 1987; Rogers & Lewis, 1989; Rogers & DiLalla, 1991). The Denver Model has also been implemented by personnel within inclusive early childhood programs in a variety of public settings, addressing both the special learning needs of young children with ASD and enhancing the learning environment for all the children.

A group setting that uses the ESDM does not, at first glance, look or feel different from any other well-designed and well-structured toddler or preschool classroom. We have found that the needed specialization for young children with autism can be embedded into a typical environment. Furthermore, setting up the classroom in a typical way supports children's inclusion in typical settings.

Our goals for individual child learning in a group environment involve broad developmental goals. Children will learn to do the following:

1. Follow daily routines and negotiate transitions independently.
2. Participate independently in large- and small-group activities.
3. Communicate intentionally with peers and adults in a group environment.
4. Engage in purposeful play and appropriate use of objects.
5. Develop personal independence in managing belongings, daily living, and safety skills (e.g., put away coats and backpacks, clear cup and plate after meals, put away toys, dressing, hand washing, toileting, eating).
6. Interact spontaneously with peers and adults.

7. Expand developmental skills in all areas.
8. Acquire the needed skills to participate in the next learning environment.

Classroom activities are designed to achieve these general developmental goals as well as each child's individual learning objectives identified through the assessment process. Each child's individual objectives are addressed every day, generally embedded in ongoing activities, and taught either in brief 1:1 exchanges or in small groups during the activity, but also in scheduled individual teaching times once or twice per day if needed in order to achieve progress.

The teaching of many content areas have already been addressed in this book—communication, play, and imitation. The teaching procedures and content are exactly the same in a group setting as those described earlier. The adult who is interacting with the child at the moment creates interesting joint activity routines within existing classroom activities, using the same materials and themes that the other children and adults are using. The adult attracts the child's attention and then creates learning opportunities. The interaction styles described earlier occur in the group setting, and are part of the scheduled group activities listed on the classroom schedule. When the activity is a group activity (e.g., a book activity) rather than a more individual activity (e.g., centers), the adult works with a small group of three to four children, moving very quickly from one child to the next and interacting with each child sequentially to maintain a high rate of participation and many learning opportunities for each child. One or more supporting adults sit behind the children, ready to intervene or support (silently) when needed, but "invisible" to the children, so that the children's attention to the leader is not interrupted, and also so that it is quite clear to the children to whom they should be looking and listening.

This chapter describes methods for designing and implementing ESDM-based instruction for young children with ASD in group classroom settings, both center-based and inclusive, using the planning and teaching strategies already described.

CONSIDERING CHARACTERISTICS OF AUTISM IN CLASSROOM ORGANIZATION

Planning for a successful classroom learning environment for young children with autism is aided by considering certain learning characteristics. Three learning needs require particular attention: assisting attention by reducing competing sensory stimuli, supporting communication by using both verbal and visual–auditory input, and supporting temporal sequencing.

Focusing Attention

Multisensory, highly enriched environments are common practice in preschool settings, but some children with ASD have difficulty screening out extraneous, unimportant information, selectively attending to primary information that is central to a task at hand, and shifting attention smoothly (Courchesne et al., 1993; Frith & Baron-Cohen, 1987). The physical environment of the classroom itself needs to highlight the important learning task of the moment and lowlight other sources of stimulation. It is quite helpful to have a classroom environment that is neat and well organized, with places for everything in an area to be put away and out of sight.

Communicating Via Multiple Modalities

The profile of strengths in visual–perceptual learning and concomitant weaknesses in auditory learning and language processing that often characterize early autism (Schopler et al., 1995) can result in a child's difficulty in orienting to the environment and current activities. Addressing this need requires the planful and consistent use of visual and auditory cues in addition to speech to communicate to children the current and next activity.

Understanding Sequences of Events and Organizing Sequences of Behaviors

There are many temporal changes that occur in a preschool classroom day. These can be examined at four different levels:

- The overall schedule of the group.
- Major "large-group" transition strategies.
- A child's individualized transition strategies.
- Simple transitions from one activity to the next within a single, scheduled activity period.

Staff need to consider the child's sequence of activities during the day, how these will be communicated to the child, and how the child will be helped to focus on an activity once the transition has been made. Attention to these needs within the classroom is part of the planning process that will ensure that the child actually participates in the planned activity—that he or she has gotten through each transition and has had focused attention during each learning activity.

PHYSICAL ORGANIZATION

The ESDM classroom structure draws from accepted early childhood education best practices and standards, and there are many excellent resources that address the basic and well-understood principles in this area (Cook, Tessier, & Klein, 1999; Bricker, Pretti-Frontzczak, & McComas, 1998). The physical environment acts to select, focus, and organize sensory stimuli. In an ESDM classroom, within every activity:

- The physical environment highlights the center of focus for each child.
- Primary goals for the area and/or activity are clearly identified when making decisions regarding room arrangement and materials.
- The activity area is visually and functionally consistent with one primary goal.

Classrooms are divided into activity-based centers, each with a particular developmental domain in mind. A typical classroom might include areas devoted to table toys, dramatic play, block building, books, art, and sensory experiences, with quiet and noisy activities set apart from each other.

Limited, Clearly Defined Spaces and Materials

It helps to arrange the classroom with limited open spaces, with concrete physical boundaries for various activities, and with clear paths from one place to another. Physical boundaries to separate activity areas may include using furniture or movable partitions; even obstacles such as stop signs can provide needed boundaries. Delimited open space and marking clear paths helps keep children in the activity area and helps them transition independently from one area to another. (See Schopler et al., 1995, for additional ideas.)

Materials Not Relevant to an Activity Are Out of Sight

The same physical space must be utilized for different activities and materials at different times. Therefore, visually hidden or inaccessible storage becomes an important component of classroom design so that only one set of materials is made available at any particular time. Adult-level storage cupboards are ideal, although closed containers or open shelves covered with a sheet or similar material also work. This approach succeeds in focusing children on the basic, appropriate use of materials. Additional materials may be stored and brought out as needed for children who are ready for more complex activities.

For example, it is common practice for dramatic play areas to include a great variety of materials in order to facilitate elaborate symbolic play schemes involving daily life and community activities. However, an area filled with many props may simply become a jumble of unrelated materials for children who demonstrate little or no symbolic play. In the Denver Model classroom, a theme for the dramatic play activity has been selected and is clearly identified for the children by including only the basic props and materials related to that theme. Additional related materials should be stored in the area so that the adult can easily add materials to elaborate the activity as needed.

Limiting the number and complexity of materials serves to focus attention and stimulate simple levels of symbolic play. This should not mean that the area is barren or uninteresting to more advanced children. A range of materials is provided, but materials are arranged planfully. Organization of materials assists all children, not just those with autism.

Other Visual Cues

As in many preschool classrooms, activity areas are clearly labeled with printed words, pictures, or unique symbols that cue their function. For daily "sit down" group activities such as circle time or meals, children's chairs are placed in consistent locations and clearly labeled with their name and picture. For activities such as dressing for water play, a chair labeled with the child's name and a clearly labeled box or basket for clothing is set up near the water table at the appropriate time and to help support the activity. Materials needed for a specific activity are set up right before the activity and put away right after, so they provide clear cues for where the child should be and what the child should be doing.

Transition Planning

An important goal in the ESDM is for children to be intentional and goal directed in their actions so that they function independently within routines. Making independent transitions within the classroom is a clear sign that the child knows where he or she is going and what will happen next. In order for young children to make independent transitions, they need to see where they are going next, they need to know what will happen there, and they need a clear, short route to get there.

For example, the table for snacks should be fairly close to where they wash their hands, so they can move from the sink to their seat at the table independently. Likewise, the post-snack activity area should be close to the snack table so they can move to it without requiring a staff member to take them, and so they can be in sight and supervised as other children finish their meals at the table.

Questions That Can Help Planning

As we've discussed, staffing patterns, physical space, and the needs and dynamics of a particular group of children determine the classroom layout and structure. We have used the following questions to help guide our initial classroom planning and our ongoing evaluation of the adequacy of the current classroom plan:

- Does the arrangement of the physical space adequately support large-group, small-group, and 1:1 activities?
- What safety concerns need to be addressed? Are they adequately managed?
- How many consistent staff members are in the classroom on a daily basis? Is there sufficient coverage for the planned activities?
- How many children are in the whole group? Is each child accounted for in the daily plan?
- How many children are able to engage in appropriate play without special adult support?
- How many children need special support to engage in appropriate play and social interactions? Who will provide the support for each child who needs it, and in each activity in which support is needed?
- Given the overall skill level of the group as well as unique group dynamics, which activities will require less adult supervision, and could occur during staff breaks? Which activities will require more adult supervision and facilitation, and so need to occur with all staff present?
- Are there children in the group who engage in dangerous, destructive, and/or aggressive behaviors without adult support? Is the support plan for those children adequate to keep everyone safe and engaged during all group activities?
- Which additional adults help in the classroom intermittently? What are their skill levels and roles? How will their support best enhance the classroom education?

This list of questions has been helpful to our lead teachers both in setting up new classroom situations and in solving existing classroom problems. When used as a frame for classroom review by the staff, the questions can help identify possible environmental difficulties that are resulting in problems for certain children, staff, or activities.

To ensure smooth transitions in which children travel independently and purposefully from one activity to another, the physical arrangement of the room and daily schedule of activities must be planned in tandem. This kind of planning is our next topic.

PLANNING THE DAILY SCHEDULE AND ROUTINES

The classroom schedule can be organized in such a way that it facilitates the teaching staff's goals and objectives for both the group and the individuals within it. For the benefit of both staff and children, the schedule needs to provide a consistent and predictable framework from one day to the next. Finally, it also has to include three sets of needs and plans: (1) plans for the child group as a whole, (2) plans for the staff members working in the room, and (3) plans for each individual child.

Group Routines

The more precisely planned, consistent, and predictable the group's daily routine is from day-to-day, the greater sense of order and organization it provides for children who often have difficulty making sense out of many events and situations in their lives. Consistent and predictable group routines seem to help children organize goal-directed behavior and predict and plan future events. The daily routine involves consistent locations and sequences of activities. Within the daily routine, there is a balance of activities in all developmental areas and alternation between more highly structured and more adult-directed activities and more child-centered activities, and between active and quiet activities.

Staff Roles

We have found it to be most helpful when staff roles and tasks are articulated for each activity period of the day and are consistent from day-to-day in order to enhance predictability for children. For example, the same staff person may be responsible each day for facilitating hand-washing routines at the sink before a snack or meal. In this way, the location, materials, and consistent staff interactions all provide cues to children for hand washing. Given that staff members all have unique styles, this level of staff consistency also facilitates consistent teaching from day-to-day and enables data collection for individual child progress. Thus, there is a specific plan for each staff member for each activity of the day, and each transition, built into the daily schedule. Of course, staff members are sometimes ill or on vacation, so each staff member needs to know the staff "script" for each activity. Providing these scripts is addressed later in this chapter.

Individual Routines

Similarly, each child's daily routine is individually planned in order to accommodate one-to-one teaching times, OT, speech–language therapies, or other individual activities, as well as small- and large-group activities. While the group structure provides the general frame for the day, for young children with autism, many (hundreds!) of individual teaching moments must be planned into the group schedule in order to support learning. There are as many choices to be made for scheduling individual activities as there are minutes in the day. Staff availability for providing this individual instruction is one variable to consider. The child's personal experience is another variable to consider. The planning needs to also consider the schedule of each individual child. Is there an appropriate sequence of activities and locations for the individual child? Is there some time regularly available for the child to play without instruction? Does the child interact with several different people across the day? We want the sequence of each child's daily experiences to facilitate child attention and engagement.

For example, Kevin's current objectives involve dressing and undressing skills, and so he changes clothes for the water table activity. He needs 1:1 teaching involving a great deal of adult support for this activity, which occurs both before and after the water table. He loves the water table, and it provides an excellent activity for working on object imitation. However, in order to accommodate the staff time needed for Kevin's dressing program, he has been the last child to join the water table and the first child to end the water table, reducing his time there to fewer than 10 minutes. This does not allow enough time to practice his imitation and peer interaction objectives and also give him some moments of free play, and he protests his early departure every day, resulting in upsets that interfere with redressing. The following activity is his speech therapy, which cannot be easily rescheduled given the S-LP's schedule. However, the preceding activity is snack, and he is not an enthusiastic eater. After his independent eating objectives are covered, Kevin does not have much more to do with eating. The lead teacher decides to have Kevin be the first child to wash hands and get to the snack table, instead of the last child, which had been occurring before because of his support needs. He is also the first to leave the snack table, transitioning to the dressing chair/water table activity before any other child. Now, his dressing routine is finished and he is the first child at the water table. This gives him twice as much time at the water table, and with this change he now makes the transition out of the water table without difficulty.

From the individual child perspective, this part of Kevin's schedule did not fit his needs and preferences. Changing his individual routine also involved changing a staff person's schedule, since he needed 1:1 assistance in all three activities. However, making this change allowed Kevin to be fully engaged in both activities following the water table: redressing and speech–language therapy. By consciously evaluating the daily routine from the perspective of the individual child, one can identify sequences that interfere with child engagement and learning and find ways to improve them.

Fitting Individual Child Objectives into the Group Activity

The plan for each group activity period should indicate which objectives from each child's Daily Data Sheet are to be accomplished in that activity period. Posting each child's activity-related objectives on the wall in the activity location helps remind all the staff members what objectives are to be taught in that activity period. In general, developmental domains fit into certain activities nicely. Fine motor skills fit well into art, play dough, manipulative center, mealtimes, and the water table. Gross motor skills occur during playground and in group floor activities. Language and social skills are involved in every activity. Cognitive activities fit inside activity centers and small-group activities. Functional and symbolic play skills are addressed in dramatic play center.

Small-group circle activities like hello, goodbye, and music and group book activities provide opportunities for receptive and expressive language, sensory social routines, gestural and vocal imitation, and cognitive and social skills practice.

Individual Instruction Inside a Group Setting

Young children with autism who are still in the stages of early language acquisition in a group setting receive daily individual instruction periods to increase the rate of learning of acquisition skills. In both center-based and inclusion classrooms, we have delivered an individual teaching session of 15 to 20 minutes daily to each child with autism. These sessions are provided by classroom staff, may take place either in the classroom or outside of the classroom, and are in addition to individual therapy sessions from others like S-LP or OT.

The focus of 1:1 teaching, as well as classroom instruction, is acquisition steps of objectives that are not learned quickly in the group activities. As soon as a target skill is acquired in 1:1 teaching, it should be brought into other activities for generalization. In this way, the child is facilitated to generalize a mastered skill with a familiar person and identical materials in a new setting. The focus may also involve generalizing skills that have been mastered in other individual therapies to a new person and location.

How and when 1:1 teaching sessions take place may be quite varied from child to child, but they are scheduled for each child and the assigned staff member as a consistent activity within the daily routine. There may be group activities that are quite difficult to individualize for a particular child. Shortening playground activity for that child may provide a good time for 1:1 teaching. Children may arrive early to class, or stay late, to accommodate some 1:1 teaching. For older, higher-functioning children, 1:1 teaching may not be needed, given the amount of individual instruction that is embedded in the group activities. However, for beginning students and those not yet verbal, or those who need individual support for most objectives, one or more individual daily teaching times in the classroom day is essential for good progress.

Daily Record Keeping

Daily record-keeping summary sheets for each child include completing his or her Daily Data Sheet after each teaching activity, which reminds staff members of each child's objectives on a daily basis. Additional notes about behavior, reinforcers, and so on may be included at that time. At the end of the week, Daily Data Sheets are updated for the following week, identifying the new acquisition and maintenance steps for the coming week based on learning from the past week. This also identifies objectives in which there is no progress, so that the teaching plan can be altered as described earlier. Each staff member is responsible for the record keeping for two or so children, updating notebooks, data sheets, and staff plans in a team meeting to plan for the next week.

Down Times

A final issue concerning child schedules is "down time." While our goal is for children to be appropriately engaged throughout the day, a certain amount of "down time" is inevitable, and is probably as valid for children as our own coffee breaks are for us. However, many children react to the lessening of structure by becoming isolated, unengaged, or somewhat disorganized, and it will take them a little time to reengage in purposeful, structured activities. By careful observation of each child we can identify activities that provide needed breaks for each, but also support appropriate play and blend with appropriate classroom behaviors to help "reentry."

For example, Lindsay greatly prefers outside time, where she wants to dig in the sand, dump it into containers, and sift it with her hands. It is very difficult to transition her back into the classroom group activity after playground because of her love of the sand and her upset at having to leave it, and her upset lasts a long time, preventing her from participating in the group. However, playground time provides staff breaks and there are not enough staff members to keep her engaged in other activities and prevent the sand play. Lindsay also loves her OT sessions, and her time there is a highly preferred activity. She leaves OT well organized and ready for the next group activity. So, the plan is to schedule OT to occur at the end of her sand time. When the OT approaches her at the sand with a therapy ball, Lindsay eagerly joins the OT and the ball for the transition to OT. The objectives she would have worked on during the group activity are woven into the OT activity, with Lindsay fully engaged in learning.

An essential part of overall planning in the ESDM is to identify a few activities for each child that the child chooses independently, seems to enjoy, and that can also be molded into appropriate "down time" activities.

CHOREOGRAPHY OF THE CLASSROOM

The level of planning that is necessary to integrate group needs and activities, needs of individual children, and staff roles requires good team communication. To lay out this complex choreography, we have found it helpful to develop and post three types of schedules for all to see. The first is the basic group daily routine schedule, which includes the time and sequence of main activities throughout the day. Table 10.1 shows an example. The second overlays each of the children's individual schedules on the daily group schedule as seen in Table 10.2. The third type overlays the staff individual schedules on the daily group schedule, as shown in Table 10.3.

The daily group schedule is usually planned by the early childhood educator, with input from the rest of the team. It is constructed around a series of activity periods; inside each activity period is a typical preschool activity with typical materials available. Each activity period provides the elements for joint activity routines (which provide the teaching) and independent play. The latter provides practice time, opportunities to model from other children, as well as independent and social spontaneous play.

STAFF PLANNING AND COMMUNICATION

The precision of the planning and implementation involved in classroom management requires extensive staff communication. Classroom staff members meet together each day after class to write progress notes together, complete data, discuss any problems that came up that day, and review the next day's plans. One afternoon a week there is a more extended meeting to plan the following week's activities, prepare materials, and

TABLE 10.1. Sample Group Daily Schedule

Time	Activity
8:45–9:00	Arrival
9:00–9:15	Opening small groups
9:15–9:45	Hand washing → Snack
9:45–10:15	Dressing programs → Sensory experience
10:15–11:00	Center activities → Individual learning
11:00–11:15	Small-group music and movement
11:15–11:45	Playground: gross motor
11:45–12:30	Hand washing → Lunch
12:30–12:45	Books/quiet time
12:45–1:15	Second center activities
1:15–1:30	Small-group music and movement → Closing

organize the space for the coming week. Staff roles, teaching skills, and interactions are evaluated and refined on an ongoing basis.

In addition, the entire group—classroom staff and individual therapists—review each child's progress weekly in brief, 15-minute meetings during the first hour of the day, before the children arrive. These progress review meetings allow for review of data and updating of the child's plans. The child's team leader oversees the discussion and identifies new acquisition steps along with any changes that need to be made to improve

TABLE 10.2. Sample Staff Daily Schedule for First Hour of Day

Time	Activity	Mary	Jane	Joe
8:45–9:00	Arrival	Greet parents	Coats/toileting	Supervise classroom
9:00–9:15	Opening group	Lead	Backup	Backup
9:15–9:45	Hand washing → Snack	"Dismiss" children from group—staggered Assist final small group to transition to sink, make sure snack equipment and materials are set up properly, and then join snack table.	Assist first small group of children with hand washing and move to snack table. Begin "filler" activity at snack table. When all children are at the table, lead opening snack song, begin to pass food.	Back up group until first children are finished hand washing. Assist second, then third small group of children with hand washing and move to table. Individual eating program with Suzie

TABLE 10.3. Sample Individual Child Daily Schedule for First 3 Hours

Time	Activity	Johnny	Suzie	Mark
8:45–9:00	Arrival	Coat then toilet—Jane	Coat then movement activities—Joe	Coat then movement activities—Joe
9:00–9:15	Opening group	Group	Group	Group
9:15–9:45	Hand washing → Snack	Wash with Jane Table with Jane	Wash with Joe Eating program—Joe	Wash with Mary Table with Jane
9:45–10:15	Dressing programs → Sensory experience	Dress with Mary Sensory with Jane: T, Th, F Speech therapy: M, W	1:1 lesson with Joe: M–F	Dress with Mary Sensory with Jane: M, W, F Speech therapy: T, Th
10:15–11:00	Center activities Individual learning	Center until 10:45 10:45 1:1 with Mary	Center: T, Th, F Speech therapy: M, W	Center

learning rates in the functional behavioral plans or various objectives, as laid out earlier in the decision tree.

Finally, the emotional demands of this kind of work need to be acknowledged. The culture of the classroom must support ongoing discussions concerning staff morale and working relationships. Conflicts have to be resolved immediately and supportively. Personal feelings of inadequacy or failure are inevitable in this kind of work. Time and again, staff face the feeling that, "If only I did the right thing, this child would do better." Such feelings of frustration, anger, failure, and disappointment need to be aired, shared, and resolved through open, supportive discussions among the team.

SMALL- AND LARGE-GROUP INSTRUCTION

Group experiences are essential preparation for later success in school settings; thus, the main goals for group activities are developing those skills needed for children to participate in and benefit from group instruction:

- The ability to sit in a group, in close proximity to other children.
- The ability to focus and maintain attention toward one "lead" adult.
- The ability to demonstrate mastered skills within a small or large group.
- The ability to respond appropriately to the bids of other children in the group.

How does one facilitate the participation of a young child with autism in a group? There are several techniques that make this work. Pick activities for group participation that have meaning for the child with autism as well as for others: familiar songs and movement games, rhythm band activities, and show and tell that involves passing materials around. Language routines need to be accompanied by props for children who don't understand the language: photos, symbols, flannel boards, or other kinds of concrete props that are meaningful to the child.

Individualized learning interactions with a child every 30 seconds or so is a key to successful participation in a group. Maintain a lively pace so that all children are actively participating the majority of the time. A child who is inattentive or engaged in inappropriate behaviors is often demonstrating that he or she is not being given enough opportunity to participate actively, that motivating objects or activities have not been included, that they are not being delivered frequently enough, or that the design or implementation of the activity is not permitting the child to participate.

Expect the child to perform a maintenance skill in a group situation at high frequency. Position the child directly in front of the leader of the group, and in close proximity. Be sure that the activity has meaning and that child participation is reinforced through access to desired materials or activities. Especially in the early stages, group activities may not contribute as much toward acquisition skills as they do toward maintenance and generalization of social, cognitive, motor, and language skills that the child has already mastered in other settings. Building group activities on what children already know how to do supports participation and engagement.

Thus, successful group experiences depend upon several factors:

- Group activities must be kept short; no more than 10 minutes is a good rule of thumb.
- Each child must be given frequent (at least every 30 seconds or so) opportunities for active and successful participation.
- Group activities must be interesting, enjoyable, and provide opportunities for movement or object manipulation for each child. They need to move along at an interesting pace.
- Children must be asked and supported to participate in ways they are capable of doing. Passive sitting and observing is an inappropriate intervention goal for a young child.

Choosing Group Activities

The group activities are chosen with the overall skill level and interests of the group in mind as well as the adaptability of the activities to accommodate varying levels of skill within the group. One or more objectives for each child are taught in each group activity, and the group activities are planned with each individual child's objectives in mind. The group activity is thus adapted for individual children, using the same materials, to be simpler or more complex, and what each child is asked to do in the activity may be quite different, though all are related to the theme of the activity.

The activities do not change daily; instead they are maintained for a week, with appropriate variation through elaboration for children who need variation. Thus, there is enough repetition that young children with ASD can learn the expectations of the activity over the week.

For example, an activity might be planned that involves cutting out three circles to make a snowman. Some children may be ready to practice cutting out the shapes and gluing them on a piece of paper. Another child might simply be expected to match several precut circles to outlines on a piece of paper. A third child might be helped to glue many precut circles on a piece of paper in order to practice squeezing a bottle of glue and stopping at the appropriate time. The objective of the activity is very specific and unique for each child, even though the activity has been prepared for the group as a whole using similar materials.

Organizing the Staff Teaching Roles

Part of the planning for each of these activities involves deciding which staff member is to teach which objectives to which children. How is this done? Let's focus first on an activity like centers, snack, or playground, where children are working more independently with the materials than they would in other activities. Assuming a ratio of 1:2 for the children with autism, a staff member will join a child, spend 5 minutes or so in a joint activity routine targeting the planned teaching objectives, mark the Daily Data Sheet for the first trial response for all maintenance and acquisition objectives observed, and move to the next child, being sure that the child who is being left is engaged appropriately. The same staff member will do this teaching activity every day, so as the child masters the acquisition step, the staff person goes on to the next teaching step.

In a teacher-led small-group activity, like hello circle, the leader of the group will deliver all of the targeted objectives to all of the children. The other staff members are positioned behind the children, ready to prompt a child who is receiving an instruction and needs prompting to respond. However, the assisting person is silent and "invisible" to the child. The instructions, interactions, and reinforcers come from the leader, so the child is attending to the group leader. In a center-based activity, each staff member will "head" one center, delivering the individual teaching related to that center to each child who comes to that center.

Preplanning the Activity

Including the young child with autism as an active participant in a group activity requires preplanning. The lead adult has to have thought through what he or she will ask the child with autism to do in this activity, and be ready with props and ideas to act on this plan. The key is to plan specific actions or responses that will be expected from the child with autism, using the same materials as the core group activity, and in such a way that blends with the overall purpose of the group. The lead adult should think through the activity ahead of time and jot down props, objectives, and ideas. Remember that the activity will run for a week, so once the planning is done, it is done for the whole week. Table 10.4 shows an example of a plan for a flannel board activity for a group of three or four children that highlights colors, shapes, and numbers. Uses of the materials for receptive and expressive language, social skills, and cognitive skills are included in the plan.

Props for Staff

A strategy that has proven to be very useful for classroom staff, as well as drop-in therapists or volunteers, is the use of "cheat sheets." These are posted above sight level for the children in each activity area, can be read from a short distance, and contain cues

TABLE 10.4. Plan for a Flannel Board Activity

Core activity and materials

Counting: flannel board shapes including matched sets of shapes in four colors.

Strategies and possible objectives

- Simple to more complex imitation may be prompted within an accompanying song and throughout the activity.
- One-step instructions may be given to individual children (i.e., "Stand up," "Sit down," "Come here," "Give me").
- Children may be asked to hand a piece to another child and prompted to use social phrases (i.e., "Your turn," "Here").
- Some children may simply rote count while others may be encouraged toward 1:1 correspondence while counting.
- Some children may match shapes or colors on the flannel board.
- Some children may identify shapes or colors.

for each child's objectives. For example, a "cheat sheet" in the fine motor skills area might be

- Johnny—cut across 1-inch strips, imitate strokes, three- to five-piece puzzles, beads
- Mary—cut along a line, representational drawing, bead sequences
- David—make marks on paper, single-piece puzzles, shape sorter

Social and communication objectives are often posted in several appropriate places around the room near each area. These "cheat sheets" are not meant to fully explain objectives—they are simply reminders. Each child's complete set of objectives is also posted in a central location in the room and can be referred to easily, as are the data sheets.

Physical Location of the Staff

The objectives targeted for an individual child for an activity should indicate the focus of the child's attention and interaction. This determines the physical position for adult and child. Appropriate physical positioning of the adult behind, beside, or in front of the child focuses the child's attention toward key elements in an activity. For many self-care, independent, and fine motor activities, the child is prompted from behind. In this way, the child's center of focus is the activity and materials (e.g., spoon and bowl, paper and marker, sink and soap). Physical positioning directly in front of the child is necessary during activities that facilitate social exchanges and communication.

CLASSROOM BEHAVIOR MANAGEMENT

The approach to behavior management has three main goals: to maximize safety for all, to maximize a classroom atmosphere conducive to learning, and to maximize individual child learning of adaptive, acceptable behavior.

In Chapter 6, we discussed the procedures for documenting problem behaviors, gathering baseline data, conducting a functional assessment or analysis, and developing a positive behavior support plan by the behavior analyst or other staff member with such expertise. The plan is shared with all team members who will work with this child. The plan for potentially dangerous behaviors is implemented immediately. If the child's problem behavior is potentially dangerous, the plan is implemented as soon as the child begins to attend the classroom program. However, if the child's unwanted behaviors are not a source of danger to anyone, the child will enter the classroom and be assigned to an individual staff member for the first days to learn the routine, while behavior data are kept. If the data demonstrate decreasing problem behaviors, we continue to chart and manage the behavior as we have been during the baseline phase. On the other hand, if the data suggest no change or an increase in problem behaviors over the first 2 weeks, then the positive behavior plan is implemented.

We also recognize that children with ASD may have difficulty modulating their own levels of sensory arousal, becoming easily agitated, aggressive, or overly passive (Baranek, David, Poe, Stone, & Watson, 2006). If this is a continuing source of difficulty for the child, the consulting OT would be asked to assist the staff in finding sensory social activities that will help the child to be better regulated. Calming or arousing activities are then provided *proactively*. As a note of caution, we have found that calming or soothing activities may also reinforce negative behaviors if they are provided after the negative behaviors occur. This is not to say we should not attempt to calm children who have become out of control due to sensory overload. It simply underscores the importance of using proactive measures with children whose arousal levels can be moderated by well-chosen sensory social activities (Anzalone & Williamson, 2000).

TRANSITIONS AND INDIVIDUAL SCHEDULE SYSTEMS

Transitions between activities present special challenges in any classroom. A successful transition is one in which the group as a whole flows smoothly from one activity into the next, with individual children transitioning independently and starting to participate in the next activity without empty "waiting time," upset, distraction, or aimless wandering. A smooth transition maximizes teaching and learning opportunities. Ragged transitions can interrupt children's participation in learning activities for a good part of the next activity.

For example, 3-year-old Melanie is happily involved with the sand table, one of her favorite activities. As the activity approaches its ending, she is allowed to play as long as possible because she enjoys it so much, and because the staff knows she will be upset at the end. At the end of the time, Jackie, the lead teacher, approaches her and says, "All done with sandbox, Melanie, all done." She signs "all done," puts the lid on the box, and then she takes Melanie's hand to lead her away. Melanie resists, straining to stay, and Jackie picks her up and carries her away. Melanie begins to cry and struggle as Jackie carries her to circle time, places her in her seat, and crouches in front of her to try to soothe her. The other children are already in circle time and music is playing as the group awaits the teacher to lead the activity. Melanie continues to cry, scream, and struggle, hitting toward the children at either side, who have to be moved and upsetting them. The children stop attending to the music and focus on struggling Melanie, and

Jackie decides to remove Melanie from the group so the activity can continue. Jackie takes Melanie to a beanbag in the back and tries to comfort her. Meanwhile, Russell, an assistant who had put the music on, now tries to interest the children again, passing out rhythm instruments and doing his best to engage the others. However, the group is now short one assisting adult, and several children are in conflict in the back, moving their chairs away from an instigator, whom Russell reprimands. Some children shake their instruments to the music, and others watch the human drama going on. Not much learning occurs in this activity for anyone, and Melanie never calmed down enough to join it. The teacher's plans for the activity have been scrapped and the whole group has been "maintained" for the 15 minutes it takes to quiet and reengage Melanie, at which point it is time for another 10-minute transition to snack for the whole group.

In this example, we see the effects of a poor transition plan, not just on the child who is having trouble, but on the entire classroom. Every person in this classroom, both child and adult, has been affected negatively by the transition problem, and a full half hour of programming time has been affected, for Melanie and for every other child.

In the ESDM, transitions are planned with as much care and detail as other activities. Independent transitions can be complex tasks for children who have difficulty sequencing behaviors and following a mental plan. Consistency from day-to-day is one way to assist children to predict "what will happen next." As we describe below, there are many additional strategies used in the ESDM classroom that help to ensure smooth transitions. These involve multiple cues, use of adults, individual plans, and various types of supports.

Use Auditory and Visual Signals for Group Transitions

All transitions begin with concrete and specific signals that an activity is ending, including both auditory and visual cues, such as flicking the lights or ringing a bell in addition to verbal cues. Verbal directions are short, precise, and consistent from day-to-day. Consistent "ending" and "beginning" songs are particularly effective for all children and especially for those who do not understand or process verbal directions well.

Assign Staff Roles for Each Transition

Clearly defined staff roles during group transitions are critical for the transition flow. There are three main staff roles that have to be assigned: the opener, the bridge, and the closer.

The Opener

At the assigned time, one staff member opens the next activity. That person is the first to go to the new location, light it up, get the materials out, and arrange the furniture. The goal is for the opener to set up the new activity so it acts as a magnet, drawing the children who are ready to move into the new activity area. If the next activity is a center activity, that staff member can set up one center and begin the activity with each child who comes in. If the next activity is a group activity and needs the whole group present to begin, the opener can use songs and finger plays, bubbles, or other short "fillers" to engage the first children while other staff are closing and finishing the previous activity and transitioning the group. In this way, the "new" activity draws children toward the new space and facilitates independent transitions.

The Bridge

The second staff member helps children end the previous activity and move from the old activity into the new activity space. That person remains in the old activity space but assists children to finish and move along into the new space, sending them "over the bridge" to the new activity. The bridging person also helps put materials away and helps children end and move to the next activity. This person moves to the new space as the majority of the group moves, to take up his or her assigned role in the next activity, and help the opener engage the children in the activity, so the children are not waiting or wandering.

The Closer

The closer is the last adult to make the transition. This person puts away the remaining materials, shuts down the lighting, facilitates and follows the last children through the transition to the next setting, and closes down the space. Now, the old activity is closed up, shut down and put away, and all staff and children are assembled for the new activity, which is already in progress.

Individual Transition Plans

As adults, we often use schedule systems like lists, handheld devices, and daytimers to keep us moving through our day and organized for what has to be accomplished in each hour. Visual or object schedules and transition strategies serve the same purpose for children who lack internal organization, are unable to plan ahead, and may not have the language capacities to benefit from verbal cues or instructions. While the consistency of the daily schedule is enough for some children to learn the daily routine and to make independent transitions, other children need additional support. Visual schedule systems and the use of transitional objects are more tangible and concrete and less transient than verbal explanations or instructions. They are provided if needed.

In our own group settings, in the first few weeks after a child joins the group classroom, the child is walked through each transition with an assigned staff member. No individual props or supports are used at this point. Our goal is to have the child experience the flow of activities and learn about each new activity and location: where they sit or stand, what happens there, and with whom. The child is engaged in the activity 1:1 with an assigned staff member.

If it is a small-group activity, the group leader engages the child within the group, with the supporting person behind. When the new child is not able to participate any more in that activity, the child may leave the group and play with a staff member near the others. When the transition cues occur, the new child is walked to the new location. Some children learn the routine in this fashion, and are anticipating the next activity by the group transition cues alone in the next few weeks. For those children, individual adult supports are withdrawn and the general transition supports are used. Those children are now transitioning independently.

Use of Visual Supports for Independent Transitions

For children who do not anticipate the next activity after this orientation period, we move to individual visual and physical supports for independent transitions. The child would have a written objective concerning making independent transitions, and a teaching plan would be developed, as described earlier in this manual. Teaching the sequence of steps in an independent transition involves teaching a behavior chain, and we use prompting, fading, shaping, and chaining to teach children to carry out independently the four individual steps in the chain: get the support, carry it to the new location, place it where it goes, and take one's place in the new activity.

In the beginning, we use hand-over-hand assistance and physical and/or verbal prompting in order to teach the use of these transition supports. Consistent key phrases should be used as prompts, (e.g., "Check your schedule," "Time to ... ," "Go to ..."). Assistance should also be faded as soon as the child is "moving in the right direction." However, immediate assistance should again be provided if the child begins to become distracted during the transition. Through repetition, the child will begin to make a connection between the object, picture or symbol, and the activity or area to go to, and will be able to complete the transition independently. This is a skill that we would teach from "behind" the child, following the child through the transition and prompting him or her from behind, so that the child has the sense of leading or moving independently.

We have learned that children learn to use transition supports more quickly if prompts and assistance are consistently available from a familiar staff member. During group transitions, this level of individual attention toward each child is not possible without staggering transitions, as previously discussed. In some instances, it may also be appropriate for a particular child to begin to use transition objects for only one or two transitions throughout the day. These kinds of "who and when" decisions need to be made with regard to the objectives, needs, and skills of individual children, group dynamics, and staff availability.

Choosing the Best Support for Each Child

Each child's cognitive and language abilities are considered in the development of the most appropriate schedule and/or transition system for that specific child. The following represents somewhat of a hierarchy in the use of objects, pictures, symbols, and more complex schedule boards. Some children will do fine with only the basic language, auditory, and visual cues that mark all transitions; others will be helped with one or a combination of the following strategies. Child behavior determines whether children need additional supports. The goal is that children move without being led from one activity to another; that is the outcome we are seeking from the use of these supports and the standard for evaluating success.

Transitional Objects

In the closing activity, the child is given and carries an object that is functionally related to the new activity location. For example, a child might be given a spoon or cup to carry to the lunch table, toothpaste to carry to the sink, a ball to take to the playground, or a favorite book to take to the book area. Once there, the child is taught to place the object in a "receptacle" of some kind that is also clearly identified with an identical object or labeled with a picture of the object. With repetition, the child will learn this simple, concrete task and will also be able to complete the transition independently.

Object Schedule

This may be implemented after a child becomes familiar with using transitional objects. In this system, each transitional object is kept in some sort of compartmentalized box. Objects are arranged in a left–right, top–bottom sequence according to the routine. At the time of a transition, the child gets the "next" object from the schedule box and carries it to the next activity area. The child places the object in a "receptacle" of some kind that is also clearly identified with an identical object or labeled with a picture of the object. With repetition, the child will learn this simple, concrete task and will also be able to complete the transition independently. The physical location is important here. The object schedule should be centrally located so the child can get there independently from each activity. If the child has to have help to get to the object schedule box because it is not on a main route, it may not help independent transitions, which is the goal.

Picture, Symbol, and Printed Word Schedules

Photos, drawings, or printed words depicting each activity are arranged (using Velcro) on a small piece of poster board or file folder in a left–right, top–bottom sequence according to the routine. This is mounted in a central location. At the time of a transition, the child gets the "next" item, carries it to the next activity, and matches it to an identical picture, symbol, or printed word that is posted (along with a strip of Velcro) in the area of the next activity.

If children who are using some visual support system demonstrate their ability to transition independently without the need for their supports (i.e., the child consistently goes to the next activity independently following the group transition cue and has to be prompted to go back and check the schedule), we withdraw the requirement to use the schedule system. The goal is not the use of a schedule system; the goal is independent transitions. (See Dettmer, Simpson, Myles, and Ganz, 2000; Hodgdon, 1995; and Cohen and Sloan, 2007, for additional ideas about ways to develop visual supports for transitions.)

CURRICULUM FOR PEER RELATIONS AND SELF-CARE

Content areas that we have not yet discussed include peer relations and self-care skills, which are main targets for teaching in all group preschool settings. These topics are addressed next.

Peer Interactions

A great advantage of the classroom setting is the availability of peers. For children who begin intervention without interest in peers, the development of simple reciprocal social relations and imitation routines with adults will provide the behaviors needed to interact with peers. We teach children these skills in individual teaching within the classroom activity and in short 1:1 teaching activities during the day. We use the group to generalize these skills into peer interactions.

Beginning peer interaction develops from imitation and shared interest in similar toys. This shared interest in objects constitutes parallel play and leads to a greater awareness of another child and what that child may be doing with the objects. Peer awareness and interaction are encouraged through planned activities that draw children together within the same physical space, particularly emphasizing double sets of toys and face-to-face positioning to foster attention to peers, peer imitation, and parallel play. Seating children across from each other at small tables with double toys scaffolds face-to-face interaction beautifully. Water table activities, group movement games such as "Ring Around the Rosy," or blowing bubbles with a small group of children facing each other are just a few examples of such activities. While motivation is initially derived from the activity and the materials, the result is a parallel play situation.

Strategies for promoting peer awareness and interaction within parallel play situations include providing many duplicate materials, careful positioning so children are face-to-face with each other, and modeling and/or prompting the children to use all the social and communicative skills in their repertoire. If these activities have been carried out with important adults, there may well now be some social reward involved, as well as object rewards. Begin these activities using a peer partner who will provide strong social rewards. Skills that can be targeted include:

- Look at what another child is doing.
- Imitate another child.
- Show something to another child.
- Give something to another child.
- Ask for a turn.
- Request an object.

Children will need verbal scripts to accompany play interactions with peers, and these should be taught with adults within joint activity routines. These include:

- Turn-taking phrases (e.g., "My turn," "Your turn," "Give me *X*," "I want *X*.").
- Teaching children to "Wait a minute," and "Let me finish."
- Providing simple scripts for interaction and conflict resolution (e.g., "That's mine," "Give it back").
- Prompting peers to initiate and maintain interaction play (e.g., "Do this," "Do it again," "More").
- Teaching structured circle or board-type games such as "Hokey Pokey," "Ring Around the Rosy," "Lotto," or "Candyland."

For children who have learned to carry out a number of joint activity routines with an adult and can cue turns and joint attention, we create "play dates" in the classroom—two children who are interested in each other and who can each contribute to the play have a chance to play together with an adult there to scaffold the interactions. The adult may be able to scaffold the interactions within activity centers, or the children may need some protected time. This could occur during a pull-out time with a speech pathologist, OT, or other staff member. If pull-out time is needed to establish these, be sure to also practice during activity periods in the classroom, for generalization and maintenance.

Caution: We have found that adults can easily and unknowingly sabotage peer interaction by interrupting the children's exchanges or occupying their attention so that the child is not available for peer interaction. When the goal is peer-to-peer interactions, adults should be behind the children or away from them, and they should not interrupt the ongoing interactions. If prompting is needed, prompt quickly and silently from behind the child. Adult presence should be "invisible" when the goal is child-to-child interaction. Adults should work hard to allow the antecedents (and reinforcers!) for target social behaviors to emanate from the other child rather than the adult.

Daily Living/Self-Care Skills

Another great advantage of a group setting is that daily living and self-care skill development activities are integral parts of the daily routine. Many functionally appropriate opportunities naturally occur or can easily be embedded within the classroom activity structure.

Dressing

Water table activities are usually quite motivating and are typically planned to accommodate social or play objectives. However, water table activities also provide a functional reason for children to remove some items of clothing in order to stay dry. We have included some version of water table activities in the classroom routine on a daily basis to support individual dressing and undressing objectives. The dressing objectives are targeted before and after the water table activity, even when water table media happens to be some other sensory material (e.g., dry beans, rice). Specific, consistent locations for each child's dressing program are set up as part of the water table activity involving a chair labeled with each child's name and picture along with a similarly labeled basket for his or her clothing.

We have often found it useful to schedule the water table activity following a snack or mealtime. It is then somewhat easier for one staff person to quickly set up individual dressing areas just before the first children are finished with the meal but while everyone is still seated and occupied. In addition, children finish with a meal or snack at different times (or can be encouraged to do so) so that dressing programs can also be staggered in such a way as to provide as much individual attention as is needed.

For children who have already begun to develop skills with dressing, one adult can assist several children at a time. However, some children will need 1:1 direct teaching and motivational strategies in order to accomplish dressing objectives. As with all activities, dressing objectives and sequences are individualized for each child based on his or her objectives. Some children may need practice only with certain items of clothing or fasteners. Other children will need to be taught every step. Each child's data sheet and developmental task analysis will target the acquisition and maintenance teaching step for the day and the data recording process, respectively.

Hygiene

There are also several naturally occurring times within the daily classroom routine for children to learn and/or practice hand and face washing and toothbrushing. Hand washing is a typical routine before and after meals and snacks; toothbrushing, of course, follows a meal. Time and staffing needs must be considered in the schedule to accomplish these. We have found that both hand washing and toothbrushing are best taught with the adult positioned "invisibly" behind the child, using physical rather than verbal prompts, so that the child is helped to move smoothly through each motor step involved in the process. Each child's individual developmental task analysis of the skill sequence is used to determine the teaching steps for each child.

Group Mealtimes

We have found great teaching advantages to structuring meal and snack times as group learning experiences that simulate a sit-down family mealtime. Individual objectives for each child form the teaching content. One adult is positioned at each end of the table and has the "parental" role for the children near them, serving food, being a communicative partner with the children, chatting, and encouraging interaction. The food is located on a rolling cart within the adult's reach but out of all children's reach, so the adult has control over all food, as well as the dishes, cups, napkins, and so on. A third adult has no role in the group and instead circulates to work behind children on individual eating objectives for children who need physical prompting from behind to learn basic spoon use. Food is served family style and children are given a plate and cup on which very small portions are provided upon request, and children may make many requests.

The seating arrangement affects implementation of social and communication objectives. Children whose objectives include peer interaction should be seated across from each other, with adults supporting peer conversation and interaction. For children whose objectives include making requests for food, the adults should be positioned across from or "kitty-corner" from the children. Favorite available foods should be visible nearby, but not able to be reached without requesting from the adult. Mixing children of varying skill levels at each table provides social partners and models for all children. Adults at the table also have the meal and use the basic ESDM teaching procedures described earlier throughout the meal. Children participate in table setting by taking or passing placemats, napkins, bowls, silverware, and cups; by passing food containers and pitchers of drinks; and by cleaning up their own places at the end of the meal, carrying their dishes to a sink, throwing napkins away, wiping spills and hands and mouth. The expectations for children are determined by their objectives involving table-related, self-care activities and chores.

Appropriate mealtime goals may involve communication objectives including simple gestural or verbal requests; waiting; peer interaction; social language; improving use of utensils; increasing the range of foods a child eats; mastery of utensils, napkins, and serving spoons; giving when requested; serving, pouring, and passing; politeness terms; and table setting and clean-up. Other skill areas also work easily into mealtimes: receptive and expressive language; cognitive objectives including matching skills (in table setting), number skills (counting out crackers), and color and shape concepts (to request crackers by shape or fruit by color); social objectives; and fine motor objectives involved in utensil grip, cutting, or using serving tools.

The classroom schedule for each staff member and each child will determine adult teaching requirements and learning objectives for each child during meals. As mentioned earlier, we have been helped by posting little cards with child objectives for an activity on the walls by the activity to help all the adults remember what objectives should be targeted for each child. Each child can be worked with individually for 5 minutes or so at the group table and then given some freedom to continue his or her meal in the social environment, while the staff member will turn his or her attention to the next child.

Teaching Utensil Skills

We have found it very helpful to teach utensil use from *behind* the child. This person physically prompts the use of a utensil, prompts stabilizing a bowl or plate if necessary, prompts putting the utensil down appropriately, and using a napkin. This allows the adult to focus on chaining the action patterns together, and it helps prevent the adult from using verbal and social prompts to teach the chain, which may then leave the child prompt dependent. The adult who is leading the meal activity is the social partner for the child; the adult behind the child is an invisible support to prompt the actions needed. Make sure that prompts follow the child's initial action toward the food. We want to support spontaneous initiation of eating. Even if the child reaches with a hand to the food, prompt the hand to the spoon. Prompts follow antecedents; they are not the antecedent. For a spontaneous behavior, the child's desire for the food is the antecedent to his or her approach behavior, which you then shape. Withdraw prompts fast! Use least-to-most strategies, and spend minimal time manipulating the child's hands. Try to prompt at wrists, shoulder, or elbows through touches and nudges rather than full physical hand-over-hand prompts. Block unwanted behaviors—hand in plate, mouth in plate, using the second hand to shovel food on the spoon or into the mouth. Remove the plate momentarily if children persist.

To conclude, mealtimes provide particularly rich social, communicative, and skill-based teaching opportunities, but providing maximum learning opportunities within mealtimes requires clearly identifying mealtime objectives for each child, and coordinating staff roles, seating arrangement, and placement of food according to those objectives. Any number of objectives may be legitimate and valuable for mealtime experiences, but implementation requires careful planning and team communication and preparation, as is true for every activity period.

KINDERGARTEN TRANSITION

The final topic in this chapter involves the inevitable transition of children out of the preschool classroom and into kindergarten. The biggest fear about this transition is the very real potential loss of children's carefully developed skills in a new environment that neither elicits nor supports them. The receiving staff must know the child's skill repertoire, how those skills are elicited and supported, and how new learning is best stimulated. A considerable flow of information must occur, beginning as early as possible after the new classroom is identified, in order to support the child's previous learning and stimulate additional learning.

There is no substitute for having the staff who will receive the child in the next setting observe the child in his or her current setting and receive the current educational plans from the preschool staff. This is necessary so the child's entry to the new program can build from what was developed in the past program. Programming needs can be shared and the child can be thoroughly prepared for a new set of expectations and methods. If possible and appropriate, any specific materials that the child is using, such as a picture schedule system, can be adapted to the new setting before the transition.

In this way, the materials can "follow" the child to the new setting and assist the child in making the transition. Skills that will help the child be successful in the new setting can also be identified and developed. In the same way, having current staff visit the new program can give them many ideas for how to help the child prepare for the transition: what new skills the child will need in the new setting and how current skills can be best adapted to meet the demands of the new setting.

Although ongoing programming within the ESDM is based on developmental needs, there are certain kindergarten readiness skills that do not depend on developmental readiness per se. Months before an expected transition to kindergarten is to take place, these skills should be carefully evaluated to ensure that appropriate kindergarten readiness programming is taking place. It is extremely helpful to meet with the receiving staff in order to outline specific skills that are typically expected as children enter the kindergarten setting. In addition, a few initial kindergarten skills can be identified and begun to be taught. In this way, an individualized "kindergarten survival checklist" (Barnes, 1997) is developed and becomes the basis for the child's ongoing objectives. Typical kindergarten survival skills are listed in Table 10.5.

As the time for transition approaches, it may also be helpful for the child to visit the "new" school with familiar "old" staff. Making a video of the new setting (e.g., classroom, playground, bathrooms) that the child may watch at home will also help to familiarize the child with the new setting. Videotaping the child within current familiar routines is also an extremely useful tool in familiarizing the receiving staff with the child's current objectives and skills and in illustrating general strategies that have been effectively implemented with the child.

In addition, written reports, written individual programs, and record-keeping forms should be provided to and reviewed with the receiving team. In general, extensive communication between teams is essential in order to effectively prepare the child for a new setting and to provide as much consistency and familiarity as possible as the child makes the transition.

CONCLUSION

The programmatic practices that have evolved around the ESDM classroom allow the educational staff to provide a highly individualized curriculum within a consistent and predictable classroom routine, suitable for both center-based and inclusive group settings. Precision planning and focused interactions take into consideration the typical developmental and learning needs of young children with ASD. Using a developmentally focused, play-oriented, relationship-based approach, intensive individual teaching also takes place within a high degree of structure. Grounding in the principles of ABA ensures careful teaching practices and an empirical approach to educational practices via ongoing data collection and interpretation. As in all early childhood educational settings in the United States, a classroom using the ESDM emphasizes children's development of independence, encouragement of social relationships and interactions, and the development of more and more sophisticated communication skills. In addition, emphasis on quality of relationships, children's positive emotional experiences, and intensive teaching embedded in play-based activities marks the classroom model just as it does the individually based delivery.

TABLE 10.5. Typical Kindergarten Survival Skills

Behavior

- Wait in line and walk in line with a group of children
- Sit quietly while attending to a short story
- Participate in clean-up activities
- Ask for help when needed
- Work in small groups
- Attempt to complete teacher-assigned tasks
- Choose free-choice activities
- Complete free-choice activities

Self-care skills

- Use appropriate bathroom skills (flush toilet, wash hands, dressing, etc.)
- Dress self (socks, coat, attempt tying shoes)
- Take care of own belongings (put coat or lunch bag away, etc.)

Language and communication

- Verbalize his or her first and last name when asked
- Complete a two-step simple direction
- Share comments, ideas, or experiences
- Listen to a variety of stories and participate in follow-up comments
- Initiate and respond to a few socially appropriate verbal interactions ("Hi," "What's your name?")
- Participate in informal pretend play with peers (play house, puppets, role playing, etc.)
- Identify general body parts (back, stomach, head, legs, facial features, etc.)
- Ask for help by raising a hand

Preacademics

- Count 1 to 10
- Demonstrate one-to-one correspondence with one to five concrete objects
- Experience with identifying, matching, and sorting objects
- Match and sort according to color, size, and shape
- Recognize his or her printed first name
- Match printed letters and numbers
- Recognize letters of the alphabet by name
- Identify and name basic colors
- Experience singing the alphabet song

Fine motor skills

- Attempt to grip crayons, markers, and pencils correctly
- Hold scissors correctly and cut along a line
- Copy, draw, and reasonably trace a line, circle, square, and triangle
- Attempt to write his or her first name
- Able to engage in tactile experiences with water, sand, clay, rice, finger painting, and so on
- Complete simple manipulative activities such as puzzles, beads, lego, and so on
- Experience in painting at an easel

Gross motor skills

- Experience with log rolls, jumping, standing on one foot, galloping, skipping, hopping, and swinging
- Throw and catch large and small balls
- Use playground equipment (climb, go down slides, swing, etc.)
- Experience with group movement and music activities

Appendix A

Early Start Denver Model Curriculum Checklist and Item Descriptions

INTRODUCTION

The ESDM Curriculum Checklist is the tool that is used in the Early Start Denver Model for designing teaching objectives for intervention. It is administered to children every 12 weeks in a play-based fashion, similar to how an adult would carry out ESDM intervention. It is directly administered, but it also uses information gained from parents and other professionals working with the child in order to form an accurate picture of the child's current skill set across the main developmental domains that the ESDM intervention addresses: communication, social and adaptive skills, cognition and play, imitation, and fine and gross motor development. The current version of the Curriculum Checklist is the product of many years of clinical research and refinement, and the items and their order reflect our clinical experience as well as information that appears in the developmental literature and in other developmental tools.

As described in Chapter 4, the ESDM Curriculum Checklist is a criterion- referenced tool that provides developmental sequences of skills in multiple developmental domains, including receptive communication, expressive communication, social skills, play skills, cognitive skills, fine motor skills, gross motor skills, and adaptive behavior skills. The skill level ranges from the 9- to 12-month period up to the 48-month level. The Checklist is organized in four levels, which roughly correspond to the developmental age periods 12–18 months, 18–24 months, 24–36 months, and 36–48 months. However, the Curriculum Checklist was developed specifically for young children with ASD and reflects their typical developmental profile involving relatively more advanced visual motor skills and relatively less advanced social and communication skills than other children of the same developmental age. Thus, in each level, the communication and social items are developmentally more immature than the fine and gross motor items, if one uses a standard of typical development as a point of comparison. In some levels, elaborated sequences have been developed for skills that are particularly important to emphasize in ASD, like the imitation items in Level 1 and the joint attention items in Level 2. While imitation can be considered a subset of social development and joint attention a subset of communication development, these skills are so affected in ASD and so crucial for further development that they receive extra attention in the ESDM Curriculum Checklist. The sequences within a domain come from wide-ranging reviews of the literature on typical child development. The placement of the items in a specific level reflects both typical child development research and also the clinical experience of several different expert ESDM interdisciplinary teams working with hundreds of young children with ASD over the past 25 years.

ADMINISTRATION

The Curriculum Checklist is developed to be administered by early intervention professionals. It can be administered in several different formats, depending on the organization of the team and the intervention program. It can be used by a single early intervention professional from any of a number of disciplines who has cross-disciplinary knowledge of development in the various domains and has practiced the tool and its scoring. This evaluation format would be used when ESDM is delivered as a single-discipline therapy, or in an intensive 1:1 delivery format using a generalist model, with the team leader administering the Checklist. If a single disciplinarian is going to use it, that person will need cross-training in other disciplines on the items that are outside of that person's knowledge base. In group programs involving a multidisciplinary team, different domains can be administered by the various professional team members, with each disciplinarian administering the sections most relevant to their skill set.

As with other assessment tools that cover a wide range of skills, the goal is to assess the child's current levels of ability rather than to administer the entire tool. At the end of the assessment, the assessor should have identified the skills in each domain that define the child's most mature skills and those skills that are too difficult for him or her. Thus, the assessor needs to establish the child's current working skill set and the next more advanced skills that are not yet a regular part of the child's repertoire. Most children's skills will cluster in a specific level for each domain. However, for children whose skills fall in the earlier items in a level, be sure to review the final items in the previous level to identify any critical skills that the child is failing in the level below. Similarly, if a child has mostly passes in one level and only a few fails, you will need to move into the next level and assess at least the first half of the items in that domain to be sure you have good information about what the child's real repertoire is at this particular time. As with other developmental tests, your goal is to determine the child's basal and ceiling levels, and particularly to identify the range in which passes turn to failures in each domain. This will be the target area for teaching.

The Curriculum Checklist is administered in the same way that intervention occurs—in a play-based interactive style using a joint activity frame. Using play activities allows for a variety of domains to be assessed within a single activity, because most toy-based interactions between a child and adult involve motor skills, cognitive skills, communicative skills, and social skills. A play-based assessment also allows one to examine social and communication components inside typical social interaction patterns for young children. The assessor organizes a play session that includes the materials needed to complete the items, and the assessor develops play activities with the child. The level of parent participation is up to the assessor. The assessor provides some materials, provides a number of models for different skills, invites the parent to participate as will be helpful, and also asks the parent about the child's demonstration of the skill in natural settings. The assessor should engage the child in a play activity that interests the child, carry out the activity with the child until a natural ending point or until no new behaviors are being elicited, and then pause and note the items on the Curriculum Checklist that were observed, as well as those that were tried but were not elicited. The assessor then begins another play activity and proceeds as before. After each play activity, the assessor should pause, take notes, check the items, and determine what items still need to be administered. Then, the assessor chooses materials and play activities that allow the elicitation of the remaining items. For those that cannot be observed (e.g., bathtime), the parent is interviewed. If there are other therapists' reports, the assessor should use that information as well. There are columns for each of these information sources: direct observation, parent report, and other therapist or teacher reports.

The Curriculum Checklist can be completely administered within one play session of 1 to 1.5 hours. The best setting is a therapy room, with a small table and chairs, beanbag, floor area, comfortable chair for the parent, and materials that will be needed to elicit the skills on the Curriculum Checklist. A list of necessary materials is presented in the beginning of the Curriculum Checklist. It is very helpful to remove from sight materials that will not be used for the assessment, so that time is not lost and children's attention is not focused on materials that cannot provide useful information for the assessment. Video recording of the assessment is not necessary but is helpful both as a source of information later, and also as a documentation of the starting point of treatment.

SCORING

Three scoring conventions are used with the Checklist: pass or P or + (for consistent performance or mastery), pass/fail or P/F or ± (to capture inconsistent performance), and fail or F or – (to use when no examples are seen or the behavior is difficult to elicit). The Curriculum Checklist Item Descriptions specify what level of response is needed to pass an item. The assessor records the parent report and the direct assessment scores in the appropriate columns, along with any additional information provided by other team members if it is available. For both passed and failed items, the assessor needs to know whether the child displays this behavior at home and/or in other settings, and if so, how consistently. There will also be behaviors that cannot be observed in the setting, like self-care skills; the parent's information is crucial for these as well. After the assessment is complete, the assessor integrates the information into a final code for each item, indicating the child's mastery level of each item in a domain within the particular level that contains both passes and fails. (*Note:* Items that are considered mastered or passed will not be targets for any teaching objectives, so it is quite important to not optimize child performance. Passes should be reserved for skills that are consistently and reliably used as described in the item description and well generalized, if appropriate, across different settings, people, and materials.) When the assessor has a good sense of the child's working repertoire of skills and the Curriculum Checklist clearly reflects the child's current level of skills with a group of Ps, P/Fs, and Fs in each domain, the assessment is complete and it is time to write the teaching objectives.

TRANSLATING ITEMS INTO TEACHING OBJECTIVES

The process for developing teaching objectives from the Curriculum Checklist is described in Chapter 4. Refer to that chapter for detailed information about how to apply the information obtained from the ESDM Curriculum Checklist to the development of individualized teaching plans.

MATERIALS NEEDED

- Small table and two straight wooden chairs that will fit the child well
- Large beanbag for sitting
- Carts with drawers and other containers for holding toys
- If floor is not carpeted, then small rugs for floor areas
- A variety of small clear containers with lids that can be used to hold various materials

- Small box with bubbles, balloons, slinkies, animal picture book
- Set of colored blocks of different sizes
- Set of colored markers and paper
- Set of farm animals and two sets of identical pictures of farm animals
- Children's book with farm animals, children's book with vehicles
- Two or three cars and trucks
- Bucket that holds four to five balls, from 3–4" to 12" diameter, and beanbags of different sizes
- Nesting cups
- Ring stacker
- Several inset puzzles
- Shape sorter with lid
- Fat pegs and pegboard
- Set of eating objects—at least two of each—cups, plates, spoons, forks, play dough, rollers and cookie cutters, plastic knife, fork, and child scissors
- Large doll (12" or bigger) with clothes—hat, socks, etc.—and large animal (same size as doll)
- Baby blanket and small bed or box to use for bed
- Set of personal grooming objects: comb, brush, mirror, hat, necklace
- Set of popbeads
- Set of large Duplos
- Toy involving a hammer and pegs or balls, etc.
- Pop-up toy with various types of buttons to open
- Snacks for the children to assess eating skills: open cup, juice, bowl for food that requires a spoon (applesauce, yogurt, etc.)
- Fat beads to string with a fat string or cord
- Photos of family members and self

EARLY START DENVER MODEL CURRICULUM CHECKLIST FOR YOUNG CHILDREN WITH AUTISM

Name: ______________________________

Date: ______________________________

Assessor: ______________________________

Parent(s) interviewed:

____

____

Others interviewed:

____

____

Instructions: Use the Checklist to define the child's most mature skills, those skills that are currently emerging, and those skills that are currently not in the child's repertoire, in each domain. See pages 230–258 for item descriptions and Appendix B for administration practices. Use + or P (pass) for consistent performance at appropriate times. Use +/– or P/F (pass/fail) for inconsistent performance. Use – or F (fail) when the behavior is difficult to elicit. Use these codes for behavior in each column: direct observation, parent report, and teacher/other report.

For the CODE column, use the following: A (acquired)—child clearly demonstrates skill and parent reports skill is used consistently. P (partial or prompted)—child is only able to demonstrate skill inconsistently or with additional prompting and parent/other reports same, or child demonstrates some, but not all, of the steps of the skill. N—child is unable or unwilling to demonstrate the skill and parent/other reports difficulty. X—no opportunity, or not appropriate for this child.

Most children's skills will cluster in one of the four levels for each domain. However, for children whose mastered skills fall in the earlier items in a level, review the final items in the previous level to identify any critical skills where the child is failing in that level. Similarly, if a child has mostly passes in one level and only a few fails, move to the next higher level and assess the first half of the items in that domain to have a good sample of the child's current repertoire. The range in which passes turn to failures defines the target area for teaching for each domain.

Skill	Level 1	Observed	Parent Report	Other/ Teacher Report	CODE
	Receptive Communication				
1	Localizes to sounds by turning toward sound source.				
2	Looks to playful vocal sounds (raspberry, whistle).				
3	Responds to voice by turning toward person.				
4	Looks at indicated pictures as adult points to pictures in book.				
5	Follows a proximal point to place objects in containers, puzzle pieces, etc.				
6	Looks when shown an object and told, "Name, look."				
7	Looks to partner when name is called.				
8	Follows a proximal point to object or location.				
9	Follows distal point to retrieve toy.				
10	Looks, reaches, or smiles in response to adult gestures and voice in social games.				
11	Looks, reaches, smiles, and/or gestures in response to adult language/gesture in songs.				
12	Responds by stopping actions momentarily in response to inhibitory words (e.g., "no," "stop").				
13	Gives object as verbally requested when paired with adult's outstretched hand.				
14	Performs a one-step, routine instruction involving body actions paired with verbal/gesture cue (e.g., "Sit down," "Come here," "Clean up").				
15	Performs a one-step, routine verbal instruction involving body actions without accompanying gesture (e.g., "Sit down," "Come here," "Clean up").				
	Expressive Communication				
1	Uses a goal-directed reach to request.				
2	Vocalizes with intent.				
3	"Asks" for help by handing object to adult.				
4	Takes turns vocalizing with communication partner.				
5	Expresses refusal by pushing away object or giving the object back to another person.				
6	Points proximally to request desired object.				
7	Makes eye contact to obtain a desired object when adult blocks access/withholds desired object.				
8	Points to indicate a choice between two objects.				
9	Combines vocalization and gaze for intentional request.				
10	Points distally to request desired object.				
11	Points distally to indicate a choice between two objects.				
12	Vocalizes with CVCV reduplicative babbling (not necessarily word approximations).				
13	Produces five or more consonants in spontaneous vocalizations.				
14	Produces CVCV with differing CV sequences (variegated babbling).				

Skill	Level 1	Observed	Parent Report	Other/ Teacher Report	CODE
	Social Skills				
1	Accepts brief sensory social activities and touch.				
2	Uses motor prompt to initiate or continue a sensory social routine.				
3	Attends briefly to another person with eye contact.				
4	Maintains engagement in sensory social routines for 2 minutes.				
5	Responds to preferred objects/activities via gaze, reach, smiles, and movements.				
6	Watches and engages with imitative adult during parallel toy play activities.				
7	Has a repertoire of 5–10 sensory social games.				
8	Responds to greetings by looking, turning, etc.				
9	Responds to greeting by gesture or vocalization.				
10	Shares smiles with partner during coordinated play.				
	Imitation				
1	Imitates 8–10 one-step actions on objects.				
2	Imitates 10 visible motor actions inside song/game routines.				
3	Imitates invisible six motor actions on head, face inside song/game routines.				
4	Imitates six oral–facial movements.				
	Cognition				
1	Matches/sorts identical objects.				
2	Matches/sorts identical pictures.				
3	Matches/sorts pictures to objects.				
4	Matches/sorts objects by color.				
	Play				
1	Fits behavior to the qualities of five different objects.				
2	Plays independently and appropriately with 10 one-step toys.				
3	Plays independently with toys requiring repetition of the same action on various objects (ring stacker, nesting cups).				
4	Demonstrates appropriate play behaviors on a variety of one-step toddler toys: throws ball, stacks blocks, pegs in holes, rolls car.				
5	Plays independently with toys requiring two different motor actions (take out, put in).				
6	Plays independently with toys requiring several different motor actions (e.g., put in, open, remove, close).				
7	Demonstrates conventional actions on self with a range of objects.				
8	Completes play task and puts away.				

Skill	Level 1	Observed	Parent Report	Other/ Teacher Report	CODE
	Fine Motor				
1	Places one to two shapes in a shape sorter.				
2	Places rings on a ring stacker.				
3	Completes three-piece wooden handle puzzle.				
4	Puts pegs in a pegboard.				
5	Pushes buttons on five different types of cause–effect toys.				
6	Takes apart pop beads, Duplos.				
7	Uses a pincer grasp and a three-finger grasp as appropriate to toy.				
8	Stacks three big blocks in a tower (or stacking cups).				
9	Makes marks, lines, scribbles, and dots with markers/ crayons.				
10	Bangs a toy hammer with balls, pegs, etc.				
11	Scoops, rakes, pours with sand, water, rice, etc.				
12	Stacks big Legos.				
	Gross Motor				
1	Kicks big ball.				
2	Walks up and down stairs with support; nonalternating feet.				
3	Climbs one to two steps up small ladder to slide.				
4	Gets on and off pieces of equipment.				
5	Protects self when off balance.				
6	Walks around objects on floor rather than stepping on them.				
7	Throws ball and beanbags any direction.				
8	Rolls ball back and forth with another person.				
	Behavior				
1	Exhibits minimal severe behavioral difficulties.				
2	Sits in a chair or facing adult during pleasurable activities without difficulty for 1–2 minutes.				
3	Willingly engages in simple games in chair and on floor with adult for 5 minutes.				
4	Tolerates adult proximity and interaction (minimal demands) without problem behaviors for 20-minute intervals.				
5	Interacts appropriately with family members (i.e., no aggression or other inappropriate interactions).				
	Personal Independence: Eating				
1	Eats meals and snacks at the table.				
2	Eats meal independently.				
3	Uses an open cup.				
4	Uses a spoon.				
5	Uses a fork.				

Skill	Level 1	Observed	Parent Report	Other/ Teacher Report	CODE
	Personal Independence: Eating *(cont.)*				
6	Eats a variety of food textures, types, and food groups.				
7	Tolerates new foods on plate.				
8	Drinks from straw.				
	Personal Independence: Dressing				
9	Removes each piece of clothing with assistance.				
10	Pulls on each piece of clothing with assistance.				
	Personal Independence: Grooming				
11	Puts hands under running water.				
12	Dries hands on towel.				
13	Rubs washcloth on body, towel on body.				
14	Tolerates hair combing, nose wiping, and toothbrushing.				
15	Helps with hairbrush/comb.				
16	Puts toothbrush in mouth.				
	Personal Independence: Chores				
17	Puts dirty clothes in hamper.				
18	Puts tissues in trash.				

Skill	Level 2	Observed	Parent Report	Other/ Teacher Report	CODE
	Receptive Communication				
1	Follows instructions to "stop" or "wait" without prompts or gestures.				
2	Follows 8–10 one-step verbal instructions involving body actions and actions on objects.				
3	Identifies by pointing or showing several named body parts on self or other person.				
4	Responds to verbal instruction to give/point/show for 8–10 specific objects in natural play, dressing, eating routines (e.g., baby, chair, car, block, cup, bear).				
5	Identifies by pointing and visually attends to three named pictures in a book (including cup, car, dog, cat, baby).				
6	Understands early spatial concepts (e.g., in, on).				
7	Looks to people and photos of people when named—family, pets, teachers.				
8	Retrieves 8–10 verbally requested objects in room but not directly in front of child, requiring some search.				
9	Upon verbal request (with gesture cues), completes two actions with one object.				
10	Points to named body parts in picture.				

Skill	Level 2	Observed	Parent Report	Other/ Teacher Report	CODE
	Expressive Communication				
1	Uses target signs or gestures with vocalizations to express (request, all done, share, help, protest).				
2	Produces 6–10 single words or approximations within the context of familiar routines, sensory–social routines, songs.				
3	Spontaneously produces multiple words associated with a play routine (roll, go, stop).				
4	Functional use of 20 or more approximations of nominals (names of objects, animals, people) and nonnominals (words that refer to actions or other relations: all gone, up, etc.).				
5	Spontaneously labels objects and pictures.				
6	Vocalizes with varied intonation during songs, etc.				
7	Requests and refuses using single words with gaze.				
8	Labels actions in context (e.g., during body movements and/or actions on objects).				
9	Approximates names of three important people (includes self).				
10	Shakes head and says "no" to refuse.				
11	Nods head "yes" and says "yes" to affirm.				
12	Asks (approximates) "What's that?" when encountering something unfamiliar.				
	Joint Attention Behaviors				
1	Responds to "Look" and offered object with gaze shift, body turn, and looks at offered object.				
2	Responds to "Look" and point by orienting to the indicated distal object/person.				
3	Gives or takes object from other person coordinated with eye contact.				
4	Responds to "Show me" by extending object to adult.				
5	Spontaneously "shows" objects.				
6	Spontaneously follows point or gaze (no verbal cue) to look at target.				
7	Spontaneously points to interesting objects.				
8	Shares smile with adult with alternating gaze during pleasurable object activity.				
	Social Skills: Adults or Peers				
1	Initiates and maintains eye contact for communication.				
2	Verbally requests or physically initiates familiar social games.				
3	Returns affection behaviors: hugs, kisses to familiar others.				
4	Uses gesture or words to attain adult's attention.				
5	Responds to social greeting with "Hi" or "Bye-bye," and waves imitatively.				

Skill	Level 2	Observed	Parent Report	Other/ Teacher Report	CODE
	Social Skills: Adults or Peers *(cont.)*				
6	Asks for help verbally or gesturally.				
7	Consistently coordinates eye contact with vocalization and/or gesture to direct communication.				
8	"Dances" with another in circle games to music.				
9	Runs with another in "chase" game.				
10	Gains communication partner's attention using name of person or game and initiates social game or activity.				
	Social Skills with Peers				
11	Gives object to peer when peer requests.				
12	Joins in with familiar songs/finger plays in a group setting.				
13	Continues with activity when peer joins in parallel play.				
14	Responds appropriately to peer's greetings.				
15	Takes turns with peer with simple action toys when peer requests; gives and takes back.				
16	Sits in group with peers and attends to adult's familiar instructions.				
17	Takes object from peer when peer offers.				
18	Passes objects to peers at table or in group when requested.				
19	Imitates peer's behavior occasionally in play activities.				
20	Plays picture-matching games (Memory, Lotto, etc.) alone and with peer.				
	Imitation				
1	Imitates a variety of vowel and consonant sounds during verbal approximations in meaningful communications.				
2	Imitates animal sounds and other sounds.				
3	Imitates recognizable single words spontaneously and frequently in interactions.				
4	Imitates motions to five songs; imitates at least 10 different actions.				
5	Imitates/approximates novel actions in songs.				
6	Imitates actions on objects—multiple steps (play actions).				
7	Imitates pretend play acts to self and partner with miniatures.				
8	Imitates two movement sequences in song/game routines.				
9	Imitates two-word phrases.				
	Cognition				
1	Matches/sorts by shapes.				
2	Matches/sorts by size.				
3	Matches/sorts designs, line drawings.				
4	Sorts similar objects into like groups.				

Skill	Level 2	Observed	Parent Report	Other/ Teacher Report	CODE
	Cognition *(cont.)*				
5	Sorts related common objects into functional groups.				
6	Searches/requests for missing object.				
7	Matches/sorts in two dimensions.				
8	Matches by quantities one through three.				
	Play: Representational				
1	Combines related objects in play (cup on saucer, spoon in dish).				
2	Imitates/produces sound effects with play (vocalizes on phone, makes car noises, animal sounds with animals).				
3	Carries out single action with a prop on a doll or animal.				
4	Combines functionally related actions on a play theme (feeds and gives drink, puts to bed and covers up).				
5	Demonstrates a trial-and-error approach to problem solving with constructive toys; schemas are flexible, not repetitive.				
	Play: Independent Play				
6	Plays appropriately and flexibly for 10 minutes with only occasional adult attention.				
7	Can occupy self appropriately with open-ended materials for at least 10 minutes at a time with occasional adult guidance.				
8	Gets materials, brings to table, completes play task, and puts away.				
	Fine Motor				
1	Puts three or more shapes in shape sorter accurately.				
2	Stacks 8–10 1-inch blocks.				
3	Copies three or more simple block designs.				
4	Puts together five or more Duplos, pop beads, Tinker Toys, bristle blocks in varied ways.				
5	Imitates five or more simple actions on play dough (roll, poke, pat, squeeze).				
6	Puts multiple stickers on sheets.				
7	Opens and closes a variety of containers, including screw-on lids.				
8	Zips and unzips large zipper.				
9	Strings large objects with rope, thick string, or aquarium tubing.				
10	Imitates strokes, scribbles, and dots with marker, crayon.				
11	Snips paper with scissors.				
12	Places checkers and pennies in a slot.				
13	Strings a variety of beads on different types of string.				
14	Completes four- to six-piece single-inset puzzles.				

Skill	Level 2	Observed	Parent Report	Other/ Teacher Report	CODE
	Gross Motor				
1	Imitates gross motor actions in a variety of positions (sitting, standing, moving).				
2	Jumps off step and over obstacles on ground.				
3	Uses some equipment on playground (climbs, slides).				
4	Sits on tricycle and pushes with feet or begins to pedal.				
5	Pulls wagon or pushes wheelbarrow.				
6	Kicks ball into target.				
7	Digs with shovel.				
	Personal Independence: Eating				
1	Uses a napkin when cued.				
2	Serves self food from bowl with utensil.				
3	Passes containers when instructed.				
4	Carries plate, cup, and silverware to sink or counter when finished.				
5	Stays at table with companion for duration of child's meal.				
6	Eats and behaves appropriately at fast food restaurants.				
7	Will touch or taste a new food that has been introduced multiple times.				
8	Eats from all food groups.				
9	Gets drink of water independently.				
	Personal Independence: Dressing				
10	Removes all clothing independently and puts in hamper (no fasteners).				
11	Completes some steps of putting on each piece of clothing independently (needs help with fasteners).				
12	Takes off jacket, hat (no fasteners), and puts on hook.				
	Personal Independence: Hygiene				
13	Wipes face with warm cloth when instructed.				
14	Wipes nose when instructed.				
15	Participates in all steps of hand washing.				
16	Cooperates with hair washing/cutting.				
17	Plays with five bath toys appropriately.				
18	Puts toys away when requested at end of bath.				
19	Helps with lotion.				
20	Brushes toothbrush over teeth.				
21	Goes to sleep independently after bedtime ritual.				
22	Shows knowledge of sequence of bedtime routine.				
	Personal Independence: Chores				
23	Sorts silverware from dishwasher tray to silverware tray.				
24	Unloads dryer into basket.				
25	Matches socks.				
26	Pours water/food into pet dish.				

Skill	Level 3	Observed	Parent Report	Other/ Teacher Report	CODE
	Receptive Communication				
1	Attends and joins in with interest for 5–10 minutes as adult reads familiar books using simple sentences.				
2	Follows one-step novel commands involving familiar objects/actions.				
3	Identifies many common objects and their pictures: clothing items, objects related to meals, hygiene, play, foods.				
4	Responds appropriately to "yes/no" questions regarding preferences.				
5	Identifies five or more actions in pictures and books.				
6	Follows two or more instructions given in situational routines (bedtime: get a book and get in bed; tooth brushing: get your toothbrush and the toothpaste).				
7	Understands spatial relationships involving objects (e.g., under, next to).				
8	Differentiates early size concepts—big/little.				
9	Differentiates at least four different colors upon request.				
10	Identifies 20 items by sound (e.g., animals, telephone; "What animal says 'meow meow'?").				
11	Comprehends the function of common objects (ride, cut, eat, sleep, put on feet, drink, etc.).				
12	Understands pronoun referents "mine" and "yours."				
13	Identifies 10 actions via pictures, choices, acting out.				
14	Follows two or more unrelated instructions in novel context.				
	Expressive Communication				
1	Produces two- to three-word combinations for a variety of communicative intentions (e.g., requesting, greeting, gaining attention, protesting).				
2	Produces two or more word utterances to comment to another person.				
3	Labels actions in pictures and books.				
4	Comments and requests on location (up, down, in, on top).				
5	Comments and requests using early possessive forms (mine, yours).				
6	Gestures or vocalizes "I don't know" in context.				
7	Consistently uses other people's names to get their attention.				
8	Delivers a simple message to another person ("Go tell Mommy 'Hi'").				
9	Says "Hi" and "Bye-bye" appropriately, both initiating and in response.				
10	Uses pronouns for self and other (me and you variants).				
11	Uses simple words and gestures to describe personal experiences.				

Skill	Level 3	Observed	Parent Report	Other/ Teacher Report	CODE
	Expressive Communication *(cont.)*				
12	Names one to two colors.				
13	Responds appropriately to "What?" questions.				
14	Responds appropriately to "Where?" questions.				
15	Responds appropriately to "Who?" questions.				
16	Asks simple "yes/no" questions using rising intonation (can be one-word utterance with rising intonation).				
17	Asks "What?" and "Where?" questions.				
18	Answers simple information questions: name, age, color of shirt, etc.				
	Social Skills: Adults and Peers				
1	Plays simple gross motor games (e.g., ball, "Hide and Seek," "Ring-around-the-Rosy").				
2	Shares and shows objects when partner requests.				
3	Imitates and carries out novel songs/finger plays in group situation.				
4	Responds appropriately to simple requests/instructions from peers.				
5	Initiates interactions and imitations of peers.				
6	Plays in familiar dramatic play routine with peer in parallel play.				
7	Takes turns with simple board games.				
8	Uses politeness terms: "Please," "Thank you," "Excuse me."				
9	Imitates a variety of novel gross motor actions in standing and while moving, such as in "Follow the Leader" or animal walks.				
10	Participates in play activities involving verbal scripts.				
11	Frequently draws others' attention to objects verbally and gesturally to comment, show, share, and request.				
12	Responds to others' bids for joint attention by looking and commenting.				
13	Receptively identifies affect (happy, sad, mad, scared) from photos, in others, and/or in line drawings.				
14	Expressively identifies affect from photos, in others, and/or in line drawings.				
15	Makes own face reflect affect (happy, sad, mad, scared).				
	Cognition				
1	Matches letters in own name.				
2	Matches letters.				
3	Matches words.				
4	Matches numbers.				
5	Receptively and expressively identifies some letters, numbers, shapes, and colors.				
6	Plays games involving memory for hidden objects.				

Skill	Level 3	Observed	Parent Report	Other/ Teacher Report	CODE
	Cognition *(cont.)*				
7	Categorizes objects/pictures into eight classes.				
8	Understands relationship between quantities and number symbols through number 5.				
9	Counts correct number of objects to five.				
10	Sequences three or more pictures in correct order and narrates sequence from pictures using "first, then" language.				
	Play				
1	Constructive play involves sequencing complex schemas with multiple coordinated objects (e.g., trucks on road, blocks make building, beads make a necklace).				
2	Links three or more related actions in a play sequence.				
3	Performs two or more linked actions on a doll or animal when instructed.				
4	Physically places figures on miniature furniture, vehicles, etc., when appropriate.				
5	Carries out actions on doll or animal figures spontaneously.				
6	Arranges props for the theme.				
	Fine Motor				
1	Completes five- to six-piece interlocking puzzle.				
2	Imitates drawing circle, cross, square, diagonal line.				
3	Imitates and builds different block structures using a variety of building materials (blocks, Legos, Tinker Toys, etc.).				
4	Laces a running stitch.				
5	Traces lines and curves with finger and writing tool.				
6	Uses a variety of tools to pick up and release objects: tongs, fork.				
7	Traces a variety of shapes.				
8	Uses scissors with appropriate grasp and uses opposite hand to stabilize and turn paper.				
9	Cuts on a line—straight and curved lines.				
10	Carries out simple two-step art projects (cut and paste, stamp with ink pad; folds paper and cuts on line).				
11	Carries out several different schemas with play dough—uses a variety of tools.				
	Gross Motor				
1	Rides tricycle well (pedals and steers, follows a route).				
2	Kicks with good form and balance.				
3	Uses all playground equipment with supports.				
4	Plays chase game with adults and peers, running smoothly, changing direction with good balance.				
5	Imitates gross motor actions with movement to songs and music.				

Skill	Level 3	Observed	Parent Report	Other/ Teacher Report	CODE
	Gross Motor (*cont.*)				
6	Throws underhand at target.				
7	Jumps forward with two feet together.				
8	Hops on one foot.				
	Personal Independence				
1	Uses spoon, fork, and cup neatly and without spilling.				
2	Behaves appropriately at sit-down restaurant.				
3	Uses icons or other symbol systems for choices, schedules, etc. independently, if needed at home and at school.				
4	Carries own materials to and from car, school, and home.				
5	Opens and closes backpack independently; puts in and removes objects when requested.				
6	Dresses and undresses when appropriate (unfastens clothing fasteners—zippers and snaps).				
	Personal Independence: Hygiene				
7	Uses toilet independently, all steps, when taken or sent.				
8	Manages clothing at toilet except for fasteners.				
9	Completes all the hand-washing steps independently.				
10	Wipes face with warm washcloth when handed to child.				
11	Runs brush or comb through hair.				
12	Covers mouth when coughing and sneezing.				
13	Assists actively in bathing and drying self after bath.				
14	Brushes teeth with toothbrush, using at least a few strokes.				
	Personal Independence: Chores				
15	Feeds/waters a pet.				
16	Helps clear table.				
17	Helps empty dishwasher.				
18	Puts clean clothes in drawers.				
19	Picks up belongings when asked.				

Skill	Level 4	Observed	Parent Report	Other/ Teacher Report	CODE
	Receptive Communication				
1	Understands a variety of descriptive physical relationship concepts.				
2	Retrieves 10–15 items using two to three multiple cues (e.g., size, quantity, color, object label).				
3	Understands gender pronouns.				
4	Understands comparatives: bigger, shorter, smaller, most, least, few, many, etc.				

Skill	Level 4	Observed	Parent Report	Other/ Teacher Report	CODE
	Receptive Communication *(cont.)*				
5	Understands spatial relationships involving objects and prepositions: behind, in back of, in front of.				
6	Understands negatives (e.g., the box with no balls, the boy who is not sitting).				
7	Understands possessives and part–whole relations.				
8	Demonstrates attention to short stories and comprehension of parts of the story by responding to simple "wh" questions (what and who).				
9	Responds to "yes/no" questions for identity.				
10	Answers questions about physical states.				
11	Responds to personal information questions.				
12	Understands "same" and "different."				
13	Understands quantity concepts.				
14	Identifies features of objects.				
15	Responds to questions regarding category membership of objects/pictures.				
16	Understands past and future tense.				
17	Understands passive voice.				
18	Understands temporal relations.				
19	Follows three-part unrelated verbal instructions.				
	Expressive Communication				
1	Responds to complex "wh" questions ("Why?", "How?").				
2	Describes object functions in response to question (e.g., "What do you do with a spoon?").				
3	Speaks in three- to four-word utterances consistently.				
4	Uses a variety of noun phrases.				
5	Uses prepositional phrases (e.g., under, next to, behind, in back of, in front of).				
6	Uses a variety of verb phrases (e.g., he cries, she likes him, he fell, he was happy, he is happy, could, should, would).				
7	Demonstrates accurate production of at least 80% of all consonants and consonant blends within connected speech.				
8	Describes recent experience using three- to four-word sentence.				
9	Requests permission to pursue an activity.				
10	Uses plural forms.				
11	Uses later possessives (e.g., his, hers, Mommy's hat).				
12	Uses regular past tense.				
13	Uses articles such as *a, an, the.*				
14	Uses comparatives/superlatives.				
15	Uses negation with auxiliary verbs.				
16	Uses present progressive verb form.				

Skill	Level 4	Observed	Parent Report	Other/ Teacher Report	CODE
	Expressive Communication *(cont.)*				
17	Uses words to describe physical states.				
18	Responds to questions about physical states: "What do you do when you are ...?"				
19	Uses category names for familiar objects.				
20	Describes features of objects.				
21	Uses reflexive pronouns.				
22	Answers telephone appropriately, including getting person.				
23	Participates in a conversation that is initiated by an adult for two to three consecutive turns involving a variety of functions (e.g., reciprocal commenting, responding to and requesting information).				
24	Initiates and maintains a conversation on a self-generated topic of conversation with an adult.				
25	Describes a two- to three-event sequence of activities (e.g., going to visit Grandma).				
26	Expresses "I don't know" paired with gesture.				
27	Asks for clarification if doesn't understand what is said.				
28	Engages in a variety of topics during conversation.				
29	Repairs own communication when listener does not understand.				
30	Answers questions about self and others.				
	Social Skills				
1	Invites peers to play.				
2	Uses polite forms such as "Excuse me," "Sorry."				
3	Seeks out others for comfort in a group situation.				
4	Expresses own feelings appropriately.				
5	Takes turns in informal play independently.				
6	Describes an event or experience to peer.				
7	Identifies what makes self feel happy, sad, mad, scared.				
8	Identifies others' emotions based on situational factors.				
9	Begins to develop coping strategies when feeling upset, mad, or scared.				
	Cognition				
1	Counts rotely to 20.				
2	Counts objects with 1:1 correspondence to 10.				
3	Gives "one," "some," "a lot," "a little," "all of them," "more," and "most."				
4	Gives quantities through 10.				
5	Knows terms for quantity concepts.				
6	Knows terms for spatial relations.				
7	Matches and understands 5–10 word/object associations.				
8	Can read some words.				

Skill	Level 4	Observed	Parent Report	Other/ Teacher Report	CODE
	Cognition *(cont.)*				
9	Can identify written name out of a field of five.				
10	"Reads" signs and symbols.				
11	Identifies numbers and letters.				
12	States opposites and analogies.				
	Play				
1	Demonstrates actions of figures in play.				
2	Uses placeholder items to symbolize props in play.				
3	Labels actions and pretend props in play.				
4	Spontaneously links three or more related behaviors in a play theme.				
5	Directs partner in play.				
6	Plays out several life events (e.g., birthday party, McDonald's, doctor), including use of verbal scripts.				
7	Plays out several story themes in play.				
8	Takes on a character role and plays it out.				
9	Follows another's lead in play.				
	Fine Motor				
1	Colors in a picture with accuracy using different colors.				
2	Imitates triangle, letters using appropriate drawing utensil.				
3	Draws lines and shapes and some letters and numbers from memory.				
4	Imitates and copies a variety of letters, numbers, and shapes.				
5	Writes first name without a model.				
6	Traces shapes and letters.				
7	Colors in shapes that are outlined.				
8	Connects dots with drawing tool.				
9	Draws lines to and from corresponding pictures, words, or shapes.				
10	Copies a variety of simple representational drawings (e.g., face, tree, house, flower).				
11	Folds paper in half and puts in envelope.				
12	Cuts out angles, straight lines, and curves.				
13	Cuts out simple shapes.				
14	Completes three-step art projects—cut, color, and paste.				
15	Uses paintbrush, stamps, markers, pencils, erasers to complete art activities.				
16	Uses a tripod grasp with drawing tool.				
17	Builds with a variety of building materials with own design and copies simple models from pictures or 3-D models.				

Skill	Level 4	Observed	Parent Report	Other/ Teacher Report	CODE
	Fine Motor *(cont.)*				
18	Puts together interlocking puzzles, floor puzzles, tray puzzles.				
19	Uses tape, paper clips, keys appropriately.				
	Gross Motor				
1	Plays catch with playground-sized ball with a peer.				
2	Throws tennis ball or baseball to another person with directionality using overhand throw.				
3	Uses all playground equipment independently, including swing, merry-go-round.				
4	Kicks a moving ball.				
5	Plays various games with balls: Throws ball in basket, hits T-ball with bat, bounces ball, golf club, beanbag toss.				
6	Rides bicycle confidently with training wheels; able to control speed, maneuver, and brake.				
7	Gallops and skips.				
8	Walks without falling off balance beam, railroad ties, sidewalk curbs.				
9	Plays typical motor games (e.g., "Red Light, Green Light," "Red Rover," "Freeze Tag").				
	Personal Independence				
1	Manages all steps involved in toileting independently at the level of peers.				
2	Takes self to toilet as needed.				
3	Washes hands independently at level of peers.				
4	Washes face with washcloth independently.				
5	Independently brushes or combs hair.				
6	Actively assists with bathing, dries self after bath.				
7	Carries out all steps for toothbrushing independently, though adult may also brush teeth for thoroughness.				
8	Fastens own clothing—buttons, snaps, and zippers.				
9	Blows nose when cued, uses tissue to catch sneezes, covers cough and sneeze.				
10	Stops at street; crosses after looking both ways when accompanied.				
11	Walks safely beside adult independently in parking lots, stores, etc.				
12	Helps with table setting.				
13	Uses knife to spread.				
14	Cleans up after spills.				
15	Pours self drink from small container.				
16	Places dishes in sink, counter, or dishwasher.				
17	Makes a two-step snack.				
18	Assists with cooking activities: stirs, pours, etc.				

Early Start Denver Model Curriculum Checklist: Item Descriptions

Skill	Level 1	Description
Receptive Communication		
1	Localizes to sounds by turning toward sound source.	Demonstrates awareness of sound by turning eyes and head.
2	Looks to playful vocal sounds (raspberry, whistle).	Demonstrates awareness of sound by becoming more active, turning eyes and head, and looking at person.
3	Responds to voice by turning toward person.	Demonstrates awareness of voice by turning eyes and head and looking at person.
4	Looks at indicated pictures as adult points to pictures in book.	Follows adult point to picture with gaze and/or gesture (e.g., touching picture).
5	Follows a proximal point to place objects in containers, puzzle pieces, etc.	Responds to proximal point by looking and placing object in indicated location.
6	Looks when shown an object and told, "Name, look."	Turns eyes and head in direction of object.
7	Looks to partner when name is called.	Turns eyes and head toward partner's body.
8	Follows a proximal point to object or location.	Responds to proximal point by turning head in direction of object or location.
9	Follows distal point to retrieve toy.	Responds to distal point by approaching and picking up the toy.
10	Looks, reaches, or smiles in response to adult gestures and voice in social games.	Attends and responds for one or more rounds. Social games include "Peek-a-Boo," "Creepy Fingers," "Tickle."
11	Looks, reaches, smiles, and/or gestures in response to adult language/gesture in songs.	Same as above. Attends and responds during songs for one or more verses.
12	Responds by stopping actions momentarily in response to inhibitory words (e.g., "no," "stop").	Stops an ongoing activity when told "No, stop," or demonstrates awareness by pausing temporarily, turning eyes and head toward adult, or showing distress (e.g., crying).
13	Gives object as verbally requested when paired with adult's outstretched hand.	Responds to adult gesture or words by placing or attempting to place the object in hand.
14	Performs a one-step, routine instruction involving body actions paired with verbal/gesture cue (e.g., "Sit down," "Come here," "Clean up").	Performs action with verbal/gesture cue. A pass is at least five actions at first opportunity. Examples include adult repeating instruction, using gestures to highlight action (e.g., patting chair to sit down, holding up bucket to clean up), or partially prompting the child through the action.
15	Performs a one-step, routine verbal instruction involving body actions without accompanying gesture (e.g., "Sit down," "Come here," "Clean up").	Completes instruction by performing action without adult gestures or physical guidance. Adult may repeat instructions a second time without gesture cue.

Skill	Level 1	Description
Expressive Communication		
1	Uses a goal-directed reach to request.	Reaches toward desired object in adult's hands to indicate request. Gesture need not be accompanied by eye contact or vocalizations/words. Does not include reaching just to grab.
2	Vocalizes with intent.	Vocalizes in conjunction with eye contact and/or gesture (e.g., reaching) to request desired item or object.
3	"Asks" for help by handing object to adult.	Indicates help by placing object in adult's hand, offering object to adult, verbalizing, or looking to adult. Gesture need not be accompanied by eye contact or vocalizations/words.
4	Takes turns vocalizing with communication partner.	Babbles and/or vocalizes with eye contact for at least two rounds.
5	Expresses refusal by pushing away object or giving the object back to another person.	Gestures need not be accompanied by eye contact or vocalizations/words. Give credit for other conventional gestures (shaking head, sign "all done") or words ("no").
6	Points proximally to request desired object.	Touches or points to object within 6–12 inches with first or index finger (not open hand) to indicate request. Object may be in adult's hand or in reach of the child.
7	Makes eye contact to obtain a desired object when adult blocks access/withholds desired object.	Turns head and eyes to adult and makes eye contact for 1–2 seconds with or without a gesture (e.g., reaching, grabbing) to request object. Eye contact and gesture need not be accompanied by vocalizations/words.
8	Points to indicate a choice between two objects.	Adult holds up two objects, one in each hand. Touches or points toward desired object with first or index finger (not open hand). Gesture need not be accompanied by eye contact or vocalizations/words.
9	Combines vocalization and gaze for intentional request.	Turns head and eyes to adult and makes eye contact while vocalizing to request desired item. Vocalization may be an approximation. Examples include "aah" for ball or "ooh" for go.
10	Points distally to request desired object.	Uses first or index finger (not open hand) to point toward desired object, 3 feet or more away from child.
11	Points distally to indicate a choice between two objects.	Adult holds up two objects, one in each hand but out of reach of child and shows and names each object to child. Points toward desired object that is out of reach with first or index finger (not open hand). Gesture need not be accompanied by eye contact or vocalizations/words.
12	Vocalizes with CVCV reduplicative babbling (not necessarily word approximations).	Examples include "ba-ba," "ma-ma." Vocalization need not be accompanied by eye contact or gesture.
13	Produces five or more consonants in spontaneous vocalizations.	Vocalizations occur with or without adult verbal models. Vocal play counts.
14	Produces CVCV with differing CV sequences (variegated babbling).	Examples include "ba-bu," "ma-wa," and strings of jargon.
Social Skills		
1	Accepts brief sensory social activities and touch.	Child shows no avoidance, withdrawal, or negative affect.
2	Uses motor prompt to initiate or continue a sensory social routine.	Examples of motor prompts include reaching, imitating the adult's movement, handing an item or object to adult. Motor prompt need not be accompanied by eye contact.

Skill	Level 1	Description
	Social Skills *(cont.)*	
3	Attends briefly to another person with eye contact.	Attends by looking and sustaining eye contact with another person for 2 seconds.
4	Maintains engagement in sensory social routines for 2 minutes.	Shows interest in sensory social routine by approaching, observing, or actively participating, and requesting continuation of the routine through eye contact, gestures (e.g., reaching, imitating adult's movement), or vocalizations.
5	Responds to preferred objects/activities via gaze, reach, smiles, and movements.	Response need not be accompanied by eye contact.
6	Watches and engages with imitative adult during parallel toy play activities.	Shows interest in activity by observing and imitating adult play acts and continues the play schema being imitated.
7	Has a repertoire of 5–10 sensory social games.	Participates two or more times in any active behavior (reach, imitate, vocalize) in a game. Eye contact and smiles alone are not enough. Examples include "Peek-a-Boo," rhymes/songs ("Eensy-Weensy Spider," "If You're Happy and You Know It"), games ("Ring-around-the-Rosy," "Patty-Cake"), bubbles, balloons, books, airplane, "Here comes a mousey."
8	Responds to greetings by looking, turning, etc.	Demonstrates awareness of greeting by turning head and body and looking at adult for 2–3 seconds. Response need not be accompanied by gesture or vocalization.
9	Responds to greeting by gesture or vocalization.	Demonstrates awareness of greeting by turning head and body and waving or vocalizing "Hi/Bye" with eye contact for 2–3 seconds.
10	Shares smiles with partner during coordinated play.	Shares smiles with eye contact for 2–3 seconds during play activity with adult.
	Imitation	
1	Imitates 8–10 one-step actions on objects.	Imitates eight or more actions on object within 5 seconds of adult's model. Examples include banging two objects together, placing an object in its container, or rolling an object.
2	Imitates 10 visible motor actions inside song/game routines.	Imitates 10 different motor actions within 5 seconds of adult's model. Imitates two different actions per song and four to five different routines to pass. Examples include gestures from songs (e.g., "Five Little Monkeys," "Eensy-Weensy Spider"), motor games (e.g., "Motor Boat," "Ring-around-the-Rosy"), or other play routines (e.g., Peek-a-Boo).
3	Imitates invisible six motor actions on head, face inside song/game routines.	Imitate six different actions that child cannot see him- or herself make. Examples are hands on head, ears, or patting cheeks.
4	Imitates six oral–facial movements.	Imitates oral–facial movement within 5 seconds of adult's model. Examples include wiggling tongue, blowing raspberries, or puffing cheeks.
	Cognition	
1	Matches/sorts identical objects.	May be in response to adult verbal (e.g., "Put here") or physical cue (e.g., hand-over-hand) for first few trials, but child needs to complete matching/sorting independently for at least five different objects. Examples include matching/sorting trains and tracks, crayons and paper, or sticks and circles in separate containers.

Skill	Level 1	Description
		Cognition *(cont.)*
2	Matches/sorts identical pictures.	May be in response to adult verbal (e.g., "Put here") or physical cue (e.g., hand-over-hand) for first few trials, but child needs to complete matching/sorting independently for at least five different pictures.
3	Matches/sorts pictures to objects.	May be in response to adult verbal (e.g., "Put here") or physical cue (e.g., hand-over-hand) for first few trials, but child needs to complete matching/sorting independently for at least five different object/picture pairs.
4	Matches/sorts objects by color.	Match/sort five or more colors. May be in response to adult verbal (e.g., "Put here") or physical cue (e.g., hand-over-hand) for first few trials, but child needs to complete matching/sorting independently. Examples include matching/sorting red versus blue blocks, orange versus green pegs, or yellow versus purple balls into separate containers.
		Play
1	Fits behavior to the qualities of five different objects.	Action needs to be initiated by child and not in response to adult model. Behavior fits the affordance of the object. Examples include shaking maraca, banging hammer, rolling or bouncing ball, or stacking blocks.
2	Plays independently and appropriately with 10 one-step toys.	Play is developmentally appropriate (i.e., not restricted or repetitive), relates to the object/activity, and involves one-step actions of objects. Examples include placing blocks in a block sorter, putting balls in a ball maze, placing pegs in holes, or taking apart pop beads.
3	Plays independently with toys requiring repetition of the same action on various objects (ring stacker, nesting cups).	Play involves independent completion of the object/activity. Pass with five or more toys. Examples include placing rings on a ring stacker, taking nesting cups in/out, stacking blocks, or placing pegs in holes.
4	Demonstrates appropriate play behaviors on a variety of one-step toddler toys: throws ball, stacks blocks, pegs in holes, rolls car.	Play relates to the object/activity and involves one-step actions of objects. Pass with 8–10 toddler toys. Example toys include throwing balls, rolling cars, or hitting drum.
5	Plays independently with toys requiring two different motor actions (take out, put in).	Play involves independent completion of the object/activity. Pass with 8–10 toys. Examples include taking blocks in/out of container, rolling and smashing play dough, or putting pop beads together and taking apart.
6	Plays independently with toys requiring several different motor actions (e.g., put in, open, remove, close).	Play involves independent completion of the object/activity. Pass with six to eight toys. Examples include opening/closing containers, taking objects in/out, performing different actions with objects.
7	Demonstrates conventional actions on self with a range of objects.	Actions are socially conventional and directed toward self. May be in response to adult model but independent, spontaneous use is necessary for at least one action. Examples include placing phone to ear, brushing hair with hairbrush/comb, putting spoon/fork to mouth, wiping nose with a tissue, cup to lips, put beads on.
8	Completes play task and puts away.	Appropriately finishes activity and shows some attempt to clean up (e.g., puts an object in container, hands materials to adult). May be in response to adult verbal or gesture cue to start routine but needs to participate without physical prompts.

Skill	Level 1	Description
		Fine Motor
1	Places one to two shapes in a shape sorter.	May be in response to adult cue to start routine but needs to place one to two shapes independently.
2	Places rings on a ring stacker.	May be in response to adult cue to start routine but places three or more rings independently.
3	Completes three-piece wooden handle puzzle.	May be in response to adult cue to start routine but places three or more pieces independently.
4	Puts pegs in a pegboard.	May be in response to adult cue to start routine but needs to place three or more pegs independently.
5	Pushes buttons on five different types of cause–effect toys.	May be in response to adult cue to start routine but needs to push buttons independently.
6	Takes apart pop beads, Duplos.	May be in response to adult cue to start routine but needs to take apart 3 or more beads or Duplos independently.
7	Uses a pincer grasp and a three-finger grasp as appropriate to toy.	Adult may place toys in child's reach but no other facilitation.
8	Stacks three big blocks in a tower (or stacking cups).	May be in response to adult cue to start routine but needs to stack at least three blocks/cups independently.
9	Makes marks, lines, scribbles, and dots with markers/crayons.	May be in response to adult cue to start routine but needs to hold and make marks independently. Marks need not be a recognizable form.
10	Bangs a toy hammer with balls, pegs, etc.	May be in response to adult cue to start routine but needs to hold and bang toy independently.
11	Scoops, rakes, pours with sand, water, rice, etc.	May be in response to adult cue to start routine but needs to hold object and scoop/rake/pour independently.
12	Stacks big Legos.	May be in response to adult cue to start routine but needs to stack at least three Legos independently.
		Gross Motor
1	Kicks big ball.	May not hold onto adult or object (table, chair) to kick ball. Maintains balance; does not fall; may be clumsy.
2	Walks up and down stairs with support; nonalternating feet.	May hold railing or adult's hand, putting both feet on each step. May not put hands or knees on steps.
3	Climbs one to two steps up small ladder to slide.	Must do so unassisted.
4	Gets on and off pieces of equipment.	Must do so unassisted. Examples include riding toy, rocking horse, child or adult-sized chairs.
5	Protects self when off balance.	Uses protective reactions or equilibrium reactions (e.g., puts hands out, reaches out, protects head).
6	Walks around objects on floor rather than stepping on them.	Shows awareness of body in relation to objects by stepping over or walking around objects.
7	Throws ball and beanbags any direction.	Must do so unassisted and with forward thrust.
8	Rolls ball back and forth with another person.	Adult may start the routine but child shows interest by rolling ball in direction of person.
		Behavior
1	Exhibits minimal severe behavioral difficulties.	Examples include self-injurious behavior, aggression, frequent and/or severe tantrums.
2	Sits in a chair or facing adult during pleasurable activities without difficulty for 1–2 minutes.	Sits calmly/happily for at least 60 seconds while interacting with adult.

Skill	Level 1	Description
	Behavior *(cont.)*	
3	Willingly engages in simple games in chair and on floor with adult for 5 minutes.	Games may include "Peek-a-Boo," song, or physical routine (e.g., tickle, up/down on adult's lap).
4	Tolerates adult proximity and interaction (minimal demands) without problem behaviors for 20-minute intervals.	Adult's requests are within child's current set of skills. Fussing may occur but no aggressive behavior.
5	Interacts appropriately with family members (i.e., no aggression or other inappropriate interactions).	No aggression or other inappropriate interactions observed by parent report.
	Personal Independence: Eating	
1	Eats meals and snacks at the table.	Sits at the table through a meal (i.e., does not get up or walk to and from table during child's meal; does not need to sit throughout family meal).
2	Eats meal independently.	Adult sets out food but no other assistance is needed.
3	Uses an open cup.	Holds and places cup to mouth without assistance. Some spilling while drinking may occur.
4	Uses a spoon.	Holds and puts spoon to mouth without assistance for most bites. Occasional spilling may occur.
5	Uses a fork.	Holds and puts fork to mouth without assistance for most bites. Occasional spilling may occur.
6	Eats a variety of food textures, types, and food groups.	Parent report is sufficient.
7	Tolerates new foods on plate.	Allows new food to stay on plate and may attempt to eat it (e.g., touches, smells, or places to mouth). Does not have to eat it.
8	Drinks from straw.	Adult may place straw to child's mouth if never given.
	Personal Independence: Dressing	
9	Removes each piece of clothing with assistance.	Does not need to unbutton or unzip clothing but can take off items (e.g., shirt, pants, shoes, socks) with assistance. Examples include adult helping child pull arms out of shirt and child pulls shirt off of head, adult unties shoes and child pulls off of foot, or adult unzips pants and child pulls down to feet.
10	Pulls on each piece of clothing with assistance.	Does not need to button or zip clothing but can pull on item (e.g., shirt, pants, shoes, socks) with assistance. Examples include adult rolling up shirt and child pulling head through shirt, adult holding shoe and child stepping into shoe, or adult helps child step into pants and child pulling up pants.
	Personal Independence: Grooming	
11	Puts hands under running water.	May be cued if necessary but is able to place hands under water for at least 5 seconds. Parent report is sufficient.
12	Dries hands on towel.	May be cued if necessary but uses towel to dry both hands. Parent report is sufficient.
13	Rubs washcloth on body, towel on body.	May be cued if necessary but uses washcloth/towel on most body parts (e.g., face, hands, stomach, legs). Parent report is sufficient.
14	Tolerates hair combing, nose wiping, and toothbrushing.	May fuss but adult is able to complete routine without aggressive, self-injurious, or severe behavior problems.

Skill	Level 1	Description
	Personal Independence: Grooming *(cont.)*	
15	Helps with hairbrush/comb.	Examples include holding hairbrush/comb, or taking a turn to brush/comb hair.
16	Puts toothbrush in mouth.	Places toothbrush in mouth, tastes toothpaste. Does not have to brush teeth.
	Personal Independence: Chores	
17	Puts dirty clothes in hamper.	May be reminded or physically cued (e.g., adult hands clothes, points to hamper) if necessary, but is able to drop clothes in hamper.
18	Puts tissues in trash.	May be reminded or physically cued (e.g., adult hands tissues, points to trash) if necessary, but is able to drop tissues in trash.

Skill	Level 2	Description
	Receptive Communication	
1	Follows instructions to "stop" or "wait" without prompts or gestures.	Child responds to verbal instruction alone; stops activity completely, looks to adult, and waits for adult instruction.
2	Follows 8–10 one-step verbal instructions involving body actions and actions on objects.	Child responds to verbal instructions involving verbs (e.g., shake maraca, bang sticks, hug baby, poke dough, cut, stand up, clap hands, wiggle ears; has to follow both types—body actions and actions on objects).
3	Identifies by pointing or showing several named body parts on self or other person.	Pass requires identification of five or more body parts.
4	Responds to verbal instruction to give/point/show for 8–10 specific objects in natural play, dressing, eating routines (e.g., baby, chair, car, block, cup, bear).	Self-explanatory.
5	Identifies by pointing and visually attends to three named pictures in a book (including cup, car, dog, cat, baby).	Responds to "Where is...?" or "Show me...?" with index finger point and look.
6	Understands early spatial concepts (e.g., in, on).	Pass requires that the child demonstrates generalized understanding of three or more prepositions by following verbal instructions using objects.
7	Looks to people and photos of people when named—family, pets, teachers.	Pass involves responses to four or more different names. If the named person/pet is present, child clearly looks at the person or pet when named (may also point). If pictures, child touches or points to picture when named.
8	Retrieves 8–10 verbally requested objects in room but not directly in front of child, requiring some search.	In response to the verbal direction, "Get the...," child retrieves objects in room but out of line of sight. The task involves remembering the request long enough to conduct a visual search of the room, and retrieving the object from floor, table, chair, or shelf.

Skill	Level 2	Description
Receptive Communication *(cont.)*		
9	Upon verbal request (with gesture cues), completes two actions with one object.	Child sequences two actions together on an object in response to verbal instruction with gesture. Must demonstrate three or more different sequences to pass (e.g., "Get your shoes and bring them to me").
10	Points to named body parts in picture.	Identifies five or more body parts in a large photo or line drawing when asked.
Expressive Communication		
1	Uses target signs or gestures with vocalizations to express (request, all done, share, help, protest).	Child combines specific gesture and vocalization or word approximation to communicate all four of these functions.
2	Produces 6–10 single words or approximations within the context of familiar routines, sensory–social routines, songs.	Produces five or more differentiated word approximations inside familiar social routines. These can be spontaneous or spontaneously imitated but not prompted.
3	Spontaneously produces multiple words associated with a play routine (roll, go, stop).	Produces three or more differentiated word approximations for verbs involving actions on self or objects—spontaneous or imitated but not prompted.
4	Functional use of 20 or more approximations of nominals (names of objects, animals, people) and nonnominals (words that refer to actions or other relations: all gone, up, etc.).	These involve word approximations used spontaneously to request actions or objects. Both nouns and nonnominals must be used to pass.
5	Spontaneously labels objects and pictures.	Pass if child labels five or more objects and five or more pictures spontaneously.
6	Vocalizes with varied intonation during songs, etc.	Child varies intonation as he or she produces some words to songs or chants, demonstrating awareness of the intonation patterns involved.
7	Requests and refuses using single words with gaze.	Child routinely uses single words with gaze to convey both requesting and protest, refusal, or negation.
8	Labels actions in context (e.g., during body movements and/or actions on objects).	Child produces 10 or more verbs both imitatively and spontaneously to label actions on self, other, or objects.
9	Approximates names of three important people (includes self).	Child uses names to label people in pictures, mirror, and real life or to get their attention. Can be in response to question "Who is that?"
10	Shakes head and says "no" to refuse.	Child spontaneously combines head shake with word "no" to refuse an offer.
11	Nods head "yes" and says "yes" to affirm.	Child spontaneously combines head nod with the word "yes" to accept an offer.
12	Asks (approximates) "What's that?" when encountering something unfamiliar.	Child spontaneously looks to adult and gestures to object via manual gesture or gaze shift while asking "What's that?" in several different contexts.
Joint Attention Behaviors		
1	Responds to "Look" and offered object with gaze shift, body turn, and looks at offered object.	Self-explanatory.
2	Responds to "Look" and point by orienting to the indicated distal object/person.	Self-explanatory.

Skill	Level 2	Description
	Joint Attention Behaviors *(cont.)*	
3	Gives or takes object from other person coordinated with eye contact.	This involves a spontaneous give or take. If it is a take, the adult should not offer the object. The gaze communicates a "request."
4	Responds to "Show me" by extending object to adult.	Self-explanatory.
5	Spontaneously "shows" objects.	This involves routine acts of showing—positioning the toy toward the adult's face, looking to the adult, and waiting for a comment. Pass if this is seen several times in an hour of play.
6	Spontaneously follows point or gaze (no verbal cue) to look at target.	Get child's gaze in face-to-face interaction, and then turn to look at object. Pass if child shows head turn and some search. Does not need to find the target.
7	Spontaneously points to interesting objects.	This involves routine acts—several per hour. Child must point to target and look to adult and wait for comment to pass.
8	Shares smile with adult with alternating gaze during pleasurable object activity.	This involves clear gaze shifts from object to adult eyes and back to object to share pleasure. Should be seen several times in a 10-minute period of social play to pass.
	Social Skills: Adults or Peers	
1	Initiates and maintains eye contact for communication.	Child routinely begins communicative exchanges (of any type) with gaze and maintains gaze in natural way throughout the exchange.
2	Verbally requests or physically initiates familiar social games.	Child initiates and cues social gazes through body movements, gestures, or vocal patterns that are specific to a certain game. Must cue three or more games to pass.
3	Returns affection behaviors: hugs, kisses to familiar others.	Child spontaneously and consistently hugs back to familiar adults with arms and body, kisses back with pucker on cheek or lips.
4	Uses gesture or words to attain adult's attention.	Child seeks adult eye contact using either words or clear gestures of any type (wave, show, turn face, pat, etc.).
5	Responds to social greeting with "Hi" or "Bye-bye," and waves imitatively.	Child responds to greetings with both words and gestures, without prompting.
6	Asks for help verbally or gesturally.	Child initiates requests for help using either conventional signs or word approximations combined with gaze. Manipulating hands and bodies do not count unless accompanied by both gaze and appropriate words.
7	Consistently coordinates eye contact with vocalization and/or gesture to direct communication.	Child consistently accompanies spontaneous communicative acts with eye gaze.
8	"Dances" with another in circle games to music.	Child plays several different circle games and imitates dance movements to music ("Hokey Pokey," "Ring-around-the-Rosy," "London Bridge").
9	Runs with another in "chase" game.	Child chases another person and catches him or her while playing "chase," and also runs to be caught, during "chase."
10	Gains communication partner's attention using name of person or game and initiates social game or activity.	Child spontaneously initiates familiar social games toward a partner by establishing eye contact and using an associated gesture and their name or an action word (e.g., "tickle," "chase").

Skill	Level 2	Description
Social Skills with Peers		
11	Gives object to peer when peer requests.	Child consistently responds to peer verbal request for an object by looking and handing it to peer.
12	Joins in with familiar songs/finger plays in a group setting.	Child participates in familiar songs and social games with appropriate movement patterns in small-group setting (one to two other children) without any special cuing.
13	Continues with activity when peer joins in parallel play.	Child continues activity when peer joins, acknowledging and accepting peer approach. Child does not "protect" materials or reject approach.
14	Responds appropriately to peer's greetings.	Child spontaneously responds to "Hi" and "Bye" from a peer with look, gesture, and appropriate words.
15	Takes turns with peer with simple action toys when peer requests; gives and takes back.	In a parallel play situation, child routinely responds to peer bids for a turn-taking exchange by both giving object when requested and asking for a turn either verbally or nonverbally, both accompanied by some gaze.
16	Sits in group with peers and attends to adult's familiar instructions.	Child sits in a small group without special seating or adult assistance, attends to lead adult, and follows verbal instructions that are within the child's repertoire. Adult may use child name to deliver instruction but no other prompting.
17	Takes object from peer when peer offers.	Child routinely takes object with eye contact when a peer offers it.
18	Passes objects to peers at table or in group when requested.	Child consistently responds appropriately to object requests in small-group situations (e.g., circle time, snack table, art table, dramatic play corner).
19	Imitates peer's behavior occasionally in play activities.	During parallel play activities, child will imitate a few peer actions spontaneously.
20	Plays picture-matching games (Memory, Lotto, etc.) alone and with peer.	Pass if child can take turns with partner and complete the match. These are the only skills needed to pass this item.
Imitation		
1	Imitates a variety of vowel and consonant sounds during verbal approximations in meaningful communications.	Includes four to five different vowel sounds and four to five different consonant sounds.
2	Imitates animal sounds and other sounds.	Imitates at least five different sounds.
3	Imitates recognizable single words spontaneously and frequently in interactions.	Produces 10 or more word approximations.
4	Imitates motions to five songs; imitates at least 10 different actions.	These are familiar actions; no prompts.
5	Imitates/approximates novel actions in songs.	Approximates at least five novel actions at first model.
6	Imitates actions on objects—multiple steps (play actions).	This involves imitating a sequence of three or more related actions (e.g., taking off the shape-sorter cover, taking out the shapes, putting the lid on, and putting the shapes through).
7	Imitates pretend play acts to self and partner with miniatures.	Child consistently imitates four or more naturalistic actions with miniatures, on self and also offered to partner.

Skill	Level 2	Description
	Imitation *(cont.)*	
8	Imitates two movement sequences in song/game routines.	Child spontaneously imitates two or more actions within a single song without any prompting or waiting.
9	Imitates two-word phrases.	Child routinely imitates a variety of two-word utterances.
	Cognition	
1	Matches/sorts by shapes.	Matches and sorts at least five different shapes.
2	Matches/sorts by size.	Matches and sorts at least three different sizes of identical objects.
3	Matches/sorts designs, line drawings.	Child matches and sorts line drawings and design patterns.
4	Sorts similar objects into like groups.	Child matches and sorts nonidentical objects by identity (e.g., cars, horses, balls, socks, shoes, cups).
5	Sorts related common objects into functional groups.	Child groups objects by function: eating, clothing, toys, drawing.
6	Searches/requests for missing object.	Child recognizes when one object out of a set is missing and asks for it or searches for it (e.g., a missing puzzle piece, a missing shoe, a missing cup).
7	Matches/sorts in two dimensions.	Child matches/sorts objects by color and shape, or shape and size, etc.
8	Matches by quantities one through three.	Child matches a variety of objects in quantity groups involving the quantities one to three (e.g., domino pieces, animal crackers on a plate).
	Play: Representational	
1	Combines related objects in play (cup on saucer, spoon in dish).	Child demonstrates awareness of functional relations of multiple sets of objects in his or her play and in clean-up.
2	Imitates/produces sound effects with play (vocalizes on phone, makes car noises, animal sounds with animals).	Pass if child makes five or more such sounds in play.
3	Carries out single action with a prop on a doll or animal.	Requires spontaneous action; do not pass for imitation only.
4	Combines functionally related actions on a play theme (feeds and gives drink, puts to bed and covers up).	Requires spontaneous actions involving at least two related acts in a row. Do not pass for imitation only.
5	Demonstrates a trial-and-error approach to problem solving with constructive toys; schemas are flexible, not repetitive.	Pass if child routinely demonstrates trial-and-error problem solving in object play.
	Play: Independent Play	
6	Plays appropriately and flexibly for 10 minutes with only occasional adult attention.	Adult can lay out several sets of constructive or visual spatial materials, but the child needs to play alone using mostly appropriate play acts, without more than two verbal interactions, to pass this item. Do not penalize if some repetitive or stereotypic acts occur within the appropriate play.
7	Can occupy self appropriately with open-ended materials for at least 10 minutes at a time with occasional adult guidance.	Adult can lay out the material (play dough, art, books, pretend play props), but the child needs to play alone using mostly appropriate play acts, without more than two verbal interactions, to pass this item. Do not penalize if some repetitive or stereotypic acts occur within the appropriate play.

Skill	Level 2	Description
Play: Independent Play *(cont.)*		
8	Gets materials, brings to table, completes play task, and puts away.	Child plays independently including getting the materials, moving into a space for play, and cleaning up and putting away materials at the end. This can involve open-ended or closed-ended activities.
Fine Motor		
1	Puts three or more shapes in shape sorter accurately.	Child completes the shape sorter independently; may use trial and error but no prompts or supports of any type.
2	Stacks 8–10 1-inch blocks.	The child independently builds a block tower of 8–10 blocks that balances.
3	Copies three or more simple block designs.	The child copies several different arrangements involving at least three blocks (e.g., vertical tower, horizontal line, bridge).
4	Puts together five or more Duplos, pop beads, Tinker Toys, bristle blocks in varied ways.	Child uses multiple types of interlocking objects and assembles five or more pieces in several ways.
5	Imitates five or more simple actions on play dough (roll, poke, pat, squeeze).	Self-explanatory.
6	Puts multiple stickers on sheets.	The adult may have to peel up a corner so the child can grasp, but the child takes the sticker off the sticker sheet and places it on a sheet of paper independently.
7	Opens and closes a variety of containers, including screw-on lids.	This is not a test of strength—the tops should be easy to remove.
8	Zips and unzips large zipper.	Child can independently unzip a zipper all the way down; the child can pull a zipper all the way up, though an adult will have to connect the two pieces for the child.
9	Strings large objects with rope, thick string, or aquarium tubing.	The child strings five or more beads, pieces of pasta, rings, etc. onto a fat string without help or prompts.
10	Imitates strokes, scribbles, and dots with marker, crayon.	The child imitates at least three different types of actions with writing tools.
11	Snips paper with scissors.	The snip need not cut off a piece of paper. May use children's or adults' scissors. Adult may show how to hold scissors but child cuts independently. Does not need to hold scissors perfectly. Must make three snips.
12	Places checkers and pennies in a slot.	The child independently picks up five or more pieces from the table and places each into a slot, both horizontal and vertical, without prompts or reminders, and is successful with pennies.
13	Strings a variety of beads on different types of string.	Child can string multiple objects on various types of cords.
14	Completes four- to six-piece single-inset puzzles.	Child completes the puzzle independently; may use trial and error but no prompts or supports.
Gross Motor		
1	Imitates gross motor actions in a variety of positions (sitting, standing, moving).	Child consistently and spontaneously imitates gross motor actions (can be instructed) regardless of location. These can be approximations; it is the consistency, not the precision, that is important.
2	Jumps off step and over obstacles on ground.	Child jumps and moves forward in space, from a low step to the ground, as well as from the ground.

Skill	Level 2	Description
	Gross Motor *(cont.)*	
3	Uses some equipment on playground (climbs, slides).	Child consistently initiates multiple appropriate actions on several pieces of low playground equipment.
4	Sits on tricycle and pushes with feet or begins to pedal.	Child independently places self on tricycle in correct position for riding and tries to pedal but may need assistance to do so.
5	Pulls wagon or pushes wheelbarrow.	Child independently operates wagon or wheelbarrow to move things on the playground.
6	Kicks ball into target.	Child kicks large ball with directionality.
7	Digs with shovel.	Child digs with shovel, scoops up material, and deposits in container independently, multiple scoops.
	Personal Independence: Eating	
1	Uses a napkin when cued.	When instructed but without further assistance, child picks up napkin and wipes the appropriate body part as per instruction. Does not have to be thorough but has to be more than cursory.
2	Serves self food from bowl with utensil.	When adult holds or positions serving bowl or plate for child, child uses the serving utensil to move food to child's plate independently. May be clumsy. Adult may cue amounts.
3	Passes containers when instructed.	At the table, when another person asks child to pass an item, child looks for item, picks it up, and passes it to the person on left or right. Child must respond to the request by searching for object and trying to pick it up independently. If someone passes a container to the child and instructs child to pass to the next person, child follows instruction without prompts.
4	Carries plate, cup, and silverware to sink or counter when finished.	When child leaves table, child follows adult instructions to take specified items to specified location without prompts.
5	Stays at table with companion for duration of child's meal.	Child sits throughout meal and stays in seat without prompts or other supports until child is finished eating and adult indicates child may go.
6	Eats and behaves appropriately at fast food restaurants.	Child participates in all steps of fast food meal—waiting, ordering, carrying, sitting, eating, clean-up, and exit, without needing full physical prompts. Child sits until finished and until adult ends meal. Child willingly walks with adult to door and table. Does not need to have hand held to stay with adult.
7	Will touch or taste a new food that has been introduced multiple times.	Child will respond willingly to instruction to taste or take a bite or a drink of a familiar food.
8	Eats from all food groups.	Child eats some items from fruits/vegetables, dairy, grains, and meats (unless there are familial restrictions) spontaneously.
9	Gets drink of water independently.	Child spontaneously gets glass and gets water from sink, shelf, or refrigerator door without any instructions or help from adult. If sink is used, child turns off water spontaneously.

Skill	Level 2	Description
	Personal Independence: Dressing	
10	Removes all clothing independently and puts in hamper (no fasteners).	When instructed, child removes shirt, pants, underwear, socks, and shoes without help other than with fasteners and places all clothes in appropriate container. Child may be verbally or gesturally reminded once or twice throughout routine but without physical prompts, either full or partial.
11	Completes some steps of putting on each piece of clothing independently (needs help with fasteners).	Self-explanatory.
12	Takes off jacket, hat (no fasteners), and puts on hook.	Takes off loose jacket and hat independently; may be prompted to place on hook.
	Personal Independence: Hygiene	
13	Wipes face with warm cloth when instructed.	After adult provides damp washcloth and instruction to "Wash your face," child rubs the entire surface of face without further help and gives cloth back or sets it down when finished.
14	Wipes nose when instructed.	When instructed to blow or wipe nose, child routinely goes to tissue box, gets tissue, blows or wipes nose, and throws tissue away with no more than one verbal, and no manual, prompts.
15	Participates in all steps of hand washing.	Child routinely carries out manual action for each step of handwashing, other than turning water on, without needing full physical prompts. Adult may prompt some steps through gesture or partial physical prompt.
16	Cooperates with hair washing/ cutting.	Child does not fight, cry, or otherwise protest during hair washing or cutting. Child participates by helping rub shampoo, towel. May use strong reinforcers during routine.
17	Play with five bath toys appropriately.	Self-explanatory—for conventional bath toys.
18	Puts toys away when requested at end of bath.	Child must routinely put all bath toys in proper container without further prompts after initial instruction to pass.
19	Helps with lotion.	Child assists parent in rubbing lotion on hands, arms, legs, belly.
20	Brushes toothbrush over teeth.	Child rubs toothbrush over lower teeth and upper teeth, front and back, when instructed. All prompt levels other than full physical prompts can be used.
21	Goes to sleep independently after bedtime ritual.	Child routinely sleeps in own bed and goes to sleep without an adult present in the room after the bedtime routine ends and lights are turned out. Child seldom gets out of bed or comes out of room after being put to bed.
22	Shows knowledge of sequence of bedtime routine.	Child demonstrates awareness of bedtime routine by initiating one or more activities, and participating in various steps of routine without need for full prompts.
	Personal Independence: Chores	
23	Sorts silverware from dishwasher tray to silverware tray.	Adult may set up the situation, but after the set up and initial instruction, child takes as many as 20 utensils from dishwasher container and places them in silverware tray without any adult help.

Skill	Level 2	Description
	Personal Independence: Chores (*cont.*)	
24	Unloads dryer into basket.	When parent opens dryer door and provides basket, child will pull all items out of dryer into basket without need for further prompts. Child may need some help with a difficult item.
25	Matches socks.	Working from a group of 10 or more socks in a basket or pile, child places socks in pairs, folds or clips them, and stacks them in a container.
26	Pours water/food into pet dish.	Adult may provide materials and direct instruction, but child carries out the act without further help.

Skill	Level 3	Description
	Receptive Communication	
1	Attends and joins in with interest for 5–10 minutes as adult reads familiar books using simple sentences.	Stays with adult, pays full attention, and participates in a story the adult is reading. Examples include alternating eye contact between book pages and adult, pointing to pictures in book, turning book pages, vocalizing the names of pictures in book.
2	Follows one-step novel commands involving familiar objects/actions.	Completes instruction by looking at adult and performing action without adult gestures or physical guidance. Adult may repeat instructions a second time without gesture cue.
3	Identifies many common objects and their pictures: clothing items, objects related to meals, hygiene, play, foods.	Identifies 50 or more common objects to pass.
4	Responds appropriately to "yes/no" questions regarding preferences.	Uses "yes/no" in the appropriate requesting and refusal contexts. Must include eye contact, though need not be accompanied by gestures (i.e., nodding/shaking head). May use politeness phrases: "yes, please," "no, thanks."
5	Identifies 5 or more actions in pictures and books.	Vocalizes and/or gestures (e.g., points) in response to adult's questions. Examples are "Show me the baby sleeping?" or "Do you see the dog running?" Response need not be accompanied by eye contact.
6	Follows two or more instructions given in situational routines (bedtime: get a book and get in bed; toothbrushing: get your toothbrush and the toothpaste).	Routinely follows two- to three-part routine instructions involving actions and objects in well-practiced routines.
7	Understands spatial relationships involving objects (e.g., under, next to).	Examples are using concepts appropriately when asked ("Put the ball *next to* the car" or "Put the ball *under* the table").
8	Differentiates early size concepts—big/little.	Vocalizes or gestures (e.g., points, hands object) in response to adult's questions. Examples are "Where is the big ball?" or "Show me the little car." Response need not be accompanied by eye contact.
9	Differentiates at least four different colors upon request.	Vocalizes or gestures (e.g., points, hands object) in response to adult's request. Examples are "Which is the blue crayon?" or "Show me the red truck." Response need not be accompanied by eye contact.

Skill	Level 3	Description
	Receptive Communication *(cont.)*	
10	Identifies 20 items by sound (e.g., animals, telephone; "What animal says 'meow meow'?").	Vocalizes or gestures (e.g., points, hands object) in response to adult's question. Examples are "What animal says 'meow meow'?," "What does the doggie say?," or "What do you hear?" Response need not be accompanied by eye contact.
11	Comprehends the function of common objects (ride, cut, eat, sleep, put on feet, drink, etc.).	Vocalizes or gestures (e.g., points, hands object) in response to adult's question. Examples are "What do we ride in?" or "What do we use to take a drink?" Response need not be accompanied by eye contact. Identifies three or more object functions to pass.
12	Understands pronoun referents "mine" and "yours."	Vocalizes or gestures (e.g., points, hands object) in response to adult's question. Adult may use an object belonging to child to probe understanding. Examples are "Whose turn is it?" or "Whose shoe is this?" Response need not be accompanied by eye contact.
13	Identifies 10 actions via pictures, choices, acting out.	Vocalizes or gestures (e.g., points, hands picture, acts out) in response to adult's question. Examples are "Show me how you throw a ball" or "Show me the pig eating."
14	Follows two or more unrelated instructions in novel context.	Completes instruction by looking at adult and performing action without adult gestures or physical guidance. Adult may repeat instructions a second time without gesture cue. Examples are "Give me the car and close the book" or "Put the ball in the bucket, and put the doll on the table."
	Expressive Communication	
1	Produces two- to three-word combinations for a variety of communicative intentions (e.g., requesting, greeting, gaining attention, protesting).	Verbalizations must include eye contact. Examples are "Want more juice," "Bye, Sally," "Help me open," or "No ball." Articulation need not be perfect.
2	Produces two or more word utterances to comment to another person.	Verbalizations must include eye contact and are not related to requests to comment on objects or actions. Examples are "See cow," "Airplane go fast," or "Doggie." Articulation need not be perfect.
3	Labels actions in pictures and books.	Verbalizations need not be accompanied by eye contact. Examples are "Baby eating" or "Bird flying." Articulation need not be perfect.
4	Comments and requests on location (up, down, in, on top).	Verbalizations must include eye contact. Examples are "Bunny on chair" or "Ball in da (there)." Articulation need not be perfect.
5	Comments and requests using early possessive forms (mine, yours).	Verbalizations must include eye contact. Adult may use an object belonging to child. Examples are "That's (sippy cup) mine," "Your turn," or "My baby." Articulation need not be perfect.
6	Gestures or vocalizes "I don't know" in context.	Verbalization or gesture (e.g., shrugging shoulders, holds up hands) must include eye contact.
7	Consistently uses other people's names to get their attention.	Verbalization must include eye contact. Articulation need not be perfect.
8	Delivers a simple message to another person ("Go tell Mommy 'Hi'").	Verbalization must include eye contact. Examples are "Go tell Mommy 'Hi'," or "Go tell Daddy to come here." Articulation need not be perfect.

Skill	Level 3	Description
	Expressive Communication *(cont.)*	
9	Says "Hi" and "Bye-bye" appropriately, both initiating and in response.	Verbalization must include eye contact.
10	Uses pronouns for self and other (me and you variants).	Verbalization must include eye contact. Adult may want to use a mirror to probe. Response may include me and you variants. Examples are "That's me" or "I see you."
11	Uses simple words and gestures to describe personal experiences.	Verbalization and/or gestures (e.g., acting out) must include eye contact. Child may use single words or simple phrases. Examples are "Doggie," "Catch ball," or "Balloon goes up." Articulation need not be perfect.
12	Names one to two colors.	Verbalization need not be accompanied by eye contact. Adult may ask "What color is the car?" but child must initiate answer ("red car"; "it's a blue balloon"). Approximation may be accepted.
13	Responds appropriately to "What?" questions.	Verbalization need not be accompanied by eye contact. Adult may ask a second time.
14	Responds appropriately to "Where?" questions.	Verbalization need not be accompanied by eye contact. Adult may ask a second time.
15	Responds appropriately to "Who?" questions.	Verbalization need not be accompanied by eye contact. Adult may ask a second time.
16	Asks simple "yes/no" questions using rising intonation (can be one-word utterance with rising intonation).	Verbalization must include eye contact. Question may be one-word utterance with rising intonation. Examples are "Cookie?" or "Go bye-bye?"
17	Asks "What?" and "Where?" questions.	Verbalization must include eye contact. Must ask both questions to pass.
18	Answers simple information questions: name, age, color of shirt, etc.	Verbalization need not be accompanied by eye contact. Examples are "What's your name?", "How old are you?", or "What color is your shirt?"
	Social Skills: Adults and Peers	
1	Plays simple gross motor games (e.g., ball, "Hide and Seek," "Ring-around-the-Rosy").	Participates two or more times in any active behavior (reach, imitate, vocalize) in three or more games. Eye-contact and smiles alone are not enough. Examples are "Hide and Seek," "Ring-around-the-Rosy," playing ball.
2	Shares and shows objects when partner requests.	Responds within 3 seconds of partner's request. Partner may repeat a second time. Response may include verbalization (e.g., "baby") or gesture (e.g., brings object to partner, holds up object in hand).
3	Imitates and carries out novel songs/finger plays in group situation.	Participates two or more times in any active behavior in two or more routines. Eye contact and smiles alone are not enough. Examples are "Creepy Fingers," "Tickle," or "Eensy-Weensy Spider."
4	Responds appropriately to simple requests/instructions from peers.	Parent report may be accepted. Examples are "Get the ball," "You be the mommy," or "Put this there."
5	Initiates interactions and imitations of peers.	Parent report may be accepted. Initiates/imitates two or more rounds in three or more age-appropriate games (e.g., "chase," "Hide and Seek," playing with trains, dress up).
6	Plays in familiar dramatic play routine with peer in parallel play.	Parent report may be accepted. Participates in two or more rounds. Behaviors may include verbalizations (e.g., "Baby's hungry"), imitating, or observing partner's play. Examples of routines are playing house, dress up, role play.

Skill	Level 3	Description
	Social Skills: Adults and Peers *(cont.)*	
7	Takes turns with simple board games.	Participates in two more rounds in three or more age-appropriate games. Examples are "Connect Four," "Caribou," or "Lucky Ducks."
8	Uses politeness terms: "Please," "Thank you," "Excuse me."	Examples are "Please," "Thank you," or "Excuse me," spontaneously and appropriately. Approximations may be accepted. Pass if frequently uses two of the three.
9	Imitates a variety of novel gross motor actions in standing and while moving, such as in "Follow the Leader" or animal walks.	Examples are "Follow the Leader," "Simon Says," or pretending to move as animals. Spontaneously imitates 10 or more novel actions. Can be imprecise.
10	Participates in play activities involving verbal scripts.	Participates in three or more activities with active behaviors (verbalizes, acts out, imitates). Eye contact and smiles alone are not enough. Examples are playing house, being teacher, or putting baby to bed.
11	Frequently draws others' attention to objects verbally and gesturally to comment, show, share, and request.	Initiates behaviors three or more times with eye contact. Examples are verbalizations (e.g., "Mama, look, kitty," "Blocks fall down," or "More crackers, Daddy") with gestures (e.g., gives or holds up object to adult, points to item).
12	Responds to others' bids for joint attention by looking and commenting.	Responds within 3 seconds of adult's bid. Adult may repeat a second time.
13	Receptively identifies affect (happy, sad, mad, scared) from photos, in others, and/or in line drawings.	Responds within 3 seconds of adult's bid. Adult may repeat a second time. Identifies two or more affective feelings (e.g., happy, sad, mad, scared, surprised). Verbalization need not be accompanied by eye contact.
14	Expressively identifies affect from photos, in others, and/or in line drawings.	Identifies two or more affective feelings (e.g., happy, sad, mad, scared, surprised). Verbalization need not be accompanied by eye contact.
15	Makes own face reflect affect (happy, sad, mad, scared).	Reflects two or more affective feelings (e.g., happy, sad, mad, scared, surprised). Response need not be accompanied by eye contact.
	Cognition	
1	Matches letters in own name.	Matches all letters in first name.
2	Matches letters.	Matches five or more letters. May be in response to adult verbal cue (e.g., "Where's A?") or demonstrate first few trials, but child needs to match independently at least five trials.
3	Matches words.	Match/sort five or more words. May be in response to adult verbal cue (e.g., "Where's *c-a-t*?") or demonstrate first few trials, but child needs to match independently at least five trials.
4	Matches numbers.	Match/sort five or more numbers. May be in response to adult verbal cue (e.g., "Where's 6?") or demonstrate first few trials, but child needs to match independently at least five trials.
5	Receptively and expressively identifies some letters, numbers, shapes, and colors.	Identifies five or more in each category. May be in response to adult verbal cue (e.g., "Where's 6?", "Show me the blue crayon.", or "What letter?") or demonstrate first few trials, but child needs to identify independently at least five trials.

Skill	Level 3	Description
	Cognition *(cont.)*	
6	Plays games involving memory for hidden objects.	Identifies three or more hidden objects. Adult may probe by showing three objects (e.g., penny, small ball, stick) to child and then placing a cup over each item. Adult waits 7 seconds and then shows a second copy of one of the hidden objects (e.g., small ball) and asks "Where's the other ball?" Response may be verbalization ("There") and/or gesture (e.g., points/picks up cup). Eye contact is not necessary. Adult should set up three or more trials.
7	Categorizes objects/pictures into eight classes.	Will sort into sets of three, for up to eight classes.
8	Understands relationship between quantities and number symbols through number 5.	Understands relationship either verbally (e.g., counts out five objects) or gesturally (e.g., touches or groups five objects).
9	Counts correct number of objects to five.	Assigns value up to five or more objects. Adult may have child count preferred objects, such as checkers, candy, trains, or blocks. Adult may count the first item to begin but child needs to continue and end independently.
10	Sequences three or more pictures in correct order and narrates sequence for pictures using "first, then" language.	May be in response to adult verbal cue (e.g., "What's next?"). Child needs to sequence independently and narrate when asked "Tell me about it" for three or more different sequences.
	Play	
1	Constructive play involves sequencing complex schemas with multiple coordinated objects (e.g., trucks on road, blocks make building, beads make a necklace).	Construct three or more schemas. Multiple objects may be trucks on road, blocks make building, beads make a necklace.
2	Links three or more related actions in a play sequence.	Examples are building track, pushing trains, and crashing trains, or taking out play dough, using shape cutter, taking out shape. (Note: These can form the picture sequence for #10 alone.)
3	Performs two or more linked actions on a doll or animal when instructed.	Examples are pretending to pour juice and feeding baby, picking up blanket and putting doll to bed, or putting animal in car and pushing car.
4	Physically places figures on miniature furniture, vehicles, etc., when appropriate.	Places figures in appropriate context during play. Examples are seating dad in chair to watch TV or putting mom in car to drive to store.
5	Carries out actions on doll or animal figures spontaneously.	Completes three or more actions without adult prompts.
6	Arranges props for the theme.	Arranges two or more prompts in three or more different play schemas. Examples are setting out fork and plate to feed baby, putting hat on self and other to play dress up.
	Fine Motor	
1	Completes five- to six-piece interlocking puzzle.	Self-explanatory.
2	Imitates drawing circle, cross, square, diagonal line.	Imitates each one at least once. Adult models and may use verbal cue (e.g., "Draw this").
3	Imitates and builds different block structures using a variety of building materials (blocks, Legos, Tinker Toys, etc.).	Uses five or more blocks to build three or more different structures. Building materials may be blocks, Legos, Tinker Toys, etc.

Skill	Level 3	Description
	Fine Motor *(cont.)*	
4	Laces a running stitch.	Laces through three or more loops/holes. Adult may use verbal cue (e.g., "Put it in there") or demonstrate first trial.
5	Traces lines and curves with finger and writing tool.	Traces at least three-fourths of line and curve with finger and writing tool. Adult may model first trial.
6	Uses a variety of tools to pick up and release objects: tongs, fork.	Uses two or more tools to pick up and release two or more objects. Examples are using a large spoon to pick up/release a piece of food or tongs to pick up/release blocks.
7	Traces a variety of shapes.	Traces three or more shapes (e.g., square, circle, triangle, rectangle). May use plastic frame or trace lines on paper.
8	Uses scissors with appropriate grasp and uses opposite hand to stabilize and turn paper.	The cut need not follow a line but cuts off a strip of paper in two. Adult may show how to hold scissors and cut through paper.
9	Cuts on a line—straight and curved lines.	Cuts along the line fairly accurately. Adult may model first trial.
10	Carries out simple two-step art projects (cut and paste, stamp with ink pad; folds paper and cuts on line).	Adult may use verbal cue (e.g., "First do this, then do this") or demonstrate steps on first trial. Examples are cut and paste, stamp ink pad and paper, folds paper and cuts on line.
11	Carries out several different schemas with play dough—uses a variety of tools.	Carries out three or more schemas. Uses two or more tools to pass. Examples are rolling dough with pin and cutting with knife to make a snake, or rolling dough into ball and pretending to eat with fork.
	Gross Motor	
1	Rides tricycle well (pedals and steers, follows a route).	Pedals and steers, follows a route independently and with good coordination.
2	Kicks with good form and balance.	Kicks without holding onto object/person. Does not stumble or fall down. Makes contact three or more times.
3	Uses all playground equipment with supports.	Climbs and uses low-play (e.g., swings, small slides, seesaws) and high-play equipment (e.g., jungle gyms, monkey bars, high slides). May hold on to railings.
4	Plays chase game with adults and peers, running smoothly, changing direction with good balance.	Plays for at least 5 minutes.
5	Imitates gross motor actions with movement to songs and music.	Imitates five or more actions in three or more different songs. Examples are imitating body movements in "If you're happy and you know it..." or "The wheels on the bus..." Imitations are spontaneous and immediate.
6	Throws underhand at target.	Throws underhand three or more times. Does not have to hit target perfectly. Adult may demonstrate up to two trials.
7	Jumps forward with two feet together.	Jumps forward three or more times.
8	Hops in one foot.	Hops on one foot at least once. May hop while holding on to another person or stable object, without falling.
	Personal Independence	
1	Uses spoon, fork, and cup neatly and without spilling.	Need not hold spoon or fork correctly.
2	Behaves appropriately at sit-down restaurant.	Family is able to eat entire meal without serious problem behavior (e.g., throwing, hitting, crawling under table, running away). Child may occasionally fuss but can be redirected to activities to occupy attention (e.g., drawing at table, playing with small toys).

Skill	Level 3	Description
Personal Independence *(cont.)*		
3	Uses icons or other symbol systems for choices, schedules, etc. independently, if needed at home and at school.	Finds icon/picture/symbol book, selects appropriate icon, and completes choice or activity without assistance. Completes independently at least 80% of time at home and at school. If none are used by child, pass the item.
4	Carries own materials to and from car, school, and home.	Carries at least one material by self. Examples are backpack, lunchbox, jacket, etc.
5	Opens and closes backpack independently; puts in and removes objects when requested.	Puts in/removes at least three objects by self on request. Examples are lunchbox, folder, toy, etc.
6	Dresses and undresses when appropriate (unfastens clothing fasteners—zippers and snaps).	Unfastens zippers and snaps independently.
Personal Independence: Hygiene		
7	Uses toilet independently, all steps, when taken or sent.	May ask for help with washing hands if cannot reach sink.
8	Manages clothing at toilet except for fasteners.	Pulls down/up underwear and pants. Adult may hold item for child to step in to (if taken off) but child pulls down/up by self.
9	Completes all the hand-washing steps independently.	Turns on/off faucet, uses soap, rubs hands, and dries hands. May be reminded.
10	Wipes face with warm washcloth when handed to child.	Places washcloth on face and wipes. May be reminded.
11	Runs brush or comb through hair.	May be reminded.
12	Covers mouth when coughing and sneezing.	Covers mouth with hand or tissue. May be reminded.
13	Assists actively in bathing and drying self after bath.	Adult may provide towel, soap, and washcloth or put soap on washcloth but child helps wash and dry body parts (e.g., face, stomach, arms, legs).
14	Brushes teeth with toothbrush, using at least a few strokes.	Brushes up/down at least five or more strokes for top and bottom teeth. Adult may put toothpaste on toothbrush. May be told to keep brushing.
Personal Independence: Chores		
15	Feeds/waters a pet.	Puts food/water in bowl and brings to pet. Adult may assist (e.g., opens can, measures amounts) or remind.
16	Helps clear table.	Takes at least two or more items (e.g., plate, cup, bowl, etc.) to sink. May be reminded.
17	Helps empty dishwasher.	Puts away five or more items. Adult may show where item goes. Takes at least two or more items (e.g., plate, cup, bowl, etc.) to sink. May be reminded.
18	Puts clean clothes in drawers.	Places three or more folded clothes neatly in drawers, but need not fold them. May be reminded.
19	Picks up belongings when asked.	Picks up possessions (e.g., clothes, toys, shoes, etc.) and puts away in appropriate location when asked. May be reminded.

Skill	Level 4	Description
	Receptive Communication	
1	Understands a variety of descriptive physical relationship concepts.	Picks up, gives, points, or shows correct item out of choice of two to adult. Child identifies five different concepts correctly. Examples: hot/cold, empty/full, wet/dry, hard/soft, heavy/light, tall/short, long/short, large/small.
2	Retrieves 10–15 items using two to three multiple cues (e.g., size, quantity, color, object label).	Picks up, gives, points, or shows correct item to adult. Example: Adult asks, "Can I have the broken blue crayon?" and child references the correct item.
3	Understands gender pronouns.	Child picks up, gives, points, or shows male or female character, figurine, or live person correctly in response to instructions involving "him or her" or "he or she." Example: "Put him in the car" or "She wants some ice cream." Child must pass at least one female and one male gender pronoun to pass item.
4	Understands comparatives: bigger, shorter, smaller, most, least, few, many, etc.	Picks up, gives, points, or shows correct item to adult out of a field of four to five choices. To pass, child must comprehend three or more comparative sets.
5	Understands spatial relationships involving objects and prepositions: behind, in back of, in front of.	Child demonstrates understanding of these concepts: behind, in back of, in front of by placing objects in correct configurations or looking to correct location when directed (e.g., "Look behind the sofa").
6	Understands negatives (e.g., the box with no balls, the boy who is not sitting).	Picks up, gives, points, or shows correct item that identifies the absence of an object (bowl with no cherries) or feature (child who does not have blue eyes) or a nonoccurring action (one who is not sleeping).
7	Understands possessives and part–whole relations.	In objects and pictures, child points to or shows the part of an item when requested (e.g., bunny's nose, tricycle's wheel, door of the car).
8	Demonstrates attention to short stories and comprehension of parts of the story by responding to simple "wh" questions (what and who).	Child listens to simple stories as they are read (five pages). Child demonstrates attention by looking at book with adult and accurately responding to what and who questions, verbally or by pointing, page by page. Answers two to three questions at end.
9	Responds to "yes/no" questions for identity.	Answers correctly by verbalizing and shaking/nodding head when adults asks, "Is this a ____________?" or "Is your name Sam?"
10	Answers questions about physical states.	Child responds correctly with a phrase to questions "What do you do if…?" for four or more: hurt, tired, hungry, thirsty.
11	Responds to personal information questions.	Responds correctly to three or more personal information questions. Examples: "What's your name?" (first and last), "What's your telephone number?", and "What's your address?"
12	Understands "same" and "different."	Picks up, gives, points, or shows pictures/items correctly given instructions involving finding objects that are the same and pictures/items that are different.
13	Understands quantity concepts.	Picks up, gives, points, or shows objects or pictures correctly in response to these quantity words: *one, some, all, few, most.* Must pass all to pass item.

Skill	Level 4	Description
	Receptive Communication *(cont.)*	
14	Identifies features of objects.	Picks up, gives, points, or shows the item with the feature that the adult indicates. Example: Adult says "Show me the dog with the long tail" and child indicates correct answer. Features should involve size, shape, texture, physical state. Pass requires comprehension of 10–15 features.
15	Responds to questions regarding category membership of objects/ pictures.	Child understands object categories involving all of these: color, shape, size, or function; the blue ones, the round ones, the big ones, the ones you eat with.
16	Understands past and future tense.	Child identifies by past tense construction something that has occurred in the past (e.g., "Show me the boy who jumped"). Same for future tense. Child must respond accurately to both past and future, with both regular and irregular verbs.
17	Understands passive voice.	Child demonstrates understanding of passive voice through object manipulations or picture selections (e.g., "The dog was hit by the ball," "The girl is being chased by the boy").
18	Understands temporal relations.	Child accurately responds to instructions involving these three temporal relations: first/last, before/after, at the same time.
19	Follows three-part unrelated verbal instructions.	Complies with adult request that contains three or more components. Example: Adult says "Give me the cup," "Kiss the bear," and "Close the box." Pass requires correct performance on five probes.
	Expressive Communication	
1	Responds to complex "wh" questions ("Why?", "How?").	Child answers questions regarding these concepts correctly (e.g., "Why do we wash hands?" "How do you brush teeth?").
2	Describes object functions in response to question (e.g., "What do you do with a spoon?").	Can describe functions of five or more common objects using simple phrases.
3	Speaks in three- to four-word utterances consistently.	Across a variety of contexts, partners, and activities.
4	Uses a variety of noun phrases.	Child combines a variety of words to make noun phrases that can be as long as four words in length, including articles, possessives, adjectives, and quantifier (e.g., "The little horse," "My red pen," "This truck," "Two cookies," "The big red square," "A chocolate milkshake," "Some more fries").
5	Uses prepositional phrases (under, next to, behind, in back of, in front of).	Child produces all of these prepositions listed above to describe object arrangements, answer questions, and instruct others in both natural and structured formats.
6	Uses a variety of verb phrases (e.g., he cries, she likes him, he fell, he was happy, he is happy, could, should, would).	Self-explanatory.
7	Demonstrates accurate production of at least 80% of all consonants and consonant blends within connected speech.	Child demonstrates accurate production of 80% of sounds within conversation; speech intelligibility is judged to be good by a naïve listener.

Skill	Level 4	Description
	Expressive Communication *(cont.)*	
8	Describes recent experience using three- to four-word sentence.	When asked, child describes a recent experience with at least two components of the experiences (who, what, where, when). Examples: "What did you do at your birthday party?" "I got presents from David."
9	Requests permission to pursue an activity.	Child asks permission before beginning a regulated activity: "Can I stir?" (pan on stove) "Can I do it?" (using an adult tool). Also used if child wants to switch activities: "Can we listen to music?"
10	Uses plural forms.	Child uses regular plurals consistently and spontaneously and also uses two irregular forms (e.g., children, mice).
11	Uses later possessives (e.g., his, hers, Mommy's hat).	Child uses these regularly.
12	Uses regular past tense.	Child uses regular past tense forms spontaneously and regularly.
13	Uses articles such as *a, an, the.*	Child uses these routinely in sentences and phrases.
14	Uses comparatives/superlatives.	Uses five or more correctly: better, best, bigger, biggest, smaller, smallest, fatter, fattest.
15	Uses negation with auxiliary verbs.	Examples: "I am not crying," "I did not hit him," "I will not sit down."
16	Uses present progressive verb form.	Verbalizes a phrase including a verb form combining am/is/are with a verb ending in *–ing.* Example: The boy is riding.
17	Uses words to describe physical states.	Child uses five or more words to describe own states: "I'm hungry, cold, thirsty, tired, hurt."
18	Responds to questions about physical states: "What do you do when you are ...?"	Child responds correctly to five or more.
19	Uses category names for familiar objects.	Refers to an item or group of items by its category name. Examples include animals, vehicles, food, clothing.
20	Describes features of objects.	Child can name three or more features of five common objects when asked "Tell me about a ____________."
21	Uses reflexive pronouns.	Uses two or more reflexive pronouns, including *myself, yourself, himself, herself, itself, oneself, ourselves, yourselves, themselves.*
22	Answers telephone appropriately, including getting person.	Walks to the ringing phone, picks up receiver and puts it to his or her ear, issues a verbal greeting, and gets person who the caller requests.
23	Participates in a conversation that is initiated by an adult for two to three consecutive turns involving a variety of functions (e.g., reciprocal commenting, responding to and requesting information).	Child keeps conversations going by adding elements, asking questions, commenting, sharing experiences, etc. Can use phrase speech but keeps the conversation going through two to three turns on the child's part.
24	Initiates and maintains a conversation on a self-generated topic of conversation with an adult.	Child begins a conversation with a partner with a comment or questions and maintains the topic through at least four conversational turns.
25	Describes a two- to three-event sequence of activities (e.g., going to visit Grandma).	In response to an open-ended question (e.g., "Tell me about your trip to Grandma's"), the child will describe two or three activities or events using phrase speech.

Skill	Level 4	Description
	Expressive Communication *(cont.)*	
26	Expresses "I don't know" paired with gesture.	When asked a question that the child does not know the answer to, the child responds appropriately.
27	Asks for clarification if doesn't understand what is said.	Child says "What?" or a similar response when child did not hear or understand a comment, question, or instruction directed to the child.
28	Engages in a variety of topics during conversation.	Child initiates conversations on a variety of topics and engages in conversations on a variety of topics.
29	Repairs own communication when listener does not understand.	Child demonstrates use of repair strategies (e.g., repeats, rephrases, combines verbalization with gesture, adds emphasis) to clarify communication when not understood by partner.
30	Answers questions about self and others.	Child can answer a variety of simple questions about the self and can also answer questions about very familiar others—family members, pets, best friend, etc.
	Social Skills	
1	Invites peers to play.	Makes one or more verbal or gestural play bids to a peer ("Come play with the train!," "Let's play chase," or waving a peer over).
2	Uses polite forms such as "Excuse me," "Sorry."	Uses several politeness terms including "No thank you," "Thank you," "You're welcome," "Excuse me," and "Sorry."
3	Seeks out others for comfort in a group situation.	When child is scared, hurt, or frustrated, child moves closer to adult or makes physical contact with adult (hugging, sitting on lap, holding hand).
4	Expresses own feelings appropriately.	Verbalizes own feelings by saying "I'm mad," etc.
5	Takes turns in informal play independently.	Takes turns with adult/peer when engaged in a play activity without clearly defined turns.
6	Describes an event or experience to peer.	Verbally retells a story to a peer or sibling, including at least three details.
7	Identifies what makes self feel happy, sad, mad, scared.	Verbalizes one or more examples for each concept (e.g., happy, sad, mad, scared). Example: Adult says, "Why are you sad?" and child says, "She took my book and I'm sad."
8	Identifies others' emotions based on situational factors.	During reading activities or conversation, child answers appropriately when asked, "Why is she crying?" or "Why is he scared?"
9	Begins to develop coping strategies when feeling upset, mad, or scared.	Engages in one or more coping strategies. Examples: requests a break, asks for help, comes for a hug, gets a comfort object.
	Cognition	
1	Counts rotely to 20.	Counts out loud from 1 to 20 in correct sequential order.
2	Counts objects with 1:1 correspondence to 10.	Touches or points to pictures or objects while counting in sequence, touching or pointing once for each number.
3	Gives "one," "some," "a lot," "a little," "all of them," "more," and "most."	Hands correct number of items to adult when adult requests.
4	Gives quantities through 10.	Hands correct number of items to adult when adult requests ("Give me five cookies" or "Can I have two pillows?").

Skill	Level 4	Description
	Cognition *(cont.)*	
5	Knows terms for quantity concepts.	Verbalizes two or more concepts, including "one," "some," and "all."
6	Knows terms for spatial relations.	Verbalizes two or more concepts, including behind, in back of, and in front of.
7	Matches and understands 5–10 word/object associations.	Matches five or more objects with the associated written three- to four-letter word.
8	Can read some words.	Reads and pronounces 10 or more three- to four-letter words for common actions and objects.
9	Can identify written name out of a field of five.	Gives, points, shows, or goes to his or her own name when name is shown in an array of three names that includes one name that begins with the same letter as the child's name.
10	"Reads" signs and symbols.	States the meaning of three or more common signs and symbols. Example: stop sign, green light, universal "no" symbol.
11	Identifies numbers and letters.	Receptively identifies and expressively states the names of all letters of the alphabet and numbers 0–30.
12	States opposites and analogies.	When adult states a concept, child names the concept for the opposite. Example: Adult says "A mouse is little, but an elephant is ___________" and child says, "big."
	Play	
1	Demonstrates actions of figures in play.	Has figures carry out five or more actions in three or more play scenarios. Example: Mommy driving to store, brother chasing sister, or doggie eating food.
2	Uses placeholder items to symbolize props in play.	Uses three or more neutral placeholder items. (Neutral = no identity of its own). Examples: using a block as a phone, a tube as a bottle, or a small box as a car.
3	Labels actions and pretend props in play.	Labels 10 or more pretend actions and/or pretend props in three or more play activities spontaneously and in response to questions.
4	Spontaneously links three or more related behaviors in a play theme.	Examples: pouring water in pot, stirring food, and pouring food in bowl; putting on firefighter hat, "driving" fire engine truck; and putting out fire.
5	Directs partner in play.	Provides three or more relevant instructions directed to partner to carry out some aspect of play theme across two or more play episodes.
6	Plays out several life events (e.g., birthday party, McDonald's, doctor), including use of verbal scripts.	Plays out three or more life events, each containing at least three embedded activities (see item 4 above), interacting with partner through verbal scripts and object actions.
7	Plays out several story themes in play.	Plays out three or more story themes with partner using multiple actions and scripts as described in the item above: Examples: *Little Red Riding Hood, Three Little Pigs, Billy Goats Gruff.*
8	Takes on a character role and plays it out.	States role (e.g., "I'm the Mommy") and plays out a life scene with verbal script, activities, and gestures appropriate to role, with three or more exchanges to partner.
9	Follows another's lead in play.	Follows partner's play directives verbally or nonverbally five or more times by imitating partner's acts or responding to partner's instructions.

Skill	Level 4	Description
Fine Motor		
1	Colors in a picture with accuracy using different colors.	Child colors mostly inside shapes and chooses different colors to complete picture on coloring book-type page.
2	Imitates triangle, letters using appropriate drawing utensil.	Child copies circle, square, triangle, and some alphabet letters recognizably.
3	Draws lines and shapes and some letters and numbers from memory.	Child initiates drawing several shapes and letters/ numbers that are recognizable.
4	Imitates and copies a variety of letters, numbers, and shapes.	Child both copies and generates four to five shapes, four to five letters, and several numbers that are recognizable.
5	Writes first name without a model.	Self-explanatory.
6	Traces shapes and letters.	Self-explanatory.
7	Colors in shapes that are outlined.	Child keeps coloring generally inside borders.
8	Connects dots with drawing tool.	Child can follow dot-to-dot patterns and can follow the number sequence.
9	Draws lines to and from corresponding pictures, words, or shapes.	Child can connect matching or related pictures of objects with a line (as in a child workbook activity).
10	Copies a variety of simple representational drawings (e.g., face, tree, house, flower).	Child copies five or more different line drawings and makes two to three recognizable pictures spontaneously.
11	Folds paper in half and puts in envelope.	Self-explanatory, following model.
12	Cuts out angles, straight lines, and curves.	Child cuts out corners and edges of large shapes (3 inches or more) using child scissors independently.
13	Cuts out simple shapes.	Child successfully cuts out 3-inch shapes.
14	Completes three-step art projects—cut, color, and paste.	Once adult models the activity, child can sequence the activity and complete it independently as long as each step involves a skill at which child is fully competent.
15	Uses paintbrush, stamps, markers, pencils, erasers to complete art activities.	Child uses a variety of art materials in an open-ended art activity to create products. Child can also imitate an adult's model using each of these tools.
16	Uses a tripod grasp with drawing tool.	Child consistently holds writing implements with a mature tripod grasp.
17	Builds with a variety of building materials with own design and copies simple models from pictures or 3-D models.	Child assembles a variety of building materials into complex designs and can also copy other's designs, both from 3-D models and from photos and line drawings. Child can demonstrate five or more different models.
18	Puts together interlocking puzzles, floor puzzles, tray puzzles.	Self-explanatory.
19	Uses tape, paper clips, keys appropriately.	Uses all these tools independently.
Gross Motor		
1	Plays catch with playground-sized ball with a peer.	Can keep a catch game going through six or more turns.
2	Throws tennis ball or baseball to another person with directionality using overhand throw.	Self-explanatory.

Skill	Level 4	Description
	Gross Motor (*cont.*)	
3	Uses all playground equipment independently, including swing, merry-go-round.	Self-explanatory, for all age-appropriate equipment.
4	Kicks a moving ball.	Child adjusts body and successfully kicks a ball in motion.
5	Plays various games with balls: Throws ball in basket, hits T-ball with bat, bounces ball, golf club, beanbag toss.	Plays five or more games with balls.
6	Rides bicycle confidently with training wheels; able to control speed, maneuver, and brake.	Self-explanatory.
7	Gallops and skips.	Imitates both and performs smoothly.
8	Walks without falling off balance beam, railroad ties, sidewalk curbs.	Self-explanatory; walks relatively smoothly and not too slowly.
9	Plays typical motor games (e.g., "Red Light, Green Light," "Red Rover," "Freeze Tag.").	Plays five or more such games—knows the rules and participates actively through the game and without prompting or coaching.
	Personal Independence	
1	Manages all steps involved in toileting independently at the level of peers.	Uses potty as needed (though adult may prompt trips to the toilet), pulls own pants/underwear up and down, flushes, and washes hands.
2	Takes self to toilet as needed.	Takes self to toilet as needed (no adult prompting needed).
3	Washes hands independently at level of peers.	Child turns on faucet, puts hands under water, applies soap to hands, rubs soaped hands together, rinses soap off, turns off water, and dries hands on towel.
4	Washes face with washcloth independently.	During bathtime, child wets washcloth, applies soap, and scrubs face with a washcloth.
5	Independently brushes or combs hair.	When adult asks child to comb/brush hair, child gets tool and runs tool throughout hair. May be age-appropriate exceptions for difficulties with long or curly hair.
6	Actively assists with bathing, dries self after bath.	Rubs body with washcloth, applies soap to body, and scrubs own scalp when shampoo is applied. Dries self reasonably well; may need "touch-up."
7	Carries out all steps for toothbrushing independently, though adult may also brush teeth for thoroughness.	From the time the child enters bathroom until toothbrush and toothpaste are returned to proper place, child can carry out all steps independently.
8	Fastens own clothing—buttons, snaps, and zippers.	Fastens own buttons, snaps, zippers, and clips when they are present on child's outfit.
9	Blows nose when cued, uses tissue to catch sneezes, covers cough and sneeze.	When adult says, "Blow your nose," child retrieves a tissue and blows nose into tissue. When child sneezes, he or she covers mouth with hand or arm.
10	Stops at street; crosses after looking both ways when accompanied.	When approaching a curb or street with partner, child automatically stops, waits, looks, and waits for partner to indicate that child may cross.
11	Walks safely beside adult independently in parking lots, stores, etc.	Child walks without holding hands and stays close to adult, monitoring adult location and maintaining proximity on own initiative.

Skill	Level 4	Description
	Personal Independence *(cont.)*	
12	Helps with table setting.	Child can place plates, cups, napkins, and utensils at the correct places independently and relatively neatly. Adult may need to mark what places to set and can provide child with the materials on the table.
13	Uses knife to spread.	Child can spread jelly-type consistencies over the surface of a piece of bread without tearing the bread.
14	Cleans up after spills.	Child cleans up spills at a table on own initiative and does a thorough job of it.
15	Pours self drink from small container.	Child can pour from a 2–4 cup pitcher into a small cup neatly and independently.
16	Places dishes in sink, counter, or dishwasher.	After meals, the child routinely cleans up his or her place and puts eating implements in correct location independently.
17	Makes a two-step snack.	Gets out two different items, places from container to plate, places at table. Examples: sets out cut-up veggies and dip, cheese and crackers, spreads cream cheese on crackers, fixes cereal and milk.
18	Assists with cooking activities: stirs, pours, etc.	Child participates in multiple steps of multistep cooking activity like making cookies, pancakes, scrambled eggs.

Appendix B

Early Start Denver Model Teaching Fidelity Rating System

Administration and Coding

PROCEDURE FOR CODING FIDELITY OF TREATMENT IMPLEMENTATION

Instructions to Raters

1. If rating from a video recording, watch the recording in a confidential setting with minimal verbal or visual distractions.
2. Review the child's objectives and the teaching plans just prior to coding, and keep them available to check as needed. The treatment being delivered should correspond to the treatment objectives and plans.
3. Read the language defining each behavior and anchor for every score, to be sure that your codes are well anchored by the scale. Don't rely on your memory or knowledge of the teaching practices or coding definitions.
4. If it is not clear what the teaching goals of the segment are, attend to what is being reinforced. Assume that the behavior being reinforced is the behavior being taught during the segment. There is often, or usually, more than one behavior targeted for teaching in any segment.
5. Take brief notes during the activity segment that you are observing, in order to remember objectives, child communications, affect, and so on. Note delivery of antecedents, reinforcers, prompts, communications and their varied functions, and elaborations, and so on, since you should not replay the recording to observe more than once.
6. When rating, be aware of rater biases including halo or recency effects that problem in one aspect of the teaching does not then bias your ratings of other behaviors in that segment or other segments you observe.
7. An activity involves an extended interaction with a particular set of materials or an extended social interaction. An activity generally has a beginning, when the activity structure is set up, a middle, containing the exchanges that are the teaching interactions, and an ending in which the materials are removed or the sensory social routine ends and a whole new activity begins. The segment to be coded is defined by the activity, not the location. If the materials

and teaching tasks change, it is a new activity. Activities are sometimes aborted after a minute or two because the adult was unable to engage the child in the activity, and no teaching has occurred. Do not code these—instead mark the times and write "aborted" in the scoring column.

8. Coding an activity requires coding the transition that precedes or follows it. In general, begin the observation after the transition into a new activity routine has occurred and continue through the transition into the beginning of the next activity before you stop the recording. You will code the transition that occurs at the end of each activity in the transition item. However, if for some unexpected reason there is no transition recorded, then code the initial transition into the activity.
9. Observe each activity one time through without stopping. Make notes as needed and begin to code. You may replay to observe something a second time as needed, especially to capture child communications and adult responses, if notes are not sufficient. Do not use slow motion and do not replay more than once.
10. When a teaching problem has occurred, decide what the main difficulty is and code the item most closely related to the problem accordingly. Do not let one problem teacher behavior be coded in multiple items. However, if one problem then leads to another (e.g., insensitivity to cues leads to a child upset, and then there is a problem modulating the negative child arousal that ensues), then both should be coded. If you are not sure where to code the problem, just code it in one of the related items. As long as you don't count it twice, the scoring will not be affected by having it in one rather than another row.
11. If you are caught between two codes, then give the higher code. However, if the reason for the two codes is that the therapist behavior changed over the activity, then the problematic teaching behavior should not be cancelled out by improvements later in the session. Rather, both aspects are important to capture and a score assigned that reflects both the less adequate and the more adequate aspects.
12. Codes:

    5—Represents the best possible example of this teaching behavior. These are optimal examples of the teaching skill, in which the coder does not see anything that the adult could have added to the situation to optimize it. This is expert level.

    4—Represents a quite competent example of this aspect of teaching, without mistakes. The episode could have been taken farther by a master teacher, but there are no flaws or mistakes in the execution of this skill and it represents good, competent display of this skill. This is a fully competent level.

    3—Represents a teacher behavior with some strengths but also some weaknesses. Overall there are more strengths than weaknesses, but there are evident oversights or mistakes according to the criteria specified. A person at this level in most of his or her teaching needs more refinement of his or her skills. The individual may continue to work with children but requires additional supervision and feedback to improve competency in the marked areas. This is a mixed level of competence.

    2—Represents flawed display of this teaching behavior. There is some effort to use some specific teaching practices but there are more weaknesses than strengths. This is a flawed level of competence and a person at this level needs more training and supervision in the basic procedures before working alone.

    1—Represents lack of an effective display of the practices specified. There are no strengths.

This is a poor and unacceptable level in this teaching behavior. A person at this level needs full training in the model before working alone.

13. Fidelity. In our training programs, a therapist is considered to have achieved fidelity to the model if they have no scores under 3 and a mean score of 80% or above on three consecutively coded joint activity routines for two to three consecutive children.

EARLY START DENVER MODEL

A. Management of Child Attention

Note: This item targets the child's visual and auditory attention to the adult and to the materials; that is, the ability of the adult to get the child's attention on a teaching activity and then "step into the spotlight"—the center of the child's visual attention, so that the child attends to the adult. If there are potential distractions in the environment, but they are not in the way and the child is not distracted by them and is attending nicely to the teaching targets, do not reduce the score.

1—Adult does not have child attention initially, either due to poor choice of activity or due to environmental problems (distracted by materials, or uncomfortable and poorly seated, or the child and adult are not positioned well in relation to each other). The therapist does not take any steps to alter the situation and continues, either fully prompting an inattentive child or having a child escape or otherwise not participate.

2—Adult does not have child attention initially, due to style of presentation of activity or environment, but appears aware of the problem. Adult tries to attain child attention but is unsuccessful and does not find a solution that results in a teaching episode. The activity continues unsuccessfully or is aborted and is not replaced by a more successful teaching activity.

3—Adult has child attention on self or materials at start of activity but does not sustain attention through the teaching task due to problems of timing, pacing, or teaching techniques. Or, the adult does not have child attention at the start of the activity but recognizes the problem, corrects it, and gains the child's attention so that some teaching can occur. Or, the child is solely focused on the materials and does not attend to the adult's face or body. However, the quality of the teaching activity in terms of opportunities for child learning has been compromised.

4—Adult has child attention at the beginning of the episode and sustains it for enough time to conduct the teaching activity. However, adult could have extended attention further or supported better attentional distribution between adult and task with additional techniques.

5—Adult has child attention at the beginning of the episode and maximizes and sustains it through a well-developed teaching activity and needed adjustments through multiple practice opportunities. The child shows coordinated or alternating attention to adult and teaching activity. Demonstrates optimal management of attention.

B. ABC Format—Quality of Behavioral Teaching

This item rates the clarity of the teaching interactions, frequency of teaching interactions, and the appropriate use of repetitions during the activity. The following elements go into the score:

• ABC format: Did the therapist use a clear ABC format in the teaching episodes? In skillful teaching, the therapist's antecedents, child behaviors, and delivery of appropriate consequences: Reinforcement or correction stands out clearly. It is clear to the observer what behavior the therapist is trying to elicit. Direct reinforcement is delivered contingently and quickly.

• Teaching trials occur frequently during the play—at least every 30 seconds on average.

• Number of repetitions: Were the number of repetitions for each skill appropriate for child learning or maintenance? The adult shows good judgment about how often a skill should be repeated based on learning needs and child motivation. New skills receive more repetition than mastered skills without loss of child motivation. The purpose of the repetitions is to shape more accurate performances.

1—The child is or is not watching the very active adult with interest, but there are very few teaching exchanges in the activity—less than one per minute. Use this code if the adult is "entertaining" the child by creating interesting spectacles that do not require many child responses.

2—Adult provides some teaching trials and is trying to teach rather than entertain. The adult has the child's attention and motivation. However, the majority of trials lack a clear ABC structure.

3—Adult provides a number of teaching trials and they occur at least every 30 seconds. The majority of trials have a clear ABC structure, though there is room for improvement in control of the ABC structure. Or, repetitions are not well matched to learner needs.

4—Adult provides many teaching trials, more than one every 30 seconds. Most teaching trials have a clear ABC structure. Repetitions appear appropriate to needs. This is competent teaching.

5—Many teaching exchanges occur during the activity—on the average they occur every 10–20 seconds. The A, B, and C segments are quite clear, and it is obvious what child behavior the adult is trying to elicit and what behaviors are being reinforced. The number of repetitions is well matched to the child's learning needs. This is optimal teaching.

C: Instructional Techniques Application

Efficacious application of instructional techniques: Did the therapist use shaping, fading, prompting, and/or chaining techniques appropriately, and was error correction managed well to elicit and teach new behaviors?

Definitions

• *Prompting and fading:* Therapist consistently applies skillful prompting (typically least to most) and fading and reinforcement techniques to support successive approximations toward target skill. Child becomes more independent in the teaching episode, demonstrating teacher's skillful use of prompt fading and choice of target behavior. Prompts are faded quickly and provide "invisible" support for new learning.

• *Chaining:* Child flows through teaching sequences smoothly and in response to the desired Sd's. The steps of the task analysis are at appropriate steps, prompts and reinforcers are handled skillfully, and the timing allows the child to participate maximally in the process.

Chaining often occurs to teach clean-up and set-up activities, and in multistep play and language objectives.

- *Management of errors:* Child makes very few errors, because adult is handling the task well. Adult generally uses a least-to-most prompting hierarchy and quickly adapts the teaching to minimize errors, generally after two sequential failures. Adult chooses target behaviors of appropriate levels of difficulty so that child performs correct responses independently rapidly and consistently.

1—Consistently poor quality teaching. There are marked problems in the three areas listed above and they occur throughout the episode.
2—The teaching is problematic in that it is inconsistent in its quality, with two of the targeted areas showing marked weaknesses.
3—Some aspects of the teaching appear satisfactory but the teaching contains marked problems in one area or mild to moderate problems in two targeted areas. The child is learning but the problems detract somewhat from child learning and there is room to improve quality of teaching.
4—Good application of principles. There is room for refinement in one or two of the areas but it does not detract from child learning.
5—This segment contains optimal examples of the principles above. The adult skillfully uses fading, shaping, prompting, and chaining techniques to increase the child's independent performance of the learning objectives during the learning activity.

D. Adult Ability to Modulate Child Affect and Arousal

Use this item to address adult management of child emotional state, or activity level: such characteristics as a tired, lethargic, or underaroused child, a passive, perhaps avoidant child, a child who is whining, escaping, frustrated, distressed, upset with someone's coming and going, upset because a favorite toy was put way, *or* an overactive, high-energy child who is not settling into an activity. This is not about overt behavior problems—those get coded in a different item. This is about optimizing a child's mood, state, or activity level for participation in learning. Did the therapist skillfully modulate problems with child affect and arousal through choice of activities, tone of voice, level of adult activity, and other interventions? If there are no problems with child affect or arousal, score 5: rationale—the adult skills are maintaining optimal learning state.

1—The child demonstrates affect/arousal problems that prevent participation. Child state or activity level prevents participation with the learning activity, and the adult does not attempt to alter the child's state, or makes such poor choices that the adult actually aggravates the child's problem.
2—The child demonstrates affect/arousal problems that impair participation. The adult attempts to alter the child's state but is not successful due to lack of skill or missed opportunities. Child state continues to limit learning opportunities in this episode.
3—The child displays problems with affect or arousal. The adult uses strategies that improve child's state or activity level so that some teaching exchanges occur. However, child continues to show less than optimal learning state throughout the episode due to some lack

of skill or missed opportunities on the therapist's part and this limits teaching opportunities.

4—Child displays problems with affect or arousal during activity. Adult management did not contribute to the affect/arousal problems, and the adult modulates problems with child affect and arousal in the episode in ways that reestablish child engagement for learning. Or, the adult appears sensitive to the child's needs and tries every conceivable way imaginable to help the child modulate states.

5—Child does not display any problems with arousal or affect during this episode. Or, the child shows some affect/arousal problems and the therapist shows great skill in finding ways to optimize the child's state quickly resulting in a very successful learning activity with many learning opportunities and a happy, engaged child.

E. Management of Unwanted Behaviors

When a problem behavior occurs, does the therapist seek or demonstrate a clear understanding of the function of behavior and use appropriate techniques to elicit more appropriate behavior? Unwanted behaviors involve aggressive acts to others, self-injury, crying, marked fussing or screaming, significant stereotypies, throwing or destroying materials, and active, oppositional refusal to follow instructions. Lack of cooperation, poor attention, overactive avoidance, whining, and passivity would not be coded.

1—The therapist compounds the problem through overt reinforcement of unwanted behavior, or by ignoring early evidence of difficulty and waiting until a bigger problem erupts. The therapist misses many clear opportunities to appropriately manage the behaviors to redirect and reengage the child.

2—The therapist does not compound the problem through reinforcing unwanted behaviors, and the therapist attempts to manage the behavior. However, the behavior does not improve because of poor management strategies.

3—The therapist does not compound the problem and applies strategies that help the child return to a learning state and participate in the activity. However, the therapist has missed more than one clear opportunity or lacks clear strategies for regaining child cooperation and/or appropriate behavior. Use this code also if the unwanted behavior goes on too long before being managed.

4—The therapist manages the behavior competently and the situation improves through the episode. Child learning occurs, and the therapist has not missed intervention opportunities or techniques. However, there is an obvious additional step the therapist could have taken to improve the situation faster or further. Use this code also if adult management did not contribute to the behavior problem, the adult understands the function of the behavior, or tries to, and the adult applies appropriate strategies for redirecting, eliciting a more appropriate behavior, and not reinforcing the unwanted behavior, even if the behavior problem continues through the episode.

5—No unwanted behaviors as defined above occurred during this episode, or, they occur but adult management did not contribute to the unwanted behaviors. The adult manages the behavior skillfully and uses positive techniques that successfully redirect child, elicit a more appropriate behavior, and reestablish child engagement and positive affect for learning as soon as possible. This represents optimal management of the situation.

F. Quality of Dyadic Engagement

This involves a type of social engagement in which adults and children are acting in a coordinated fashion. At its best, the child is aware of the adult's activities and the adult is an interactive partner, and the child demonstrates this through shared gaze, directed, intentional communicative exchanges, and smiles. Both partners lead, and both follow. In a more structured, material-based activity, dyadic exchanges may not occur throughout the activity, but rather in moments of socially engaged, enjoyable, reciprocal acts. These are expected to occur somewhere in every teaching episode.

1—There is no example of dyadic engagement. Adult never takes a turn, other than to model the first instruction. The adult directs the teaching episode but does not join in the activity. There is no socially engaged or reciprocal exchange. *Requiring the child to perform a skill is not a turn for this code.*

2—There is one example of turn taking or dyadic exchange, but there are several missed opportunities for more and the teaching episode would have been improved by adding them.

3—There is more than one example of turn taking and/or reciprocal, dyadic exchange, but the adult misses a clear opportunity for turn taking, resulting in the adult being too much of an onlooker or director. Or, child does not seem aware of adult turn; does not give materials to adult or watch adult's turn.

4—Turn taking or reciprocal engagement occur multiple times in the episode (can be repeated acts all at once). Child and adult are aware of each others' turns and intentionally share gaze, smiles, and some communication. Adult is competent at creating turn taking and dyadic engagement exchanges.

5—Turn taking and dyadic engagement occur throughout the episode. The child is actively involved in adult turns, including giving toys, co-constructing, helping, or cuing the adult's turn. Reciprocity and social engagement permeate the teaching activity and this is an optimal example of incorporating reciprocal dyadic engagement into teaching.

G. Adult Optimizes Child Motivation for Participating in the Activity

Note: This item is not about managing child states of arousal or emotion. That is covered in an earlier item. This item refers to the child's motivation to perform this specific teaching task multiple times, through the number of trials the adult requests. If problems of motivation in this episode lead to problems with state or unwanted behaviors, then all the appropriate items would be coded. Child choices are a very important aspect of this item. In a naturalistic teaching episode, this involves child choice of materials/activity. In an activity that does not involve objects (songs, play) the adult may "offer" the activity, but adult still follows the child's lead in determining whether to continue. In an adult-directed teaching episode, this can include child choice of reinforcers, or child choice of a preferred activity in which a didactic teaching episode will be embedded. Valuing child choice does not preclude modeling a new toy or activity, or taking a child through an activity for the first time to introduce it, even if the child is mildly protesting. However, it does preclude continuing an activity in the face of marked child protest or disinterest unless the activity is necessary for child safety, hygiene, and so on. An adult who is consistently suggesting a new activity to the child—"Let's play food, okay?" is not giving adequate opportunity for choices. This is not a problem when done once in a while, but if it occurs more often than that then the adult is being too directive and not creating and following child choices and leads.

Motivation for child participation can be optimized by the following:

- Interspersing maintenance and acquisition trials.
- Good reinforcer management, including reinforcing child attempts, reinforcement schedules, use of Premack principle, and use of intrinsic reinforcers where possible.
- Giving child choices and following child leads.
- Choosing activities well and creating interesting activities with materials.
- Ending or changing activity before child becomes bored or tired.

1—The child is not motivated by this activity and the adult does not use any of the above techniques to improve motivation. Adult chooses the activity and provides no child choice. Child does not show interest in the activity, does not attempt the task, or is fully prompted through it.

2—The child is not motivated by this activity. The adult chooses the activity and uses one or more of the above strategies to try to increase motivation but is not successful and the child does not perform the teaching task under his or her own effort, or the child performs once and does not continue. The adult provides one or two choices only to the child and misses multiple opportunities to give choices.

3—The child demonstrates some motivation for the activity and makes several responses to the teaching task. Adult uses at least three of the above techniques to involve or sustain child interest and participation. Adult provides two or more opportunities for child choice but misses clear opportunities for choices. However, there are problems with motivation that adult could have addressed by better application of the above techniques.

4—The child chooses the activity or becomes motivated to perform the task due to successful adult application of principles. The adult applies the above principles in a skillful way and this results in multiple teaching opportunities. Child has several opportunities to make choices within the episode.

5—The episode demonstrates a highly motivated child who chooses the activity and is very interested in the activity. The child engages repeatedly in the learning activities that are presented, responds consistently to adult instruction, and initiates repeated communicative behaviors requesting the learning activities. The adult demonstrates optimal use of the four variables above. The adult is adept at making small adjustments and creating many child choices to maintain high motivation throughout the activity.

H. Adult Use of Positive Affect

1—Adult does not display positive affect during the episode in face, voice, or style. The adult is inappropriately business-like or the adult may display a negative affective state.

2—The adult uses unnatural, unmodulated, or otherwise inappropriate displays of positive affect—too strong or too artificial, resulting in an unnatural and/or overly intense display poorly matched to child state.

3—The adult is rather neutral or flat, or is inconsistent affectively throughout the episode, and the activity is one in which one would typically see more positive affective display. Quality of the social interaction would be enhanced by a somewhat warmer affect.

4—The adult displays genuine natural levels of positive affect, including a general background of positive feeling, during the episode.

5—The adult displays rich, genuine, and natural positive affect throughout the episode *matched by child positive affect*. Positive affect permeates the episode, is well matched to the child's needs and capacities, does not overarouse the child, and serves teaching well.

I. Adult Sensitivity and Responsivity to Child Communicative Cues

This refers to adult's attunement to child states, motives, and feelings. A sensitive and responsive adult acknowledges communicative cues, whether verbal or gestural, by verbalizing or by acting contingently according to the child's communication so that the child seems to have been "heard." Or, in the face of an affective cue, the adult responds empathically to the child's emotional state by mirroring the emotion and communicating an understanding of it. The adult does not reinforce unwanted behavior, but acknowledges the child's cues and responds appropriately given the situation. The adult uses a range of techniques including modeling, restatement, expansion of child utterances, and repetition of child utterances embedded in meaningful activities.

1—Adult appears insensitive and unresponsive to virtually all child cues in this episode. The adult carries out his or her own agenda and ignores child cues. Or, the adult uses a directive teaching style and does not provide any opportunity for child communications, so that there are no child cues or communications in this episode.

2—The adult responds to two of the child's cues but not to the majority of them, either because the adult is not attending, not interpreting, or is directing and thus overriding child communications.

3—The adult shows some sensitivity and responsivity to the majority of the child's communicative cues, but the adult does not respond sensitively and responsively to a minority of child-directed communications when optimal teaching would dictate some type of response.

4—The adult shows sensitive and contingent responding to the majority of child communications. There are one or two misses, but they are mostly due to other factors: lack of clarity of the child cue, the teaching plan, or attention to another aspect of the environment, rather than being due to lack of sensitivity or responsivity.

5—The adult demonstrates optimal sensitivity and responsivity to child cues. The adult is maximally attuned to the child's communications, both directed and undirected. The adult reads the child very well or makes every effort to interpret the child's meaning. The adult uses the full range of responses: restatement, modeling, expansion, and affirmation through repetition.

J. Multiple and Varied Communicative Opportunities Occur in the Activity

This item addresses the number of pragmatic functions expressed in child communications and elicited by the adult. Examples include requesting, commenting, naming, protesting/affirming, seeking help, being "all done," greeting, or imitating the adult's sounds or gestures with eye contact. Children's imitation of an adult action on an object, without accompanying gaze, vocalization, gesture, and so on is not considered a communication for this item.

1—Opportunity for child communication is virtually absent. Object-oriented activities do not contain a communicative component; sensory social routines involve the adult acting on the child rather than creating opportunities for child communication.

2—Opportunities to practice communication occur only for one function—like requesting or naming. Use this code also for adult-directed drill and practice format.

3—There are several communicative opportunities that occur in naturalistic communicative situations and more than one type of communication is practiced or used. However, there is overreliance on one pragmatic function (like requesting or protesting). Or, there is too much repetition of a single word where the situation clearly calls for some vocabulary expansion at least through modeling. Clear opportunities to practice existing communication objectives that apply in this activity are missed.

4—There are multiple, varied communicative opportunities in the activity. Several communication objectives are addressed, and/or several different pragmatic functions, vocabulary use, or syntactic combinations are practiced. The adult is competent in teaching varied language and using techniques to model and expand child utterances even though one or two opportunities were missed.

5—This is an optimal example of the adult scaffolding multiple communications involving several different communicative functions throughout the episode as specified in the child's objectives, including opportunities to request, protest, comment, ask for help, greet, name, expand, and so on. The range of pragmatic and communicative opportunities fit well with the child's language level. For an object-oriented activity, there are multiple child communications per minute. For a sensory social routine, child communication (including gaze and smiles) occurs approximately every 10 seconds. The adult uses a range of techniques including modeling, restatement, expansion of child utterances, and repetition of child utterances embedded in meaningful activities. No clear opportunities for child communication were missed, and the child's communication objectives are woven throughout the activity.

K. Appropriateness of Adult Language for Child's Language Level

Is the therapist's language appropriate for expanding the child's language level in terms of vocabulary, syntax, and pragmatics? This includes comments to the child, language models, and appropriate narration of the actions or themes involved in the activity.

1—Adult language is not appropriate for the child in any of the dimensions. Adult vocabulary and/or syntax is consistently too complex or too simplified. Or, pragmatics are inappropriate, with language used to instruct, direct, and name. The one-up rule is not followed.

2—Adult language is syntactically appropriate for child (one-up rule), but adult uses language only to give instructions, name objects, and praise ("good talking"), rather than to communicate in pragmatically appropriate ways.

3—Majority of adult communications are appropriate syntactically (one-up rule), semantically, and pragmatically (i.e., they fit the child's objectives), but there are several instances of obvious errors in two or more of these in an utterance or opportunities to narrate child's behavior and actions are missed.

4—Adult language is generally appropriate syntactically, semantically, and pragmatically.

Though there may be a miss here or there, the adult is generally using language that represents the child's current understanding level, with more mature language provided as models, narrates appropriately, and shows consistent use of the one-up rule.

5—Adult language is consistently appropriate developmentally and pragmatically for the child's verbal and nonverbal communicative intent and capacity. Adult generally follows the one-up rule, responds to child's communications with appropriate language, narrates child and adult acts or themes appropriately, and uses language to demonstrate a variety of pragmatic functions, semantic relations, and syntactic combinations.

L. Joint Activity Structure and Elaboration

Does the therapist develop a four-part joint activity: (1) a set-up in which child chooses activity and helps adult set up the theme; (2) a middle in which both participate equally, building, and co-constructing the theme; (3) elaboration to encourage flexible, varied use of actions and materials by using multiple materials and varied schemas, or through theme and variation; and (4) an ending in which the timing to close down the activity was fitting and the child is well supported through the transition to the next activity? Does the adult target multiple objectives from different developmental domains?

Note: If the child needs adult-directed, mass trial teaching to learn, activities can still be elaborated by having the child help take out, put away, and choose materials, or by interweaving of social exchanges. Thus, this item applies to all kinds of teaching approaches.

1—Adult focuses on teaching only one objective but is not successful. Activity does not contain a clear structure involving set-up, theme, and closure. Activity lacks elaboration component and so either ends too soon, missing teaching opportunities, or is too repetitive.

2—Adult teaches one objective successfully. Activity does not contain a clear structure involving set-up, theme, and closure. Adult tries but is unsuccessful at eliciting any other learning behaviors on multiple objectives or elaborating responses. Lack of success is due to lack of therapist skill.

3—Adult provides clear structure involving at least three parts: set-up, theme, and closure. There is some attempt at elaboration and therapist teaches more than one objective, but misses multiple opportunities to elaborate and sustain the activity or address more objectives. The activity appears overly repetitive or underdeveloped for this child.

4—Adult provides clear structure involving all four parts: set-up, theme, variation, and closure. Adult demonstrates competence in elaborating the activity sufficiently to sustain interest in the activity through all four parts. Adult creates a variety of opportunities and successfully teaches objectives from multiple domains.

5—Adult provides an optimal four-part joint activity including a well-developed closure. Adult demonstrates optimal and imaginative elaboration of this activity, targeting many objectives. Therapist supports the child's learning by combining skills from objectives in different domains in flexible teaching. (*Note:* If the child needs many repetitions to master this skill and the child is highly motivated, then do not score down due to lack of theme and variation. However, there should always be more than one child objective targeted in an activity.)

M. Transitions between Activities

Does the adult skillfully transition between activities or locations to maximize child attention, motivation, and independent physical transition to new activity? (*Note:* If no transitions are present on the video at either the beginning or the ending of the activity, then score this as N/O [no opportunity] and do not use the item to calculate level of fidelity.)

1—There is no real transition. The activity ends/begins abruptly with negative effect on child attention, motivation, or interest. The transition is abrupt because the child leaves the activity or child is physically led through the transitions. There is no effort to help the child shift attention, or to draw the child's interest and awareness to the new activity. Child may be physically moved from one location to another and wait with nothing to do while the adult gets an activity.

2—There is a transition but the adult leads the child through the transition, either by physically moving the child from one activity or location to another without encouraging independence in the transition, or by choosing the activity without any child choice and directing the child into the start of the activity without seeking child initiation.

3—Transition is accomplished by shifting child interest to a new activity without physically leading child. However, the activity choice is not optimal, either because there is not enough variation from the last activity or because the child's obvious needs or choices (quiet to active, active to calm, change of location, change of pace) are not acted upon in choosing the next activity.

4—The transition is smooth and the child moves independently in the transition. The adult engages the child in the new activity, via some type of child choice or child initiation. The new activity represents variation in terms of location, activity level, or teaching domain.

5—Transition is optimally managed. Adult scaffolds child's shift of interest by closing down one activity at the appropriate time and bringing up another, so that the child's learning in both activities is maximized and interest flows from one activity to the next with minimal down time. Child chooses and initiates the next activity.

Early Start Denver Model Fidelity Coding Sheet

Therapist ______________________________ Rater and date ____________________

Child and episode ____

Scoring rules: View one entire activity before scoring. Read the full definition of each rating before assigning score. Give a single numerical score. Note reasons for score in boxes.

Item	Activity 1	Activity 2	Activity 3	Activity 4	Activity 5	Activity 6
A. Management of child attention						
B. ABC format						
C. Instructional techniques						
D. Modulating child affect/ arousal						
E. Management of unwanted behaviors						
F. Quality of dyadic engagement						
G. Adult optimizes child motivation						

(cont.)

Early Start Denver Model Fidelity Coding Sheet *(cont.)*

Item	Activity 1	Activity 2	Activity 3	Activity 4	Activity 5	Activity 6
H. Adult use of positive affect						
I. Adult sensitivity and responsivity						
J. Multiple varied communicative opportunities						
K. Adult's language for child's level						
L. Joint activity and elaboration						
M. Transition between activities						
Comment columns for note taking						

References

Ainsworth, M. D. S., Blehar, M. C., Waters, E., & Wall, S. (1978). *Patterns of attachment.* Hillsdale, NJ: Erlbaum.

Anderson, J. R. (2000). *Learning and memory: An integrated approach* (2nd ed.). New York: Wiley.

Ansbacher, H., & Ansbacher, R. R. (1956). The style of life. In *The Individual Psychology of Alfred Adler.* New York: Basic Books.

Anzalone, M., & Williamson, G. G. (2000). Sensory processing and motor performance in autism spectrum disorders. In A. M. Wetherby & B. M. Prizant (Eds.), *Autism spectrum disorders: A transactional developmental perspective* (pp. 143–166). Baltimore: Brookes.

Baer, D. M., & Sherman, J. A. (1964). Reinforcement control of generalized imitation in young children. *Journal of Experimental Child Psychology, 1,* 37–49.

Baillargeon, R. (2004). Infants' reasoning about hidden objects: Evidence for event-general and event-specific expectation. *Developmental Science, 7,* 301–424.

Bandura, A., Ross, D., & Ross, S. A. (1963). Vicarious reinforcement and imitative learning. *Journal of Abnormal and Social Psychology, 67,* 601–607.

Baranek, G. T., David, F. J., Poe, M. D., Stone, W. L., & Watson, L. R. (2006). Sensory experiences questionnaire: Discriminating sensory features in young children with autism, developmental delays, and typical development. *Journal of Child Psychology and Psychiatry, 47*(6), 591–601.

Barnes, E. (1997). *Paving the way to kindergarten: Timelines and guidelines for preschool staff working with young children with special needs and their families.* Syracuse, NY: Center on Human Policy, Syracuse University.

Baron-Cohen, S., & Bolton, P. (1994) *Autism: The facts.* Oxford, UK: Oxford Medical Publications.

Bates, E. (1976). *Language and context: The acquisition of pragmatics.* New York: Academic Press.

Bates, E., Bretherton, I., & Snyder, L. (2001). *From first words to grammar: Individual differences and dissociable mechanisms.* Cambridge, UK: Cambridge University Press.

Bates, E., & Dick, F. (2002). Language, gesture, and the developing brain. *Developmental Psychobiology, 40,* 293–310.

Bates, E., Marchman, V., Tal, D., Fenson, L., Dale, P., Reznick, J., et al. (1994). Developmental and stylistic variation in the composition of early language. *Journal of Child Language, 21,* 85–123.

Bauman, M. L., & Kemper, T. L. (1994). Neuroanatomical observation of the brain in autism.

In M. L. Bauman & T. L. Kemper (Eds.), *The neurobiology of autism* (pp. 119–145). Baltimore: Johns Hopkins University Press.

Bauminger, N., Solomon, M., Aviezer, A., Heung, K., Brown, J., & Rogers, S. J. (2008). Friendship in high-functioning children with autism spectrum disorder: Mixed and non-mixed dyads. *Journal of Autism and Developmental Disorders, 38*(7), 1211–1229.

Beecher, H. K. (1955). The powerful placebo. *Journal of the American Medical Association, 159,* 1602–1606.

Blake, J., McConnell, S., Horton, G., & Benson, N. (1992). The gestural repetoire and its evaluation over the 2nd year. *Early Development and Parenting, 1,* 127–136.

Bondy, A. S., & Frost, L. A. (1994). The picture exchange communication system. *Focus on Autistic Behavior, 9,* 1–19.

Bricker, D. D., Pretti-Frontzczak, K., & McComas, N. (1998). *An activity-based approach to early intervention* (2nd ed.). Baltimore: Brookes.

Brown, J. R., & Rogers, S. J. (2003). Cultural issues in autism. In S. Ozonoff, S. J. Rogers, & R. L. Hendren (Eds.), *Autism spectrum disorders: A research review for practitioners* (pp. 209–226). Washington, DC: American Psychiatric Association.

Bruner, J. (1972). Nature and uses of immaturity. *American Psychologist, 27,* 687–708.

Bruner, J. (1975). The ontogenesis of speech acts. *Journal of Child Language, 2,* 1–19.

Bruner, J. (1981a). The pragmatics of acquisition. In W. Deutsch (Ed.), *The child's construction of language* (pp. 35–56). New York: Academic Press.

Bruner, J. (1981b). The social context of language acquisition. *Language and Communication, 1,* 155–178.

Bruner, J. (1995). From joint attention to the meeting of minds: An introduction. In C. Moore & P. J. Dunham (Eds.), *Joint attention: Its origins and role in development* (pp. 1–14). Hillsdale, NJ: Erlbaum.

Bruner, J. S. (1977). Early social interaction and language acquisition. In H. R. Schaffer (Ed.), *Studies in mother–infant interaction* (pp. 271–289). New York: Academic Press.

Capps, L., Sigman, M., & Mundy, P. (1994). Attachment security in children with autism. *Development and Psychopathology, 6,* 249–261.

Carpenter, M., & Tomasello, M. (2000). Joint attention, cultural learning, and language acquisition: Implications for children with autism. In A. M. Wetherby & B. M. Prizant (Eds.), *Autism spectrum disorders: A transactional developmental perspective* (pp. 31–54). Baltimore: Brookes.

Carr, E. G., Dunlap, G., Horner, R. H., Koegel, R. L., Turnbull, A. P., Sailor, W., et al. (2002). Positive behavior support: Evolution of an applied science. *Journal of Positive Behavior Interventions, 4,* 4–16.

Caselli, C., Casadio, P., & Bates, E. (1999). A comparison of the transition from first words to grammar in English and Italian. *Journal of Child Language, 26,* 69–111.

Cassuam, V. M., Kuefner, D., Weterlund, A., Nelson, C. A. (2006). A behavioral and ERP investigation of 3-month-olds' face preferences. *Neuropsychologia, 44,* 2113–2125.

Chakrabarti, S. & Fombonne, E. (2005). Pervasive developmental disorders in preschool children: Confirmation of high prevalence. *American Journal of Psychiatry, 162,* 1133–1141.

Charman, T. (1998). Specifying the nature and course of the joint attention impairment in autism in the preschool years: Implications for diagnosis and intervention. *Autism: An International Journal of Research and Practice,* 2(1), 61–79.

Charman, T., Howlin, P., Aldred, C., Baird, G., Degli Espinosa, F., Diggle, T., et al. (2003). *Research into early intervention for children with autism and related disorders: Methodological and design issues.* Report on a workshop funded by the Wellcome Trust, Institute of Child Health. November 2001. *Autism,* 7(II), 217–225.

Charman, T., Swettenham, J., Baron-Cohen, S., Cox, A., Baird, G., & Drew, A. (1998). An experimental investigation of social–cognitive abilities in infants with autism: Clinical implications. *Infant Mental Health Journal, 19*(2), 260–275.

Chartrand, T. L. & Bargh, J. A. (1999). The chameleon effect: The perception–behavior link and social interaction. *Journal of Personality and Social Psychology, 76,* 893–910.

Cipani, E. & Spooner, F. (1994). *Curricular and instructional approaches for persons with severe disabilities.* Boston: Allyn & Bacon.

Cohen, M. J., & Sloan, D. L. (2007). *Visual supports for people with autism: A guide for parents and professionals* (2nd ed.). Bethesda, MD: Woodbine House.

Cook, R. E., Tessier, M., & Klein, D. (1999). *Adapting early childhood curricula for children in inclusive settings* (5th ed.). Englewood Cliffs, NJ: Prentice-Hall.

Cooper, J. O., Heron, T. E., & Heward, W. L. (2006). *Applied behavior analysis* (2nd ed.). Upper Saddle River, NJ: Prentice-Hall.

Coulter, L., & Gallagher, C. (2001). Evaluation of the early childhood educators programme. *International Journal of Language and Communication Disorders, 36,* 264–269.

Courchesne, E., Pierce, K., Schumann, C. M., Redcay, E., Buckwalter, J. A., Kennedy, D., et al. (2007). Mapping early brain development in autism. *Neuron, 56,* 399–413.

Courchesne, E., Redcay, E., & Kennedy, D. P. (2004). The autistic brain: Birth through adulthood. *Current Opinion in Neurology, 17*(4), 489–496.

Courchesne, E., Townsend, J. P., Akshoomoff, N. A., Yeung-Courchesne, R., Press, G. A., Murakami, J. W., et al. (1993). A new finding: Impairment in shifting attention in autistic and cerebellar patients. In S. H. Broman & J. Grafman (Eds.), *Atypical deficits in developmental disorders: Implications for brain function.* Hillsdale, NJ: Erlbaum.

Crais, E., Douglas, D. D., & Campbell, C. C. (2004). The intersection of the development of gestures and intentionality. *Journal of Speech, Language, and Hearing Research, 47*(3), 678–694.

Csibra, G., & Gergely, G. (2005). Social learning and social cognition: The case for pedagogy. In M. H. Johnson & Y. Munakata (Eds.), *Processes of change in brain and cognitive development. Attention and performance.* Oxford, UK: Oxford University Press.

Dale, E., Johoda, A., & Knott, F. (2006). Mothers' attributions following their child's diagnosis of autistic spectrum disorder: Exploring links with maternal levels of stress, depression and expectations about their child's future. *Autism, 10*(5), 463–479.

Dawson, G. (2008). Early behavior intervention, brain plasticity, and the prevention of autism spectrum disorder. *Developmental Psychopathology, 20*(III), 775–803.

Dawson, G., & Adams, A. (1984). Imitation and social responsiveness in autistic children. *Journal of Abnormal Child Psychology, 12,* 209–226.

Dawson, G., Carver, L., Meltzoff, A. N., Panagiotides, H., & McPartland, J. (2002a). Neural correlates of face recognition in young children with autism spectrum disorder, developmental delay, and typical development. *Child Development, 73,* 700–717.

Dawson, G., & Galpert, L. (1990). Mothers' use of imitative play for facilitating social responsiveness and toy play in young autistic children. *Development and Psychopathology, 2,* 151–162.

Dawson, G., Rogers, S. J., Munson, J., Smith, M., Winters, J., et al. (2010). Randomized controlled trial of an intervention for toddlers with autism: The Early Start Denver Model. *Pediatrics, 125,* 17–23.

Dawson, G., Toth, K., Abbott, R., Osterling, J., Munson, J., Estes, A., et al. (2004). Defining the early social attention impairments in autism: Social orienting, joint attention, and responses to emotions. *Developmental Psychology, 40*(2), 271–283.

Dawson, G., Webb, S. J., & McPartland, J. (2005a). Understanding the nature of face processing impairment in autism: Insights from behavioral and electrophysiological studies. *Developmental Neuropsychology, 27,* 403–424.

Dawson, G., Webb, S., Schellenberg, G. D., Dager, S., Friedman, S., Aylward, E., et al. (2002). Defining the broader phenotype of autism: Genetic, brain, and behavioral perspectives. *Development and Psychopathology, 14,* 581–611.

Dawson, G., Webb, S. J., Wijsman, E., Schellenberg, G., Estes, A., Munson, J., et al. (2005b). Neurocognitive and electrophysiological evidence of altered face processing in parents of children with autism: Implications for a model of abnormal development of social brain circuitry in autism. *Development and Psychopathology, 17,* 679–697.

Dawson, G., & Zanolli, K. (2003). Early intervention and brain plasticity in autism. *Novartis Foundation Symposium, 251,* 266–274.

Dettmer, S., Simpson, R. L., Myles, B. S., & Ganz, J. B. (2000). The use of visual supports to facilitate transitions of students with autism. *Focus on Autism and Other Developmental Disabilities, 15,* 163–169.

Drew, A., Baird, G., Baron-Cohen, S., Cox, A., Slonims, V., Wheelwright, S., et al. (2002). A pilot randomized control trial of a parent training intervention for pre-school children with autism: Preliminary findings and methodological challenges. *European Child and Adolescent Psychiatry, 11,* 266–272.

Duda, M. A., Dunlap, G., Fox, L., Lentini, R., & Clark, S. (2004). An experimental evaluation of positive behavior support in a community preschool program. *Topics in Early Childhood Special Education, 24,* 143–155.

Elder, L. M., Dawson, G., Toth, K., Fein, D., & Munson, J. (2007). Head circumference as an early predictor of autism symptoms in younger siblings of children with autism spectrum disorder. *Journal of Autism and Developmental Disorders, 38*(6), 1104–1111.

Eldevik, S., & Gardner, J. (2006). *Assessment and Learning.* London: Sage.

Farrar, M. J. (1992). Negative evidence and grammatical morpheme acquisition. *Developmental Psychology, 28,* 90–98.

Ferguson, D. L., & Baumgart, D. L. (1991). Partial participation revisited. *Journal of the Association for the Severely Handicapped, 16,* 218–227.

Fergus, C. A., Menn, L., Stoel-Gamman, C. (1992). *Phonological development: Models, research, implications.* Baltimore, MD: York Press.

Fewell, R. R., & Sandall, S. R. (1986). Developmental testing of handicapped infants. *Topics in Early Childhood Special Education, 6*(3), 86–100.

Frith, U., & Baron-Cohen, S. (1987). Perception in autistic children. In D. J. Cohen & A. M. Donnellan (Eds.), *Handbook of autism and pervasive developmental disorders.* New York: Wiley.

Fuentes, J., & Martin-Arribas, M. C. (2007). Bioethical issues in neuropsychiatric genetic disorders. *Child and Adolescent Psychiatric Clinics of North America, 16*(3), 649–661.

Garber, K. (2007). Neuroscience: Autism's cause may reside in abnormalities at the synapse. *Science, 17,* 190–191.

Gardner, J. (2006). *Assessment and Learning.* London: Sage.

Geschwind, D. H. (2008). Autism: Many genres, common pathways? *Cell, 135,* 391–395.

Geschwind, D. H., & Levitt, P. (2007). Autism spectrum disorders: Development disconnection syndromes. *Current Opinion in Neurobiology, 17*(I), 103–111.

Gilkerson, L., & Stott, F. (2005). Parent–child relationships in early intervention with infants and toddlers with disabilities and their families. In C. H. Zeanah, Jr. (Ed.), *Handbook of infant mental health* (2nd ed.). New York: Guilford Press.

Goldstein, H., Wickstrom, S., Hoyson, M., Jamieson, B., & Odom, S. L. (1988). Effects of sociodramatic play training on social and communicative interaction. *Education and Treatment of Children, 11,* 97–117.

Goodman, R. (1989). Infantile autism: A syndrome of multiple primary deficits. *Journal of Autism and Developmental Disorders, 19,* 409–424.

Gray, C., & Garand, J. (1993). Social stories: Improving responses of students with autism with accurate social information. *Focus on Autistic Behavior, 8,* 1–10.

Gray, D. E. (1998). *Autism and the family: Problems, prospects, and coping with the disorder.* Springfield, IL: Charles C. Thomas.

Greenspan, S. I., Kalmanson, B., Shahmoon-Shanok, R., Wieder, S., Gordon-Williamson, G., & Anzalone, M. (1997). *Assessing and treating infants and young children with severe difficulties in relating and communicating.* Washington, DC: Zero to Three.

Griffith, E. M., Pennington, B. F., Wehner, E. A., & Rogers, S. J. (1999). Executive functions in young children with autism. *Child Development, 70,* 817–832.

Gutstein, S. E. (2005, winter). Relationship development intervention: Developing a treatment program to address the unique social and emotional deficits in autism spectrum disorders. *Autism Spectrum Quarterly.*

Gutstein, S. E., & Sheely, R. K. (2002). *Relationship development intervention with young children: Social and emotional development activities for Asperger syndrome, autism, PDD and NLD.* London: Jessica Kingsley.

Hansen, R., & Hagerman R. (2003). Contributions of pediatrics. In S. Ozonoff, S. J. Rogers, & R. L. Hendren (Eds.), *Autism spectrum disorders: A research review for practitioners.* Washington, DC: American Psychiatric.

Happe, F., Ronald, A., & Plomin, R. (2006). Time to give up on a single explanation for autism. *Nature Neuroscience, 9*(10), 1218–1220.

Harris, S. L., Wolchik, S. A., & Weitz, S. (1981). The acquisition of language skills by autistic children: Can parents do the job? *Journal of Autism and Developmental Disorders, 11,* 373–384.

Hart, B., & Risley, T. R. (1975). Incidental teaching of language in the preschool. *Journal of Applied Behavior Analysis, 8,* 411–420.

Hart, B., & Risley, T. R. (1995). *Meaningful differences in the everyday experience of young American children.* Baltimore: Brookes.

Hayden, D. (2004). A tactually-grounded treatment approach to speech production disorders. In I. Stockman (Ed.), *Movement and action in learning and development: Clinical implications for pervasive developmental disorders.* San Diego: Elsevier-Academic Press.

Higgins, D. J., Bailey, S. R., & Pearce, J. C. (2005). Factors associated with functioning style and coping strategies of families with a child with an autism spectrum disorder. *Autism, 9*(2), 125–137.

Hodapp, R. M., & Urbano, R. C. (2007). Adult siblings of individuals with down syndrome versus with autism: Findings from a large-scale U.S. survey. *Journal of Intellectual Disability Research, 51*(12), 1018–1029.

Hodgdon, L. A. (1995). *Visual strategies for improving communication.* Troy, MI: Quirk Roberts.

Hughes, C., Russell, J., & Robbins, T. W. (1994). Evidence for executive dysfunction in autism. *Neuropsychologia, 32,* 477–492.

Huttenlocher, J., Vasilyeva, M., Cymerman, E., & Levine, S. (2002). Language input and language syntax. *Cognitive Psychology, 45,* 337–374.

Iacoboni, M. (2005). Neural mechanisms of imitation. *Current Opinion in Neurobiology, 15,* 632–637.

Iacoboni, M. (2006). Understanding others: Imitation, language, empathy. In S. Hurley & N. Chater (Eds.), *Perspectives on imitation: From mirror neurons to memes: Vol. 1. Mechanisms of imitation and imitation in animals.* Cambridge, MA: MIT Press.

Iacoboni, M., & Mazziotta, J. C. (2007). Mirror neuron system: Basic findings and clinical implications. *Annals of Neurology, 62,* 213–218.

Individuals with Disabilities Act (IDEA). (1991). Pub. L. No. 101-476 §1400 et seq., 104 stat. 1142.

Ingersoll, B., & Gergans, S. (2007). The effect of a parent-implemented imitation intervention on spontaneous imitation skills in young children with autism. *Research in Developmental Disabilities, 28*(II), 163–175.

Ingersoll, B., & Schreibman, L. (2006). Teaching reciprocal imitation skills to young children with autism using a naturalistic behavioral approach: Effects on language, pretend play, and joint attention. *Journal of Autism and Developmental Disorders, 36*(4), 487–505.

Insel, T. R., O'Brien, D. J., & Leckman, J. F. (1999). Oxytocin, vasopressin, and autism: Is there a connection? *Biological Psychiatry, 45,* 145–157.

Johnson, M., Griffin, R., Cisbra, G., Halit, H., Faroni, T., deHann, J., et al. (2005). The emergence of the social brain network: Evidence from typical and atypical development. *Development and Psychopathology, 17,* 599–619.

Kaiser, A. P., Yoder, P. J., & Keetz, A. (1992). Evaluation milieu teaching. In S. F. Warren & J. Reichle (Eds.), *Communication and language intervention series: Vol. I. Causes and effects in communication and language intervention* (pp. 9–48). Baltimore: Brookes.

Kasari, C. (2002). Assessing change in early interventions programs for children with autism. *Journal of Autism and Developmental Disorders, 32*(5), 447–461.

Kasari, C., Sigman, M., Mundy, P., & Yirmiya, N. (1990). Affective sharing in the context of joint attention interactions of normal, autistic, and mentally retarded children. *Journal of Autism and Developmental Disorders, 20,* 87–100.

Kasari, C., Sigman, M., & Yirmiya, N. (1993). Focused and social attention of autistic children in interactions with familiar and unfamiliar adults: A comparison of autistic, mentally retarded, and normal children. *Development and Psychopathology, 5,* 403–414.

Kasari, C., Sigman, M., Yirmiya, N., & Mundy, P. (1994). Affective development and communication in young children with autism. In A. Kaiser & D. B. Gray (Eds.), *Enhancing children's communication: Research foundations for intervention.* Baltimore: Brookes.

Kennedy, D. P., & Courchesne, E. (2008). The intrinsic functional organization of the brain is altered in autism. *Neuroimage, 39*(IV), 1877–1885.

Kern, L., Marder, T. J., Boyajian, A. E., & Elliot, C. M. (1997). Augmenting the independence of self-management procedures by teaching self-initiation across settings and activities. *School Psychology Quarterly, 12,* 23–32.

Kjelgaard, M., & Tager-Flusberg, H. (2001). An investigation of language impairment in autism: Implications for genetic subgroups. *Language and Cognitive Processes, 16,* 287–308.

Koegel, L. K. (2000). Interventions to facilitate communication in autism. *Journal of Autism and Developmental Disorders, 30*(5), 383–391.

Koegel, L. K., Koegel, R. L., Harrower, J. K., & Carter, C. M. (1999a). Pivotal response intervention 1: Overview of approach. *Journal of the Association for Persons with Severe Handicaps, 24,* 174–185.

Koegel, L. K., Koegel, R. L., Hurley, C., & Frea, W. D. (1992). Improving social skills and disruptive behavior in children with autism through self-management. *Journal of Applied Behavior Analysis, 25,* 341–353.

Koegel, L. K., Koegel, R. L., Shoshan, Y., & McNerney, E. (1999b). Pivotal response intervention II: Preliminary long-term outcome data. *Journal of the Association for Persons with Severe Handicaps, 24,* 186–198.

Koegel, R., & Koegel, L. K. (1988). Generalized responsivity and pivotal behavior. In R. H. Horner, G. Dunlap, & R. L. Koegel (Eds.), *Generalization and maintenance: Lifestyle changes in applied settings* (pp. 41–66). Baltimore: Brookes.

Koegel, R. L., Bimbela, A., & Schreibman, L. (1996). Collateral effects of parent training on family interactions. *Journal of Autism and Developmental Disorders, 26,* 347–359.

Koegel, R. L., & Frea, W. D. (1993). Treatment of social behavior in autism through the modification of pivotal social skills. *Journal of Applied Behavior Analysis, 26,* 369–377.

Koegel, R. L., & Koegel, L. K. (1995). *Teaching children with autism: Strategies for initiating positive interactions and improving learning opportunities.* Baltimore: Brookes.

Koegel, R. L., Koegel, L. K., & Surratt, A. (1992). Language intervention and disruptive behavior in preschool children with autism. *Journal of Autism and Developmental Disorders, 22*(2), 141–153.

Koegel, R. L., O'Dell, M., & Dunlap, G. (1988). Producing speech use in nonverbal autistic children by reinforcing attempts. *Journal of Autism and Developmental Disorders, 18*(4), 525–538.

Koegel, R. L., O'Dell, M., & Koegel, L. K. (1987). A natural language teaching paradigm for nonverbal autistic children. *Journal of Autism and Developmental Disorder, 17,* 187–199.

Koegel, R. L., & Williams, J. A. (1980). Direct vs. indirect response—Reinforcer relationships in teaching autistic children. *Journal of Abnormal Child Psychology, 8*(IV), 537–547.

Kreppner, J. M., Rutter, M., Beckett, C., Castle, J., Colvert, E., Grothues, E., et al. (2007). Normality and impairment following profound early institutional deprivation: A longitudinal examination through childhood. *Developmental Psychology, 43*(4), 931–946.

Kuhl, P. K., Tsao, F. M., & Liu, H. M. (2003). Foreign-language experience in infancy: Effects of short-term exposure and social interaction on phonetic learning. *Proceedings of the National Academy of Sciences USA, 100*(15), 9096–9101.

Kylliainen, A., Braeutigam, S., Hietanen, J. K., Swithenby, S. J., & Bailey, A. J. (2006). Face and gaze processing in normally developing children: A magnetocephalographic study. *European Journal of Neuroscience, 23,* 801–810.

Legerstee, M., Markova, G., & Fisher, T. (2007). The role of maternal affect attunement in dyadic and triadic communication. *Infant Behavior and Development, 2,* 296–306.

Leonard, L. B., Newhoff, M., & Mesalam, L. (1980). Individual differences in early child phonology. *Applied Psycholinguistics, 1,* 7–30.

Lifter, K., Sulzer-Azaroff, B., Anderson, S. R., Coyle, J. T., & Cowdery, G. E. (1993). Teaching play activities to preschool children with disabilities: The importance of developmental considerations. *Journal of Early Intervention, 17*(2), 139–159.

Lord, C., Risi, S., & Pickles, A. (2005). Trajectory of language development in autistic spectrum disorders. In M. L. Rice & S. F. Warren (Eds.), *Developmental language disorders: From phenotypes to etiologies* (pp. 7–30). Mahweh, NJ: Erlbaum.

Lord, C., Wagner, A., Rogers, S., Szatmari, P., Aman, M., Charman, T., et al. (2005). Challenges in evaluating psychosocial interventions for autistic spectrum disorders. *Journal of Autism and Developmental Disorders, 35*(6), 695–708.

Losardo, A., & Bricker, D. (1994). Activity-based intervention and direct instruction: A comparison study. *American Journal of Mental Retardation, 98,* 744–765.

Lovaas, O. I. (1987). Behavioral treatment and normal educational and intellectual functioning in young autistic children. *Journal of Consulting and Clinical Psychology, 55*(1), 3–9.

Lovaas, O. I. (2002). *Teaching individuals with developmental delays: Basic intervention techniques.* Austin, TX: PRO-ED.

Lovaas, O. I., Berberich, J. P., Perloff, B. F., & Schaeffer, B. (1966). Acquisition of imitative speech by schizophrenic children. *Science, 151,* 705–707.

Lovaas, I. O., Freitag, G., Gold, V. J., & Kassorla, I. C. (1965). Experimental studies in child schizophrenia: Analysis of self-destructive behavior. *Journal of Experimental Child Psychology, 2,* 67–84.

Lynch, E. W., & Hanson, M. J. (1992). *Developing cross-cultural competence.* Baltimore: Brooks/Cole.

Macks, R. J., & Reeve, R. E. (2007). The adjustment of non-disabled siblings of children with autism. *Journal of Autism and Developmental Disorders, 37*(6), 1060–1067.

Maestro, S., Muratin, F., Cavallaro, M. C., Pei, F., Stern, D., Golse, B., & Palacio-Esposa, F. (2002). Attentional skills during the first 6 months of age in autism spectrum disorders. *Journal of the American Academy of Child and Adolescent Psychiatry, 4*, 1239–1245.

Mahoney, G., & Perales, F. (2003). Using relationship-focused intervention to enhance the social-emotional functioning of young children with autism spectrum disorder. *Topics in Early Childhood Special Education, 23*, 77–89.

Mahoney, G., & Perales, F. (2005). The impact of relationship focused intervention on young children with autism spectrum disorders: A comparative study. *Journal of Developmental and Behavioral Pediatrics, 26*, 77–85.

Mahoney, G., Wheeden, C. A., & Perales, F. (2004). Relationship of preschool special education outcomes to instructional practices and parent–child interaction. *Research in Developmental Disabilities, 25*, 539–558.

Marcus, L. M., Kunce, L. J., & Schopler, E. (2005). In F. R. Volkmar, R. Paul., A. Klin, & D. Cohen (Eds.), *Handbook of autism and developmental disorders* (3rd ed., Vol. 2, pp. 1055–1086). Hoboken, NJ: Wiley.

Mashal, M., Feldman, R. B., & Sigal, J. J. (1989). The unraveling of a treatment paradigm: A followup study of the Milan approach to family therapy. *Family Process, 28*(4), 187–193.

McCann, J., & Peppe, S. (2003). Prosody in autism spectrum disorders: A critical review. *International Journal of Language and Communication Disorders, 38*(4), 325–350.

McCleery, J. P., Tully, L., Slevc, L. R., & Schreibman, L. (2006). Consonant production patterns of young severely language-delayed children with autism. *Journal of Communication Disorders, 39*, 217–231.

McCollum, J. A., & Yates, T. J. (1994). Dyad as focus, triad as means: A family-centered approach to supporting parent–child interactions. *Infants and Young Children, 6*(4), 54–63.

McCune, L. (1995). A normative study of representational play at the transition to language. *Developmental Psychology, 31*, 198–206.

McCune-Nicholich, L. (1977). Beyond sensorimotor intelligence: Assessment of symbolic maturity through analysis of pretend play. *Merrill-Palmer Quarterly, 23*, 89–99.

McGee, G. G., Morrier, M. J., & Daly, T. (1999). An incidental teaching approach to early intervention for toddlers with autism. *Journal of the Association for Persons with Severe Handicaps, 24*, 133–146.

McIntosh, D. N. (1996). Facial feedback hypotheses: Evidence, implications, and directions. *Motivation and Emotion, 20*, 121–147.

Meltzoff, A., & Moore, M. K. (1977). Imitation of facial and manual gestures by human neonates. *Science, 198*, 75–78.

Montes, G., & Halterman, J. S. (2008). Child care problems and employment among families with preschool-aged children with autism in the United States. *Pediatrics, 122*(1), 202–208.

Mundy, P. (2003). Annotation. The neural basis of social impairments in autism: The role of the dorsal medial-frontal cortex and anterior cingulate system. *Journal of Child Psychology and Psychiatry, 44*(VI), 793–809.

Mundy, P. & Neal, R. (2001). Neural plasticity, joint attention and a transactional social-orienting model of autism. In L. Glidden (Ed.), *International review of research in mental retardation: Vol. 23. Autism* (pp. 139–168). New York: Academic Press.

Mundy, P., Sigman, M., & Kasari, C. (1990). A longitudinal study of joint attention and language development in autistic children. *Journal of Autism and Developmental Disorders, 20*, 115–128.

Mundy, P., Sigman, M., Ungerer, J., & Sherman, T. (1986). Defining the social deficits of autism: The contribution of non-verbal communication measures. *Journal of Child Psychology and Psychiatry and Allied Disciplines, 27*, 657–669.

Mundy, P., Sigman, M., Ungerer, J., & Sherman, T. (1987). Nonverbal communication and play correlates of language development in autistic children. *Journal of Autism and Developmental Disorders, 17,* 349–364.

Murias, M., Webb, S. J., Greenson, J., & Dawson, G. (2007). Resting state cortical connectivity reflected in EEG coherence in individuals with autism. *Biological Psychiatry, 62,* 270–273.

Nadel, J., Guerini, C., Peze, A., & Rivet, C. (1999). The evolving nature of imitation as a format for communication. In J. Nadel & G. Butterworth (Eds.), *Imitation in infancy* (pp. 209–234). Cambridge, UK: Cambridge University Press.

Nadel, J., & Pezé, A. (1993). What makes immediate imitation communicative in toddlers and autistic children? In J. Nadel & L. Camaioni (Eds.), *New perspectives in early development* (pp. 139–156). London: Routledge.

Nelson, K. (1973). Structure and strategy in learning to talk. *Monographs for the Society for Research in Child Development, 38*(1–2), 1–135.

Niedenthal, P. M., Barsalou, L. W., Winkielman, P., Krauth-Gruber, S., & Ric, F. (2005). Embodiment in attitudes, social perception, and emotion. *Personality and Social Psychology Review, 9,* 184–211.

O'Neill, R. E., Horner, R. H., Albin, R. W., Sprague, J. K., Storey, K., & Newton, J. S. (1997). *Functional assessment and program development for problem behavior: A practical handbook* (2nd ed.). Pacific Grove, CA: Brookes/Cole.

O'Neill, R. E., Horner, R. H., Albin, R. W., Storey, K., & Sprague, J. K. (1990). *Functional analysis of problem behavior: A practical assessment guide.* Sycamore, IL: Sycamore.

Orsmond, G. I., & Seltzer, M. M. (2007). Siblings of individuals with autism or down syndrome: Effects on adult lives. *Journal of Intellectual Disability Research, 51*(9), 682–696.

Orsmond, G. I., Seltzer, M. M., Greenberg, J. S., & Krauss, M. W. (2006). Mother–child relationship quality among adolescents and adults with autism. *American Journal on Mental Retardation, 3*(2), 121–137.

Osterling, J., & Dawson, G. (1994). Early recognition of autism: A study of first birthday home video tapes. *Journal of Autism and Developmental Disorders, 24,* 247–257.

Owens, R. E. (1996). *Language development: An introduction.* Needham Heights, MA: Allyn & Bacon.

Ozonoff, S., Pennington, B. F., & Rogers, S. J. (1991). Executive function deficits in high-functioning autistic individuals: Relationship to theory of mind. *Journal of Child Psychology and Psychiatry, 32,* 1081–1105.

Palomo, R., Belinchon, M., & Ozonoff, S. (2006). Autism and family home movies: A comprehensive review. *Developmental and Behavioral Pediatrics, 27,* S59–S68.

Pardo, C. A., Vargas, D. L., & Zimmerman, A. W. (2005). Immunity, neuroglia, and neuroinflammation in autism. *International Review of Psychiatry, 17,* 485–495.

Parten, M. B. (1933). Social play among preschool children. *Journal of Abnormal and Social Psychology, 28*(2), 136–147.

Pelphrey, K. A., & Carter, E. J. (2008). Charting the typical and atypical development of the social brain. *Development and Psychopathology, 2,* 1081–1082.

Pennington, B. F., & Ozonoff, S. (1996). Executive functions and developmental psychopathology. *Journal of Child Psychology and Psychiatry, 37,* 51–88.

Piaget, J. (1963). *The origins of intelligence in children.* New York: Norton.

Pierce, W. D., & Cheney, C. D. (2008). *Behavior analysis and learning* (4th ed.). New York: Psychological Press.

Pinkham, A. E., Hopfinger, J. B., Pelphrey, K. A., Piven, J., & Penn, D. L. (2008). Neural bases for impaired social cognition in schizophrenia and autism spectrum disorders. *Schizophrenia Research, 99,* 164–175.

Plaisted, K. C. (2001). Reduced generalization in autism: An alternative to weak central coherence. In J. A. Burack, T. Charman, N. Yirmiya, & P. R. Zelazo (Eds.), *The development of autism: Perspectives from theory and research* (pp. 149–169). Mahwah, NJ: Erlbaum.

Posey, D. J., Erickson, C. A., Stigler, K. A., & McDougle, C. J. (2006). The use of selective serotonin reuptake inhibitors in autism and related disorders. *Journal of Child and Adolescent Psychopharmacology, 16,* 181–186.

Powell, D., Dunlap, G., & Fox, L. (2006). Prevention and intervention for the challenging behaviors of toddlers and preschoolers. *Infants and Young Children, 19,* 25–35.

Premack, D. (1959). Toward empirical behavior laws: I. positive reinforcement. *Psychological Review, 66,* 219–233.

Prizant, B. M., & Duchan, J. F. (1981). The functions of immediate echolalia in autistic children. *Journal of Speech and Hearing Disorders, 46,* 241–249.

Prizant, B. M., & Wetherby, A. M. (1998). Understanding the continuum of discrete-trial traditional behavioral to social-pragmatic developmental approaches in communication enhancement for young children with autism/PDD. *Seminars in Speech and Language, 19*(4), 329–353.

Prizant, B. M., Wetherby, A. M., Rubin, E., Laurent, A. C., & Rydell, P. J. (2006). *The SCERTS Model: A comprehensive educational approach for children with autism spectrum disorders.* Baltimore: Brookes.

Redclay, E., & Courchesne, E. (2005). When is the brain enlarged in autism? A meta-analysis of all brain size reports. *Biological Psychiatry, 58,* 1–9.

Remy, F., Wenderoth, N., Lipkens, K., & Swinnen, S. P. (2008). Acquisition of a new bimanual coordination pattern modulates the cerebral activations elicited by an intrinisic pattern: An fMRI study. *Cortex, 44*(5), 482–493.

Rescorla, L. (1980). Overextension in early language development. *Journal of Child Language, 7,* 321–335.

Rivera-Gaziola, M., Silva-Pereyra, J., & Kuhl, P. K. (2005). Brain potentials to native and non-native contrasts in 7- and 11-month-old American infants. *Developmental Science, 8,* 162–172.

Rogers, S. J. (1977). Characteristics of the cognitive development of profoundly retarded children. *Child Development, 48,* 837–843.

Rogers, S. J. (1998). Neuropsychology of autism in young children and its implications for early intervention. *Mental Retardation and Developmental Disabilities Research Reviews, 4*(2), 104–112.

Rogers, S. J., & DiLalla, D. (1991). A comparative study of the effects of a developmentally based instructional model on young children with autism and young children with other disorders of behavior and development. *Topics in Early Childhood Special Education, 11,* 29–48.

Rogers, S. J., Hall, T., Osaki, D., Reaven, J., & Herbison, J. (2000). A comprehensive, integrated, educational approach to young children with autism and their families. In S. L. Harris & J. S. Handleman (Eds.), *Preschool education programs for children with autism* (2nd ed., pp. 95–134). Austin, TX: Pro-Ed.

Rogers, S. J., Hayden, D., Hepburn, S., Charlifue-Smith, R., Hall, T., & Hayes, A. (2006). Teaching young nonverbal children with autism useful speech: A pilot study of the Denver Model and PROMPT interventions. *Journal of Autism and Developmental Disorders, 36*(8), 1007–1024.

Rogers, S. J., Hepburn, S. L., Stackhouse, T., & Wehner, E. (2003). Imitation performance in toddlers with autism and those with other developmental disorders. *The Journal of Child Psychology and Psychiatry and Allied Disciplines, 44*(5), 763–781.

Rogers, S. J., Herbison, J., Lewis, H., Pantone, J., & Reis, K. (1986). An approach for enhancing the symbolic, communicative, and interpersonal functioning of young children with autism and severe emotional handicaps. *Journal of the Division of Early Childhood, 10,* 135–148.

Rogers, S. J., & Lewis, H. (1989). An effective day treatment model for young children with pervasive developmental disorders. *Journal of the American Academy of Child and Adolescent Psychiatry, 28,* 207–214.

Rogers, S. J., Lewis, H. C., & Reis, K. (1987). An effective procedure for training early special education teams to implement a model program. *Journal of the Division of Early Childhood, 11*(2), 180–188.

Rogers, S. J., Ozonoff, S., & Maslin-Cole, C. (1993). Developmental aspects of attachment behavior in young children with pervasive developmental disorders. *Journal of the American Academy of Child and Adolescent Psychiatry, 32,* 1274–1282.

Rogers, S. J., & Pennington, B. F. (1991). A theoretical approach to the deficits in infantile autism. *Development and Psychopathology, 3,* 137–162.

Rogers, S. J., & Williams, J. H. G. (2006). Imitation in autism: Findings and controversies. In S. J. Rogers & J. H. G. Williams (Eds.), *Imitation and the social mind: Autism and typical development.* (pp. 277–309). New York: Guilford Press.

Russell, J. (1997). How executive disorders can bring about an inadequate "theory of mind." In J. Russell (Ed.), *Autism as an executive disorder.* Oxford, UK: University Press.

Rydell, P., & Mirenda, P. (1994). Effects of high and low constraint utterances on the production of immediate and delayed echolalia in young children with autism. *Journal of Autism and Developmental Disorders, 24,* 719–735.

Saffran, J. R., Aslin, R. N., & Newport, E. K. (1996). Statistical learning by 8-month-old infants. *Science, 13,* 1926–1928.

Sallows, G. O., & Graupner, T. D. (2005). Intensive behavioral treatment for children with autism: Four-year outcome and predictors. *American Journal on Mental Retardation, 110,* 417–438.

Sander, E. K. (1972). When are speech sounds learned? *Journal of Speech and Hearing Disorders, 37,* 55–63.

Schieve, L. A., Blumberg, S. J., Rice, C., Visser, S. N., & Boyle, C. (2007). The relationship between autism and parenting stress. *Pediatrics, 119,* S114–S121.

Schopler, E., Mesibov, G. B., & Hearsey, K. A. (1995). Structured teaching in the TEACCH system. In E. Schopler & G. B. Mesibov (Eds.), *Learning and cognition in autism* (pp. 243–268). New York: Plenum Press.

Schopler, E., Reichler, R., & Rochen, R. B. (1988). *The childhood autism rating scale (CARS).* Los Angeles: Western Psychological Services.

Schreibman, L. (1988). *Autism.* Newbury Park, CA: Sage.

Schreibman, L., & Koegel, R. L. (2005). Training for parents of children with autism: Pivotal responses, generalization, and individualization of interventions. In E. D. Hibbs & P. S. Jensen (Eds.), *Psychosocial treatment for child and adolescent disorders: Empirically based strategies for clinical practice* (2nd ed., pp. 605–631). Washington, DC: American Psychological Association.

Schreibman, L., & Pierce, K. L. (1993). Achieving greater generalization of treatment effects in children with autism: Pivotal response training and self-management. *Clinical Psychologist, 46*(4), 184–191.

Schumann, C. M., & Amaral, D. G. (2006). Stereological analysis of amygdala neuron number in autism. *Journal of Neuroscience, 26,* 7674–7679.

Seibert, J., Hogan, A., & Mundy, P. (1982). Assessing social interactional competencies: The early social-communication scales. *Infant Mental Health Journal, 3,* 244–258.

Seligman, M. & Darling, R. B. (1997). *Ordinary families, special children: A systems approach to childhood disabilities* (2nd ed.). New York: Guilford Press.

Sendak, M. (1963). *Where the wild things are.* HarperCollins Juvenile Books.

Sherer, M. R., & Schreibman, L. (2005). Individual behavioral profiles and predictors of treatment effectiveness for children with autism. *Journal of Consulting and Clinical Psychology, 73,* 1–14.

Shonkoff, J., & Phillips, D. (2000). *From Neurons to Neighborhoods.* Washington, DC: National Academy Press.

Siegel, L. M. (2007). *The complete IEP guide: How to advocate for your special ed child.* Berkeley, CA: Nolo Press.

Sigman, M., & Mundy, P. (1989). Social attachments in autistic children. *Journal of the American Academy of Child and Adolescent Psychiatry, 28,* 74–81.

Sigman, M., & Ungerer, J. (1984). Cognitive and language skills in autistic, mentally retarded, and normal children. *Developmental Psychology, 20,* 293–302.

Siller, M., & Sigman, M. (2002). The behaviors of parents of children with autism predict the subsequent development of their children's communication. *Journal of Autism and Developmental Disorders, 32,* 77–89.

Sivberg, B. (2002). Family system and coping behaviors: A comparison between parents of children with autistic spectrum disorders and parents with non-autistic children. *Autism, 6*(4), 397–409.

Smith, T., Eikeseth, S., Klevstrand, M., & Lovaas, I. O. (1997). Intensive behavioral treatment for preschoolers with severe mental retardation and pervasive developmental disorder. *American Journal on Mental Retardation, 102,* 238–249.

Smith, T., Groen, A. D., & Wynn, J. W. (2000). Randomized trial of intensive early intervention for children with pervasive developmental disorder. *American Journal on Mental Retardation, 105*(4), 269–285.

Sparks, B. F., Friedman, S. D., Shaw, D. W., Aylward. E. H., Echelard, D., Artru, A. A., et al. (2002). Brain structural abnormalities in young children with autism spectrum disorder. *Neurology, 59,* 184–192.

Stahmer, A., & Schreibman, L. (1992). Teaching children with autism appropriate play in unsupervised environments using a self-management treatment package. *Journal of Applied Behaviour Analysis, 25,* 447–459.

Steele, H., & Steele, M. (1994). Intergenerational patterns of attachment. In K. Bartholomew & D. Perlman (Eds.), *Attachment processes in adulthood: Advances in personal relationships series* (Vol. 5, pp. 93–120). London: Jessica Kingsley.

Stern, D. N. (1985). *The interpersonal world of the infant.* New York: Basic Books.

Stone, W. L., & Caro-Martinez, L. M. (1990). Naturalistic observations of spontaneous communication in autistic children. *Journal of Autism and Developmental Disorders, 20,* 437–453.

Stone, W. L., Lee, E. B., Ashford, L., Brissie, J., Hepburn, S. L., Coonrod, E. E., et al. (1999). Can autism be diagnosed accurately in children under three years? *Journal of Child Psychology and Psychiatry, 40,* 219–226.

Stone, W. L., Ousley, O. Y., Yoder, P. J., Hogan, K. L., & Hepburn, S. L. (1997). Nonverbal communication in two- and three-year-old children with autism. *Journal of Autism and Developmental Disorders, 27*(6), 677–696.

Tager-Flusberg, H. (1993). What language reveals about the understanding of minds in children with autism. In S. Baron-Cohen, H. Tager-Flusberg, & D. J. Cohen (Eds.), *Understanding other minds: Perspectives from autism* (pp. 138–157). Oxford, UK: Oxford University Press.

Tager-Flusberg, H., Calkins, S., Nolin, T., Baumberger, T., Anderson, M., & Chadwick-Dias, A. (1990). A longitudinal study of language acquisition in autistic and Down syndrome children. *Journal of Autism and Developmental Disorders, 20,* 1–21.

Tamis-LeMonda, C. S., Bornstein, M. H., & Baumwell, L. (2001). Maternal responsiveness and children's achievement of language milestones. *Child Development, 72*, 748–767.

Tomasello, M. (1992). The social bases of language acquisition. *Social Development, 1*, 67–87.

Tomasello,M. (1995). Joint attention and social cognition. In C. Moore & P. J. Dunham (Eds.), *Joint attention: Its origins and role in development* (pp. 103–130). Hillsdale, NJ: Erlbaum.

Tomasello, M. (1998). Do apes ape? In B. F. Galef, Jr. & C. M. Heyes (Eds.), *Social learning in animals: The roots of culture* (pp.) New York: Academic Press.

Tomasello, M. (2006). Acquiring linguistic constructions. In D. Kuhn & R. S. Siegler (Eds.), *Handbook of child psychology: Vol. 2. Cognition, perception, and language* (6th ed., pp. 255–298). Hoboken, NJ: Wiley.

Tonge, B., Brereton, A., Kiomall, M., Mackinnon, A., King, N., & Rinehart, N. (2006). Effects on parental mental health of an education and skills training program for parents of young children with autism: A randomized controlled trial. *Journal of the American Academy of Child and Adolescent Psychiatry, 45*(5), 561–569.

Ungerer, J., & Sigman, M. (1981). Symbolic play and language comprehension in autistic children. *Journal of the American Academy of Child Psychiatry, 20*, 318–337.

Uzgiris, I. C. (1973). Patterns of vocal and gestural imitation in infants. In L. J. Stone, H. T. Smith, & L. B. Murphy (Eds.), *The competent infant* (pp. 599–604). New York: Basic Books.

van Ijzendoorn, M. H., Rutgers, A. H., Bakermans-Kranenburg, M. J., Van Daalen, E., Dietz, C., & Buitelaar, J. K. (2007). Parental sensitivity and attachment in children with autism spectrum disorders: Comparison with children with mental retardation, with language delays, and with typical development. *Child Development, 78*(2), 597–608.

Vidoni, E. D., & Boyd, L. A. (2008). Motor sequential learning occurs despite disrupted visual and proprioceptive feedback. *Behavioral and Brain Functions, 4*(XXXII).

Vismara, L. A., Colombi, C., & Rogers, S. J. (2009). Can 1 hour per week of therapy lead to lasting changes in young children with autism? *Autism, 13*(I), 93–115.

Vismara, L., & Rogers, S. J. (2008). Treating autism in the first year of life: A case study of the Early Start Denver Model. *Journal of Early Intervention, 31*(I), 91–108.

Vygotsky, L. S. (1978). *Mind in society: Development of higher psychological processes.* Cambridge, MA: Harvard Press.

Warren, S. F., Bredin-Olga, S. L., Fairchild M., Finestock, L. H., Fey, M. E., & Brady, N. C. (2006). Responsivity education/prelinguistic milieu teaching. In R. J. McCauley & M. Fey (Eds.), *Treatment of language disorders in children* (pp. 45–75). Baltimore: Brookes.

Warren, S. F., & Yoder, P. J. (2003). Early intervention for young children with language impairments. In L. Verhoeven & H. van Balkon (Eds.), *Classification of developmental language disorders: Theoretical issues and clinical implications* (pp. 367–382). Mahwah, NJ: Erlbaum.

Wetherby, A. M., & Prutting, C. A. (1984). Profiles of communicative and cognitive-social abilities in autistic children. *Journal of Speech and Hearing Research, 27*, 364–377.

Whiten, A. & Ham, R. (1992). On the nature and evolution of imitation in the animal kingdom: Reappraisal of a century of research. In P. J. B. Slater, J. S. Rosenblatt, C. Beer, & Milinksi (Eds.), *Advances in the study of behavior* (Vol. 21, pp. 239–283). New York: Academic Press.

Williams, D. L., & Minshew, N. J. (2007). Understanding autism and related disorders: What has imaging taught us? *Neuroimaging Clinics of North America, 17*(IV), 495–509.

Williams, J., Whiten, A., Suddendorf, T., & Perrett, D. (2001). Imitation, mirror neurons, and autism. *Neuroscience and Biobehavioral Reviews, 25*, 287–295.

Yirmiya, N., Kasari, C., Sigman, M., & Mundy, P. (1989). Facial expressions of affect in autistic, mentally retarded and normal children. *Journal of Child Psychology and Psychiatry, 30,* 725–735.

Yoder, P. J., & Layton, T. L. (1988). Speech following sign language training in autistic children with minimal verbal language. *Journal of Autism and Developmental Disorders, 18,* 217–229.

Yoder, P., & Stone, W. L. (2006). Randomized comparison of two communication interventions for preschoolers with autism spectrum disorders. *Journal of Consulting and Clinical Psychology, 74,* 426–435.

Yoder, P. J., & Warren, S. F. (2001). Intentional communication elicits language-facilitating maternal responses in dyads with children who have developmental disabilities. *American Journal on Mental Retardation, 106*(4), 327–335.

Zeanah, C. H., & McDonough, S. (1989). Clinical approaches to families in early intervention. *Seminars in Early Perinatology, 13*(6), 513–522.

Zwaigenbaum, L., Bryson, S., Rogers, T., Roberts, W., Brian, J., & Szatmari, P. (2005). Behavioral manifestations of autism in the first year of life. *International Journal of Developmental Neuroscience, 23,* 143–152.

Index

ABC format, Teaching Fidelity Rating System and, 261–262
Acquisition skills
behaviors that demonstrate, 71–72
pivotal response training (PRT) and, 23
staff training and, 49
Activity zones, 129–130. *See also* Environment
Adult language
child language learning and, 177–178
Teaching Fidelity Rating System and, 268–269
Adult response
child language learning and, 177–178
Denver Model and, 24
Teaching Fidelity Rating System and, 266–267
Advocacy for the child, parents and, 54–55
Affect
Denver Model and, 24
Early Start Denver Model (ESDM) and, 25–26
Teaching Fidelity Rating System and, 263–264, 266–267
Affective sharing, 15–16
Ages of children targeted in ESDM services, 36
Aggressive behaviors, 27
Amygdala, social brain network and, 5*f*, 10
Antecedent stimulus, 70–71
Antecedent–behavior–consequence (ABC), 21
Antecedents, staff training and, 49
Applied behavior analysis (ABA)
compared to PRT, 16–17
Early Start Denver Model (ESDM) and, 14, 18–19, 20–22, 36–37
interdisciplinary treatment team, 40–41
overview, 20–22
speech–language pathologist and, 44
staff training and, 48
Arousal
Denver Model and, 24
Teaching Fidelity Rating System and, 263–264
Articulation, vocal imitation and, 145
Assessment
Curriculum Checklist and, 58–68
organization of the treatment team and, 42
unwanted behaviors and, 121
Attachment security, 28–29
Attention
becoming a play partner and, 103–106
capturing, 20
classroom environment and, 185–186
positive, 122
sensory social routines and, 112, 113
states of, 24
Teaching Fidelity Rating System and, 261
Attention, joint. *See* Joint attention
Auditory supports, 199

B

Balanced interactions, 23
Baseline skills, task analysis and, 81–82
Behavior analyst, 41*f*, 44–45
Behavior bundles, 83–84. *See also* Learning steps
Behavior management, in a classroom setting, 197–198
Behavior plans, 121–123

Behaviors
applied behavior analysis (ABA) and, 21–22
Curriculum Checklist and, 216, 234–235
kindergarten transition and, 208*t*
of others, 7–8
that demonstrate objectives, 71–72
unwanted, 120–123, 264
Biological motion, 7
Board-certified behavior analyst (BCBA), 44–45. *See also* Behavior analyst
Brain development
brain changes and, 12
early intervention and, 13
how autism likely affects, 8–11
social-communicative skills and, 4–8, 5*f*
Broca's area, mirror neuron system and, 11

C

Cerebellum, 10
Chaining, Teaching Fidelity Rating System and, 262–263
Child psychologist, 41*f*, 43
Choices
pivotal response training (PRT) and, 23–24
spontaneous speech and, 174
Choreography of the classroom, 192, 193*t*, 194*t*
Chores, 217, 221, 225, 236, 243–244, 250
Classroom intervention
classroom management and, 197–198
environment and, 185–189
overview, 184–185
schedule and routines and, 189–192, 193*t*, 194*t*
staff planning and communication and, 192–194
Clean-up routines, 115–118. *See also* Chores
Closing phase of joint activity routines, 108
Cognitive skills
clean-up routines and, 115–116
Curriculum Checklist and, 215, 219–220, 223–224, 227–228, 232–233, 240, 247–248, 254–255
ESDM in a group setting and, 190–191
example of learning objectives for, 78, 99
play and, 26
Communication. *See also* Nonverbal communication; Verbal communication
coordinated attention and, 155–156
joint activity routines and, 109
kindergarten transition and, 208*t*
mirror neuron system and, 11
Teaching Fidelity Rating System and, 267–268
between team members, 47–48, 192–194
Communicative cues
Denver Model and, 24
Teaching Fidelity Rating System and, 267
Complex skills, 18
Conflicts with the child, 106
Consequences, applied behavior analysis (ABA) and, 21
Constructionist theory of early cognition, 2–3
Constructive play, 26. *See also* Play
Cooperation with the child, 106
Coordinated attention, 155–156
Curriculum Checklist
administration of, 210–211
assessment using, 58–68
becoming a play partner and, 105
case example of, 60–68
complete, 213–229
developmental sequences and, 82
imitation and, 139
Item Descriptions, 17, 230–258
learning objectives and, 68–69
materials needed for, 212
organization of the treatment team and, 42, 45
overview, 17, 37, 209–210
scoring of, 211
selecting skill content from, 69–70
social behavior and, 183
staff training and, 48
writing functional objectives and, 75–76, 76*t*

D

Daily Data Sheet
decision tree regarding lack of progress and, 130
ESDM in a group setting and, 190–191, 191, 196
examples of, 87*f*, 88*f*–90*f*

joint activity routines and, 135
overview, 37–38, 87–94, 87*f*, 88*f*–90*f*, 93*f*
planning the flow of joint activities in a session and, 126
treatment notebook and, 38
Daily living skills
Curriculum Checklist and, 216–217, 221, 225, 229, 235–236, 242–244, 249–250, 256
kindergarten transition and, 208*t*
teaching procedures and, 204–206
Daily schedule and routines, 189–192, 193*t*, 194*t*
Daily teaching targets. *See also* Teaching procedures
ESDM in a group setting and, 190–192
examples of, 95–100
learning steps for, 80–86
overview, 80, 94
progress tracking and, 87–94, 87*f*, 88*f*–90*f*, 93*f*
Data collection, 49, 91–92. *See also* Daily Data Sheet
Decision tree regarding lack of progress
overview, 130–134, 131*f*
speech development and, 179, 180*f*
Denver Model. *See also* Early Start Denver Model (ESDM)
delivery settings of, 35
effectiveness of, 29–32, 31*f*
overview, 14–15
teaching procedures and, 24–25
Describing the child's play, 105
Destructive behaviors, 27. *See also* Unwanted behaviors
Developmental processes
brain changes and, 12
gestural communication and, 158*t*, 160–161
infant learning and, 2–4
Developmental task analysis, 80–81, 94. *See also* Task analysis
Diagnosis, effectiveness of ESDM and, 32
Discrete trial teaching, 23
Discriminative stimulus. *See* Antecedent stimulus
Dolls, teaching symbolic play with, 149. *See also* Toys
Down times, ESDM in a group setting and, 191–192
Dressing
Curriculum Checklist and, 217, 221, 235, 243
teaching procedures and, 204
DSM-IV diagnosis, 32
Dyadic engagement
Denver Model and, 24
Teaching Fidelity Rating System and, 265

E

Early childhood special education, 18–19
Early interventions, role of, 13
Early Start Denver Model (ESDM). *See also* Classroom intervention
compared to other intervention models, 33–34
curriculum of, 17–19
delivery settings of, 35–36
effectiveness of, 29–32, 31*f*
families and, 50–55
foundations of, 14–17
generalist model to deliver intervention and, 39–40
in group settings, 184–185
interdisciplinary treatment team, 40–50, 41*f*
overview, 1–2, 13, 14, 34, 57
procedures of, 37–39
target population for services, 36
teaching procedures, 19–29
transitioning out of, 55–57
who delivers services, 36–37
Early symptoms of autism, 1–2
Eating
Curriculum Checklist and, 216–217, 221, 235, 242
teaching procedures and, 205–206
Echolalic children, adult language and, 178
Elaboration, 25, 139–140
Elaboration phase of joint activity routines, 108, 109
Electroencephalography (EEG), 6
Emotion perception, 6–7
Empathic reactions, 11
Engagement
with environment, 3–4
Teaching Fidelity Rating System and, 265
transitions and, 118–119

Environment. *See also* Setting
antecedent stimulus and, 71
becoming a play partner and, 103–104, 105
Curriculum Checklist administration and, 211
engagement with, 3–4
joint activity routines and, 124
planning the flow of joint activities in a session and, 129–130
social environment, 27–28
Errors, management of, 263
ESDM Curriculum Checklist. *See* Curriculum Checklist
Ethical issues, 38
Executive function skills, 116
Expressive communication. *See also* Verbal communication
Curriculum Checklist and, 214, 218, 222–223, 226–227, 231, 237, 245–246, 252–254
ESDM in a group setting and, 191
example of learning objectives for, 77, 95–96
play and, 26
Expressive language impairment, 177
Eye contact
becoming a play partner and, 104
gestural communication and, 158–159, 165–166
Eye gaze, 6

F

Face recognition, 6
Facial imitation. *See also* Imitation
overview, 136
teaching, 141–143
Facial movements and expressions
becoming a play partner and, 104
Early Start Denver Model (ESDM), 15
overview, 15–16, 162
Facial processing, 6–7
Fading, Teaching Fidelity Rating System and, 262
Families
effects of autism on, 51–52
involvement of, 27–29, 50–55
treatment and, 52–53
Family systems theory, 53
Fidelity Rating System, 50
Fine motor development
Curriculum Checklist and, 216, 220, 224, 228–229, 234, 241, 248–249, 257
ESDM in a group setting and, 190
kindergarten transition and, 208*t*
play and, 26
Frequency of behaviors, 84–85
Functional assessment of analysis of behavior
applied behavior analysis (ABA) and, 22
board-certified behavior analyst (BCBA), 45
parental involvement in, 28
Functional magnetic resonance imaging (fMRI), 6
Functional objectives, 75–76, 76*t*. *See also* Short-term learning objectives
Functional play acts. *See also* Play
ESDM in a group setting and, 190–191
teaching, 147–148
themes for, 151
Fusiform gyrus, 5*f*

G

Gaze of the child
becoming a play partner and, 104
gestural communication and, 158–159
Generalist model in delivery of interventions, 39–40
Generalization of skills, criterion for, 73–74
Gestural communication. *See also* Nonverbal communication
Early Start Denver Model (ESDM), 15
ESDM in a group setting and, 191
mirror neuron system and, 11
overview, 154, 166–167
teaching, 156–166, 158*t*
Gestural imitation. *See also* Imitation
overview, 137, 161
teaching, 140–141, 142–143
Gestures of others, 159–160
Giving gestures, 163–164. *See also* Gestural communication
Goodbye routines, 114–115
Greeting activities, 114–115
Grooming
Curriculum Checklist and, 217, 221, 225, 235–236, 243, 250
teaching procedures and, 204–205

Gross motor development
Curriculum Checklist and, 216, 221, 224–225, 229, 234, 241–242, 249, 257–258
ESDM in a group setting and, 190
kindergarten transition and, 208*t*
play and, 26
Group programs
classroom management and, 197–198
environment and, 185–189
interdisciplinary treatment team, 41
overview, 184–185, 194–197, 197*t*

H

Head size, 9
Hello routines, 114–115
Helping the child, 105–106
Home-based nature of the treatment, 38, 41
Hygiene
Curriculum Checklist and, 217, 221, 225, 235–236, 243, 250
teaching procedures and, 204–205

I

IFSP/IEP meetings, 54–55, 56–57
Imitation
becoming a play partner and, 106
building up, 18
Curriculum Checklist and, 215, 219, 232, 239–240
ESDM in a group setting and, 191
example of learning objectives for, 78, 98–99
overview, 15–16, 136–137
play and, 26
staff training and, 48
teaching, 136–146
vocalization and, 170, 172
Incidental teaching, 33
Individualization, 19. *See also* Teaching procedures
Infants
brain changes and, 12
early symptoms of autism and, 1
facial processing and, 6–7
interpreting behavior of others and, 7–8
learning and, 2–4
social-communicative skills and, 4–8, 5*f*
Inferior frontal cortex, 11
Inferior parietal lobe, 11
Inflammation of the brain, 9
Initiation, child's, 109
Injury threat, 121
Instructions, following, 181–182
Intensive teaching, 27, 33
Interdisciplinary approach, 18–19
Interdisciplinary teams
communication between team members, 47–48
Early Start Denver Model (ESDM), 15
organization of, 41–47, 41*f*
overview, 40–50, 41*f*
staff training, 48–50
Interpersonal development in autism model
Early Start Denver Model (ESDM) and, 14
overview, 15–16
Interpersonal engagement, 15
Intervention Session Plan
lack of progress and, 133
overview, 126–129, 127*f*–128*f*
Intervention techniques, 157–158

J

Joint activity routines. *See also* Play
communication and, 172
flow of in a session, 126–129, 127*f*–128*f*
managing unwanted behaviors and, 120–123
object-based, 109–110
organizing and planning, 123–130, 125*t*, 127*f*–128*f*
overview, 101–102, 108–120, 134–135
partner-focused, 110–114
peer relations and, 203–204
phases of, 108–109
Teaching Fidelity Rating System and, 269
teaching inside, 109
Joint attention
behaviors that demonstrate, 72
building up, 18
coordinated attention and, 155
Curriculum Checklist and, 218, 237–238
example of task analysis for, 81
how autism likely affects, 9
overview, 6
staff training and, 48
teaching, 162–163

K

Kindergarten transition, 206–207, 208*t*

L

Language development, 18
Language intervention approach in the ESDM, 18
Language learning. *See also* Learning
  acquisition of language, 30
  adult language and, 177–178
  developmentally appropriate language and, 25
  ESDM in a group setting and, 190
  overview, 25–26
  Teaching Fidelity Rating System and, 268–269
Language model, 109
Language skills, 208*t*
Language use, 18
Learning. *See also* Language learning; Short-term learning objectives; Teaching procedures
  Early Start Denver Model (ESDM) and, 25–26
  how autism likely affects, 8–11
  infants and, 2–4
  joint activity routines and, 135
  selecting skill content and, 69–70
  sensory social routines and, 112
Learning objectives. *See* Short-term learning objectives
Learning steps. *See also* Daily teaching targets
  middle learning steps, 82–86
  overview, 94
Linking behavior to new antecedents, 85–86
Living skills
  Curriculum Checklist and, 216–217, 221, 225, 229, 235–236, 242–244, 249–250, 256
  kindergarten transition and, 208*t*
  teaching procedures and, 204–206

M

Magnetoencephalography (MEG), 6
Maintenance skills
  group settings and, 195
  learning objectives and, 84–85
  pivotal response training (PRT) and, 23
  staff training and, 49
Mastery of skills, 72–74
Materials in play. *See also* Play; Toys
  becoming a play partner and, 107
  classroom environment and, 187
  Curriculum Checklist and, 212
  group transitions and, 201–202
  imitation and, 138
  interference issues with, 119–120
  joint activity routines and, 109–110
  planning the flow of joint activities in a session and, 129–130
  sensory social routines and, 112–113
Mealtimes
  Curriculum Checklist and, 216–217, 221, 235, 242
  teaching procedures and, 205–206
Mean length of utterance (MLU)
  child language learning and, 177–178
  vocal imitation and, 145–146
Mental representations, 3
Middle learning steps, 82–86. *See also* Daily teaching targets
Milieu teaching, 33
Mirror neuron system, 11
Motivation
  becoming a play partner and, 102–103
  pivotal response training (PRT) and, 22–23
  Teaching Fidelity Rating System and, 265–266
Motor cortex, 11
Motor development, 44
Mullen Early Learning Composite, 31–32, 31*f*
Multistep activities, 117
Multiword utterances
  building up, 175–176
  vocal imitation and, 145–146

N

Neurochemistry, 11
Neuroimaging, 6
New skills, learning objectives and, 86
Nonverbal communication. *See also* Gestural communication
  coordinated attention and, 155–156
  ESDM or Denver Model and, 25, 30
  mirror neuron system and, 11

overview, 154–155, 166–167
receptive language and, 179–180
staff training and, 48
teaching, 156–166, 158*t*
Nonverbal communication development, 15

O

Object imitation, 138–140. *See also* Imitation
Object permanence, 3
Object spectacles, 103
Object substitution, 149–150
Object use, 15
Object-based joint activities. *See also* Materials in play
overview, 109–110, 134–135
sensory social routines and, 112–113, 114
Occupational therapist
Early Start Denver Model (ESDM) and, 18–19, 36–37
generalist model to deliver intervention and, 39
interdisciplinary treatment team, 40–41
organization of the treatment team and, 41*f*
speech–language pathologist and, 44
"One-up" rule
child language learning and, 177–178
vocal imitation and, 145–146
Opening and closing routines, 114–115
Opening phase of joint activity routines, 108, 109
Oral–facial imitation, 141–143. *See also* Imitation
Outcomes, 13
Overgeneralization, 173
Oxytocin, 11

P

Parallel play. *See also* Play
becoming a play partner and, 106
peer relations and, 203
teaching, 148
Paraprofessionals
interdisciplinary treatment team, 40–41
organization of the treatment team and, 45–46
staff training and, 48
Parents
as advocates for their child, 54–55
effects of autism on, 51–52
involvement of, 27–29, 39, 41
organization of the treatment team and, 41*f*
parent training and, 30
parent–child play, 61
parenting practices, 28
Partial participation, 117
Partial prompts, 172
Partner-focused joint activities, 110–114
Pediatrics, 40–41
Peer relations
attachment security and, 28–29
Curriculum Checklist and, 218–219, 223, 238–239, 246–247
teaching procedures and, 202–204
Peptides, 11
Percentage statements, as a criterion for mastery, 73–74
Pervasive developmental disorder not otherwise specified (PDD-NOS), 32
Phonology, 177–178
Physician, 41*f*, 45
Picture Exchange Communication System (PECS), 133–134
Pivotal response training (PRT)
Early Start Denver Model (ESDM) and, 14, 33
overview, 16–17, 22–24
Planning, staff, 192–194
Play
becoming a play partner, 102–108
Curriculum Checklist and, 59–60, 210–211, 215, 220, 224, 228, 233, 240–241, 248, 255
ESDM in a group setting and, 190–191
example of learning objectives for, 78–79, 99–100
as the frame for intervention, 26
joint activity routines and, 101–102, 108–120
overview, 134–135
peer relations and, 203
staff training and, 48
symbolic play, 18
teaching, 19–20, 146–153
Pointing gestures, 165–166. *See also* Gestural communication
Positive affect, 24, 25–26

Positive attention, 122
Positive behavior supports, 27, 120–122
Preacademic skills, kindergarten transition and, 208*t*
Prefrontal cortex, 5*f*
Professionals delivering the ESDM of services. *See also* Behavior analyst; Board-certified behavior analyst (BCBA); Child psychologist; Occupational therapist; Paraprofessionals; Physician; Special education teacher; Speech–language pathologist
  Curriculum Checklist and, 59
  overview, 36–37
Progress tracking
  decision tree regarding lack of progress and, 130–134, 131*f*, 180*f*
  examples of, 95–100
  lack of progress in speech development and, 179, 180*f*
  overview, 87–94, 87*f*, 88*f*–90*f*, 93*f*
Prompts
  applied behavior analysis (ABA) and, 21
  gestural communication and, 159
  imitation and, 141
  Teaching Fidelity Rating System and, 262
  teaching receptive language and, 181–182
  verbal communication and, 173
Prompts for restructuring oral phonetic targets (PROMPT therapy)
  compared to the Denver Model, 30
  speech–language pathologist and, 44, 46
Proximity to the child
  becoming a play partner and, 104, 105
  during group mealtimes, 205

R

Recasts, child language learning and, 177–178
Receptive communication. *See also* Verbal communication
  Curriculum Checklist and, 214, 217, 222, 225–226, 230, 236–237, 244–245, 251–252
  ESDM in a group setting and, 191
  example of learning objectives for, 77, 96–97
  play and, 26
  teaching, 179–182
Record keeping, ESDM in a group setting and, 191
Reinforcement. *See also* Rewards
  clean-up routines and, 117–118
  lack of progress and, 130, 132–133
  managing unwanted behaviors and, 123
  pivotal response training (PRT) and, 23
  staff training and, 49
  stereotypic behaviors and, 123
  teaching receptive language and, 182
Repetitive behavior
  abnormal neurochemistry and, 11
  positive behavior approaches to, 27
  transitions and, 119
Resistant children, 119
Responding to others
  behaviors that demonstrate, 72
  teaching receptive language and, 181
Response to multiple cues, pivotal response training (PRT) and, 22–23
Restatements, 177–178
Rewards. *See also* Reinforcement
  managing unwanted behaviors and, 123
  social engagement and, 26
  stereotypic behaviors and, 123
Role in the children's play, 106–107
Role play, 151–153
Role reversal, 147–148
Roles, staff
  ESDM in a group setting and, 189
  during group mealtimes, 205
  group transitions and, 199–200
  kindergarten transition and, 206–207, 208*t*
Roles in the family, 53
Routines, 189–192, 193*t*, 194*t*

S

Safety, classroom environment and, 188
Scaffolding, 24–25
Schedule, daily
  ESDM in a group setting and, 189–192, 193*t*, 194*t*, 198–202
  group transitions and, 202
Self-care skills
  Curriculum Checklist and, 216–217, 221, 225, 229, 235–236, 242–244, 249–250, 256
  kindergarten transition and, 208*t*
  teaching procedures and, 204–206

Self-injury, 121
Sensitive response, 24
Sensorimotor play, 146. *See also* Play
Sensory development, 44
Sensory social routines
ESDM in a group setting and, 191
object-based joint activities and, 112–113, 114
overview, 15, 110–114, 134–135
Sensory social toys, 103
Sequence of activities during a session
classroom environment and, 186
example of, 125*t*
overview, 124
Session plan
lack of progress and, 133
overview, 126–129, 127*f*–128*f*
Setting, 71. *See also* Environment
Set-up phase of joint activity routines, 108, 109
Shared goals with the child, 106
Short-term learning objectives
balancing and amount of, 68–69
becoming a play partner and, 105
case example of, 76–79
constructing, 68
Curriculum Checklist and, 211
daily teaching targets and, 80–86
elements of, 70–75
examples of, 95–100
functional, 75–76, 76*t*
learning steps for, 80–86
overview, 58, 79
progress tracking and, 87–94, 87*f*, 88*f*–90*f*, 93*f*
selecting skill content and, 69–70
writing, 75–76, 76*t*
Siblings, 51–52, 53
Snack routines
Curriculum Checklist and, 216–217, 221, 235, 242
joint activity routines and, 115
teaching procedures and, 205–206
Social behavior
abnormal neurochemistry and, 11
teaching, 183
Social brain network
how autism likely affects, 10
overview, 4–8, 5*f*
Social communication, 104
Social development, 48
Social engagement, 26
Social interaction, 77–78, 97–98
Social learning, 25–26
Social motivation disorder model, 14, 16
Social rewards, 10
Social skills
Curriculum Checklist and, 215, 218–219, 223, 227, 231–232, 238–239, 246–247, 254
ESDM in a group setting and, 190–191
play and, 26
Social-communicative skills, 4–8, 5*f*
Songs, imitation and, 141
Special education
Early Start Denver Model (ESDM) and, 18–19, 36–37
interdisciplinary treatment team, 40–41
parents and, 54–55
Special education teacher, 41*f*, 42–43
Speech development. *See also* Language learning
lack of progress and, 179, 180*f*
overview, 4, 169–170
stimulating, 169–179
Speech–language pathologist
Early Start Denver Model (ESDM) and, 18–19, 36–37
generalist model to deliver intervention and, 39
interdisciplinary treatment team, 40–41
multiword utterances and, 176
organization of the treatment team and, 41*f*, 43–44
Spontaneous play, 149. *See also* Play
Spontaneous speech, moving from imitation to, 172–175
Staff planning, 192–194
Staff roles
ESDM in a group setting and, 189, 196
during group mealtimes, 205
group transitions and, 199–200
kindergarten transition and, 206–207, 208*t*
Statistical learning, 3
Stereotypic behavior, 122–123
Storyboard, 152
Substitution, object, 149–150
Superior temporal sulcus, 5*f*, 11
Symbolic combinations, 150–151
Symbolic play. *See also* Play
building up, 18
ESDM in a group setting and, 190–191

Symbolic play (*cont.*)
play and, 26
teaching, 148–151
Symptoms of autism, during infancy, 1–2
Synapses, 8–9

T

Task analysis
mapping out learning steps and, 80–81, 94
overview, 37–38
Teaching Fidelity Rating System
coding, 259–261, 271–272
Early Start Denver Model (ESDM), 261–270
sequence of activities during a session and, 126
staff training and, 48, 48–49
Teaching procedures. *See also* Daily teaching targets; Short-term learning objectives
applied behavior analysis (ABA) and, 20–22
clean-up routines and, 115–118
combining, 25–29
Curriculum Checklist and, 211
daily living/self-care skills, 204–206
decision tree regarding lack of progress and, 130–134, 131*f*
Denver Model and, 24–25
imitation and, 136–146
joint activity routines and, 109
kindergarten transition and, 206–207, 208*t*
managing unwanted behaviors and, 120–123
overview, 19–29, 37–38
peer relations and, 202–204
pivotal response training (PRT) and, 22–24
play skills, 146–153
receptive language and, 179–180
selecting skill content and, 69–70
sequence of activities during a session and, 124–126, 125*t*
speech production and, 169–179
spontaneous speech and, 174–175
staff training and, 49
Teaching Fidelity Rating System and, 259–272, 261–263
using data to inform, 92
Teaching structure, 133
Teaching trials (A-B-C chains), 49
Team leader, 41*f*, 42
Temporal lobe, 11
Temporal sequencing, 116
Termination, 55–57
Theme in play activities
joint activity routines and, 108, 109
teaching play skills and, 151
Theory of mind problems, 11
Toys. *See also* Play
becoming a play partner and, 103, 107
Curriculum Checklist and, 212
imitation and, 138
interference issues with, 119–120
joint activity routines and, 109–110
planning the flow of joint activities in a session and, 129
sensory social routines and, 112–113
teaching symbolic play with, 149
Training, 48–50
Transitional objects, 201–202
Transitions
in a classroom setting, 188, 198–202
joint activity routines and, 118–120
to kindergarten, 206–207, 208*t*
Teaching Fidelity Rating System and, 270
Treatment notebook, 38
Turn taking. *See also* Play
becoming a play partner and, 106, 107–108
Denver Model and, 24
imitation and, 137
peer relations and, 203
sensory social routines and, 113

U

Unwanted behaviors
managing, 120–123
Teaching Fidelity Rating System and, 264
Utensil skills, 206

V

Variations in play, 106
Vasopressin, 11
Verbal communication. *See also* Expressive communication; Receptive communication
Denver Model and, 25
development of, 15

mirror neuron system and, 11
overview, 168–169
speech production and, 169–179
staff training and, 48
Verbs in speech, speech production and, 175
Visual supports
classroom environment and, 187
group transitions and, 199, 200–201
lack of progress and, 133–134
Vocabulary, 174–175. *See also* Speech development
Vocal imitation. *See also* Imitation
echolalic children and, 178
ESDM in a group setting and, 191
moving to spontaneous words from, 172–175
overview, 136–137, 170, 172
teaching, 138, 143–146
Vocalizations, 170. *See also* Verbal communication